Advanced Concepts in

ARRHYTHMIAS

Advanced Concepts in
ARRHYTHMIAS

HENRY J.L. MARRIOTT, M.D., F.A.C.P., F.A.C.C.

Director of Clinical Research, Rogers Heart Foundation,
St. Petersburg, Florida; Clinical Professor of
Medicine (Cardiology), Emory University,
Atlanta, Georgia

MARY BOUDREAU CONOVER, R.N., B.S.

Critical Care Consultant and Lecturer,
Education Director, Summit Symposia,
Santa Cruz, California

SECOND EDITION

with 906 illustrations

The C. V. Mosby Company

ST. LOUIS • BALTIMORE • PHILADELPHIA • TORONTO   1989

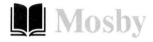

Editor: Don Ladig
Assistant editor: Audrey Rhoades
Project manager: Mark Spann
Book and cover design: Gail Morey Hudson
Editing and production: Top Graphics

SECOND EDITION

Previous edition copyrighted 1983

Printed in the United States of America

The C.V. Mosby Company
11830 Westline Industrial Drive, St. Louis, Missouri 63146

Library of Congress Cataloging-in-Publication Data

Marriott, Henry J.L. (Henry Joseph Llewellyn), 1917-
    Advanced concepts in arrhythmias / Henry J.L. Marriott, Mary
  Boudreau Conover. -2nd ed.
      p. cm.
    Includes bibliographies and index.
    ISBN 0-8016-3239-0
    1. Arrhythmia. I. Conover, Mary Boudreau, 1931-   II. Title.
    [DNLM: 1. Arrhythmia.   WG 330 M359a]
RC685.A65M369 1989
616.1'2807—dc19
DNLM/DLC
for Library of Congress   89-3208
                                          CIP

C/D/D 9 8 7 6 5 4 3 2 1

TO
GEORGE PATRICK FEE

Preface

The second edition of this book reflects the important advances made in electrocardiography in the last decade. The chapter on cellular electrophysiology has been brought up-to-date, especially regarding the function and mechanism of the sodium-potassium ATPase pump. Four new chapters have been added, which cover arrhythmogenic mechanisms and the new guidelines in the electrocardiographic and bedside recognition of ventricular tachycardia. A new chapter on altered automaticity and triggered activity elaborates on the cellular mechanism and the causes of the two types of altered automaticity and on afterdepolarizations as a cause of triggered activity. Another chapter is devoted to the recognition of digitalis-induced dysrhythmias by subjective symptoms and the ECG. In a chapter on the proarrhythmic effects of antiarrhythmic drugs, the mechanism of drug access to sodium and calcium channels is illustrated, and the antiarrhythmic, as well as the possible arrhythmogenic, effects are explained.

Using the surface ECG alone, 80% to 90% accuracy is now possible in differentiating the usually benign AV nodal reentry from the potentially lethal arrhythmias of Wolff-Parkinson-White syndrome and in differentiating ventricular tachycardia from supraventricular tachycardia with aberration. These new guidelines are clearly stated and illustrated.

As in the last edition, there is a new approach to the diagnosis of AV block and a time-tested, dependable method of tackling arrhythmias. Other chapters illustrate and explain sinus node and His bundle electrograms, phase 3 and phase 4 aberration, concealed conduction, accessory pathways, and how to draw and use laddergrams as a diagnostic and teaching aid.

This book will bring you up-to-date regarding the value of the surface ECG as a superior, reproducible, noninvasive, and economical diagnostic tool. For those who care for the critically ill, this new information is vital to patient safety and personal professional adequacy, especially in the light of treatment now available.

Henry J.L. Marriott
Mary Conover

Contents

1 Development of the conduction system, 1

Development of the sinus node, 2
Internodal conduction, 4
Development of the AV node, 6
Branching portion of the bundle of His, 8

2 Sinus node and His bundle electrograms, 12

Silent zones on surface ECG, 12
Sinus node electrogram, 14
SA conduction time, 14
His bundle electrogram, 15
HBE deflections, 15
HBE intervals and normal values, 15
Sequence of activation through the conduction system, 16
Noninvasive His bundle electrogram, 16
Indications for His bundle recordings, 17

3 Cellular electrophysiology, 19

Historical highlights, 19
Current flow in the heart: its cable properties, 20
Normal cellular electrophysiology, 21
   Resting membrane potential, 21
   Sodium pump and sodium-potassium ATPase, 21
   Sodium-potassium exchange, 22
   Sodium concentration gradient, 23
   Sodium-calcium exchange, 23
   Potassium concentration gradient, 23
   Summary of functions of sodium pump, 24
Membrane channels, 24
Electrical cardiac cycle and action potential, 25
Phase 4, 26
Phase 4 depolarization, 27
Threshold potential, 28

Phase 0 depolarization, 28
Repolarization, 28
Phase 1, 28
Phase 2, 29
Phase 3, 30
Membrane channels related to the action potential, 30
Types of action potentials, 30
Refractory periods, 32
Cardiac action potential compared to other action potentials, 33
Gating mechanism, 34
Supernormal period, 35
Membrane potential related to conduction velocity, 35
Normal automaticity, 37
Overdrive suppression, 38
Action potential of the two nodes, 40
Automaticity versus excitability, 41
Action potential related to the electrocardiogram, 42
Summary, 43

4   Altered automaticity and triggered activity, 45

Altered automaticity, 46
Enhanced normal automaticity, 46
Abnormal automaticity, 47
Enhanced normal automaticity versus abnormal automaticity, 48
Triggered activity, 52
Delayed afterdepolarizations, 52
Early afterdepolarizations, 54
Summary, 56

5   Digitalis dysrhythmias, 59

Mortality in undiagnosed digitalis toxicity, 59
Cellular basis for positive inotropy, 59
Cellular basis for digitalis dysrhythmias, 60
Digitalis and potassium, 61
Drugs that interact with digoxin, 61
ECG recognition of digitalis dysrhythmias, 62
Atrial tachycardia with block, 62
Fascicular ventricular tachycardia, 66
Bidirectional ventricular tachycardia, 70
Ventricular bigeminy, 72
Accelerated idiojunctional rhythm and junctional tachycardia, 74
Ventricular tachycardia, 75
Double tachycardia, 76
Sinus bradycardia and SA Wenckebach period, 77
AV Wenckebach period, 78
Atrial fibrillation with accelerated idiojunctional rhythm and Wenckebach
exit block, 78

Accelerated idioventricular rhythm, 80
Sinus bradycardia and junctional tachycardia, 81
Summary, 81

6 The reentry mechanism, 84

Historical background, 86
Slow conduction, 87
Depressed fast response, 87
Slow response, 87
Unidirectional block, 88
Summation, 89
Inhibition, 90
Reflection, 91
Summary, 92

7 Intraventricular reentry, 94

Reentry within terminal Purkinje fibers, 94
Reentry through ischemic myocardial tissue, 95
Reentrant extrasystolic grouping, 98
Concealed reentry, 100
Concealed bigeminy, 101
Reentry within the bundle branches and His bundle (macroreentry), 102
Summary, 104

8 SA reentry, block, and sick sinus syndrome, 105

SA node, 105
Blood supply, 107
Role of the autonomic nervous system in SA nodal function, 107
Temperature, 107
Paroxysmal sinus tachycardia caused by SA nodal reentry, 108
SA nodal reentry mechanism, 108
ECG features, 109
SA block, 110
First degree SA block, 110
Second degree SA block, 110
Third degree SA block, 113
Sick sinus syndrome, 113
History, 113
Etiology, 113
ECG features, 114
Summary, 117

9 AV nodal reentry, 120

Dual AV nodal pathways, 120
Mechanism of AV nodal reentry, 122
ECG signs of common type of AVNR tachycardia, 125

Uncommon form of AVNR, 126
Maintenance and interruption of a reentry circuit, 126
Differentiating the reciprocating supraventricular tachycardias, 129
Reciprocal (echo) beats, 129
   AV junction (V-A-V sequence), 131
   Ventricles (V-A-V sequence), 132
   RP' interval in V-A-V sequences, 136
   Atria (A-V-A sequence), 137
Summary, 139

10 Preexcitation and its arrhythmias, 141

Terminology, 141
Wolff-Parkinson-White syndrome, 142
   Historical background, 142
   Clinical significance, 143
   Anatomy, 143
   Degrees of preexcitation, 146
   ECG in overt WPW syndrome, 148
   Concealed accessory pathway, 152
   Nonevident WPW syndrome, 152
   Classification, 154
   Locating the accessory pathway, 154
   Masking and mimicking by WPW syndrome, 157
   Arrhythmias of WPW syndrome, 157
   Orthodromic circus movement tachycardia, 159
   Differential diagnosis in PSVT, 160
   Persistent circus movement tachycardia, 162
   Antidromic circus movement tachycardia, 163
   Atrial fibrillation in WPW syndrome, 164
   Differential diagnosis in irregular wide QRS tachycardia, 168
Lown-Ganong-Levine syndrome, 169
Mahaim fibers, 170
Summary, 171

11 Proarrhythmic actions of antiarrhythmic drugs, 174

Membrane channel, 175
Fast Na$^+$ channel blockade by local anesthetic antiarrhythmics, 176
Abnormal conduction caused by cardiac disease, 178
Abnormal conduction caused by antiarrhythmic drugs, 180
Proarrhythmic effects of prolonging the refractory period, 182
Drug-induced supraventricular arrhythmias, 183
Drug-induced ventricular tachyarrhythmias, 183
   Uniform spontaneous and sustained VT of new onset or increased
      frequency, 184
   New persistent VT with toxic concentrations of class IA or IC antiarrhythmics, 184
   Accelerated idioventricular rhythm, 184
   Torsades de pointes, 186

Persistent VT caused by class IC drugs, 188
Drug-induced ventricular fibrillation, 189
Risk factors, 189
Summary, 189

12 Aberrant ventricular conduction, 192

Mechanism, 193
Phase 3 aberration, 195
Phase 4 aberration, 198
Rate-dependent and critical rate BBB, 200
Phase 3 and phase 4 AV blocks, 200
Morphology of aberration, 202
  RBBB aberration, 202
  LBBB aberration, 205
Additional helpful clues, 205
  QRS duration, 205
  Preceding atrial activity, 206
  Initial deflection identical with that of conducted beats, 207
  Second-in-the-row anomaly, 208
Aberrancy in atrial fibrillation, 210
Aberrancy in atrial tachycardia, 212
Aberrancy in atrial flutter, 213
Alternating aberrancy, 214
Clinical implications, 216
Summary, 216

13 Differential diagnosis in the broad QRS tachycardia, 218

The "lidocaine reflex," 218
Overdiagnosis of aberration, 218
New findings, 219
When in doubt, 219
Hemodynamic status and age, 220
Steps in the differential diagnosis, 220
  Leads of choice, 220
  QRS configuration, 220
  QRS width, 223
  QRS axis, 223
  AV dissociation, 224
  Additional helpful clues, 224
  Bedside diagnosis of VT, 226
Clinical application, 226
Exceptions to the rules, 241
Summary, 245

14 AV block, 247

The PR interval, 247
Nonconducted beats, 247

Type I and type II block, 248
Anatomy versus behavior, 250
Wenckebach periodicity and RP/PR reciprocity, 252
2 to 1 AV block, 254
"Skipped" P waves, 256
High-grade (or advanced) AV block, 256
Complete AV block, 256
Ventricular asystole, 258
Need to reclassify, 260
Remedial measures, 265

15   Fusion, 268

Ventricular fusion, 270
   Clinical significance, 270
   Diagnosis, 270
Fusion in parasystole, 276
Fusion during accelerated idioventricular rhythm, 276
Fusion beats in the diagnosis of ventricular tachycardia, 280
Fusion with ventricular escape beats, 282
Fusion with paced beats, 284
Ventricular fusion in preexcitation, 285
Atrial fusion, 286
Summary, 287

16   Parasystole, 288

Mechanism of impulse formation, 288
Rate of discharge, 289
Entrance block through the years, 289
Exit block, 294
Classical ventricular parasystole, 294
Classical parasystole without exit block, 295
Classical parasystole with exit block, 300
Concealed parasystole, 301
Modulated ventricular parasystole, 301
Intermittent parasystole, 302
   Entrance block during the entire cycle, 302
   Entrance block only during early cycle, 302
Parasystolic accelerated idioventricular rhythm, 303
Fixed coupling in parasystole, 304
Paired ectopic ventricular beats, 305
Atrial parasystole, 305
Clinical significance of parasystole, 308
Summary, 308

17   Concealed conduction, 312

Historical background, 312
Concealed conduction in atrial fibrillation, 313
Interpolated ventricular extrasystoles with concealed retrograde conduction, 315
Concealed junctional extrasystoles, 318
  ECG clues to concealed junctional extrasystoles, 320
Concealed conduction affecting impulse formation, 321
Summary, 326

18   Supernormality, 328

The supernormal period, 328
Supernormal conduction, 330
Concealed supernormal conduction, 331
Mimics of supernormal conduction, 332
  Concealed junctional extrasystoles, 332
  Phase 4 (paradoxical critical rate), 333
  Concealed reentry, 334
  The gap phenomenon, 334
Summary, 336

19   Laddergrams, 338

Illustrating supraventricular ectopic mechanisms, 340
  Atrial premature beats, 340
  Nonconducted APBs, 341
  AV nodal reentry, 342
  Atrial flutter, 343
  Atrial flutter with Wenckebach conduction, 343
  Atrial flutter with exit block out of the flutter focus, 344
Illustrating SA block, 345
  SA Wenckebach conduction, 345
  SA Wenckebach conduction with junctional escape, 346
Illustrating junctional ectopic mechanisms, 348
  Junctional rhythm with reciprocal beats, 348
  Junctional escape, 350
  Accelerated idiojunctional rhythm with Wenckebach exit block, 351
  Concealed junctional beats, 353
Illustrating ventricular ectopic beats, 353
  Ventricular fusion, 354
  Ventricular microreentry, 356
Now it is your turn, 357

20   An approach to arrhythmias, 362

Principles of monitoring, 362
   Use a lead containing maximal information, 362
   Ensure a mechanically convenient monitoring system, 363
   One lead is not enough, 364
   Know when to use which other leads, 366
A systematic approach, 368
   Know the causes, 369
   Milk the QRS, 383
   Cherchez le P, 384
   Who is married to whom? 389
   Pinpoint the primary disturbance, 390

Glossary, 392

CHAPTER 1

Development of the conduction system

The conduction system is composed of highly specialized muscle tissue peculiar to the heart. We briefly present its fascinating embryology here in the belief that some knowledge of the development of the conduction system will facilitate an understanding of its normal and abnormal function.

The primitive straight cardiac tube is illustrated in Fig. 1-1 at 3 weeks of intrauterine development. Five segments are recognized: the truncus, bulbus, ventricle, atrium, and sinus venosus (sinus horn). Each is separated from adjacent segments by a slightly constricted ring named for the segments it separates—the sinoatrial (SA), atrioventricular (AV), bulboventricular (B-V), and bulbotruncal (B-T) rings. These rings of specialized tissue are believed to form the conducting tissues.

The SA ring, separating the sinus venosus from the atrium, is destined to form the sinus node. The B-V ring is destined to become the right bundle branch (RBB) and contribute to the left bundle branch (LBB) along with the AV ring.

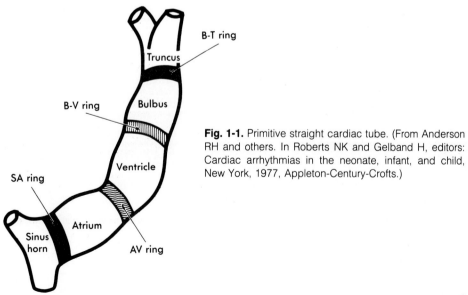

Fig. 1-1. Primitive straight cardiac tube. (From Anderson RH and others. In Roberts NK and Gelband H, editors: Cardiac arrhythmias in the neonate, infant, and child, New York, 1977, Appleton-Century-Crofts.)

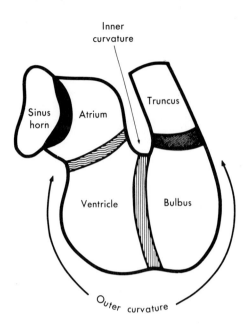

Fig. 1-2. Primitive straight cardiac tube begins to loop, bringing three rings into close apposition. (From Anderson RH and others. In Roberts NK and Gelband H, editors: Cardiac arrhythmias in the neonate, infant, and child, New York, 1977, Appleton-Century-Crofts.)

The origin of the AV node is controversial. Anderson and associates[1] believe the node has multiple origins, whereas others[2,3] believe that it is derived from the left horn of the sinus venosus and that the sinus node comes from the right horn.

As the tube begins to loop, the sinus venosus is absorbed into the right atrium so that the SA ring is in the posterior wall of the right atrium. One end of each of the remaining three rings is now in close apposition, as shown in Fig. 1-2.

Development of the sinus node

After 11 weeks of intrauterine life the SA node can be recognized. Its formation begins with a thickening of the junction between the superior vena cava and the sinus venosus in the region of the SA ring cells. This thickening is confined to the anteromedial quadrant of the junction between the superior vena cava and the atrium. By 11 weeks the thickening has aggregated around a prominent artery and is recognizable as the SA node, generally called simply the sinus node. The embryonic origin of the sinus node is illustrated in Fig. 1-3.

Blood supply. The large central sinus node artery is a branch of the right coronary artery in 55% of people and of the left coronary artery in 45%.

Ultrastructure. A wax model of the human sinus node as reconstructed from longitudinal sections is shown in Fig. 1-4.[4]

Note how nodal tissue blends with atrial tissue. These perinodal fascicles have a different refractory period from that of the sinus node and the atrial tissue. Thus they may provide reentry pathways for arrhythmias and the anatomical substrate for SA nodal blocks.

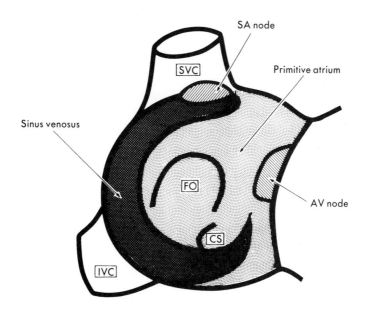

Fig. 1-3. Sinus node begins with thickening of junction between superior vena cava and sinus venosus. *SVC,* superior vena cava; *IVC,* inferior vena cava; *FO,* fossa ovalis; *CS,* coronary sinus. (From Anderson RH and others. In Roberts NK and Gelband H, editors: Cardiac arrhythmias in the neonate, infant, and child, New York, 1977, Appleton-Century-Crofts.)

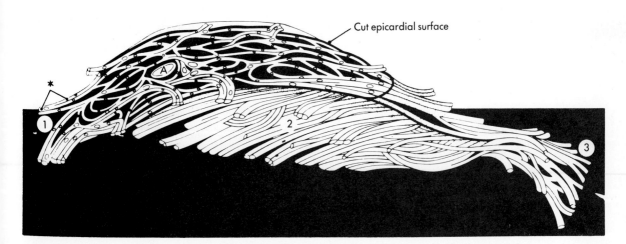

Fig. 1-4. Wax model of human sinus node. (From Truex RC. In Wellins HJJ, Lie KI, and Janse MJ, editors: The conduction system of the heart, Hingham, Mass, 1976, Martinus Nijhoff, Publishers.)

Internodal conduction

Controversy concerning the existence of specialized internodal tracts is "as old as the history of the conduction system itself,"[5] although the existence of preferential conduction implemented by the *geometrical structure* of the muscle bundles of the right atrium is well established.[5-8]

On the one hand, Sherf and James,[9] using light and electron microscopic studies of atrial tissue, have described six different types of atrial cells, with morphological evidence of specialization that, according to Hoffman,[10] is "clear and compelling."

Conversely, Anderson and Becker[5] in 1980 "strongly endorse the opinion that there are *no* histologically discrete tracts of specialized conduction tissue extending between the sinoatrial and atrioventricular nodes."

We will briefly outline the historical development of this controversy. In 1906 Wenckebach[11] described a muscle bundle extending from the area of the superior vena cava to the muscle of the right atrial appendage. This description was made before the discovery of the sinus node. He did not, therefore, describe a specialized *internodal* pathway. In 1910 Thorel[12] described "Purkinje cells" connecting the two nodes and running along the crista terminalis. This was refuted by the German Pathological Society[13] and by Aschoff[14] and Mönckeberg[15] who said that the internodal tissue was plain atrial myocardium.

In 1916 Bachman[16] described an interatrial bundle, and in 1963 James[17] proposed that there were specialized fibers within Bachman's bundle that divided at the crest of the interatrial septum to continue down the septum and enter the top of the A-V node (the anterior internodal tract). At this time James also described the middle (Wenckebach's muscle bundle) and posterior (Thorel's "specialized" pathway) internodal tracts. The impetus for his studies came from the discovery in 1961, that cells of the atria differed from each other in their electrophysiological characteristics.[18] The internodal tracts as described by James are illustrated in Fig. 1-5.

Most modern investigators[2,5-7] except James[17] believe that, without ruling out the possibility of the existence of atrial cells with different electrophysiological properties, there is no evidence of specialized internodal conduction tissue, although preferential conduction exists through muscle bundles (Fig. 1-6).

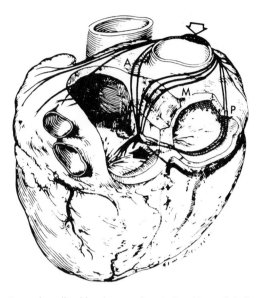

Fig. 1-5. Internodal tracts as described by James. *A,* anterior; *M,* medial; *P,* posterior. (From James TN. In Hurst JW, editor: The heart, ed 5, New York, 1982, McGraw-Hill Book Co.)

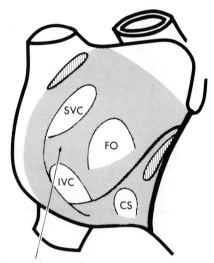

Working atrial myocardium

Fig. 1-6. Diagram of results of Anderson's investigations concerning nature of intermodal atrial myocardium. Geometry, rather than specialized tissue, favors preferential conduction. *SVC,* superior vena cava; *IVC,* inferior vena cava; *FO,* fossa ovalis; *CS,* coronary sinus. (From Anderson RH and Becker AE. In Mandel WJ, editor: Cardiac arrhythmias: their mechanisms, diagnosis, and management, Philadelphia, 1980, JB Lippincott Co.)

Development of the AV node

Controversies also exist regarding the embryology of the AV node and the bundle of His.[1,3,19] Anderson and others[20] have found specialized tissue analogous to the AV node and bundle as early as 5 to 6 weeks in the embryo and therefore consider that these structures develop in situ from multiple origins and are not a migration of tissue as proposed by some.

Blood supply. In 90% of subjects the AV node receives its blood supply from the right coronary artery (Figs. 1-7 and 1-8). In the remaining 10% the circumflex artery supplies the AV node (Fig. 1-9).

Ultrastructure. The AV node is located just beneath the endocardium in the right atrium between the coronary sinus and the medial leaflet of the tricuspid

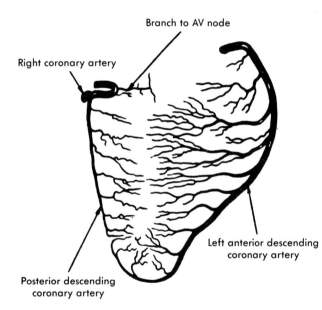

Fig. 1-7. Drawing from vinylite cast of normal blood supply of human interventricular septum. (From James TN and Burch GE: Circulation 17:391, 1958. By permission of the American Heart Association, Inc.)

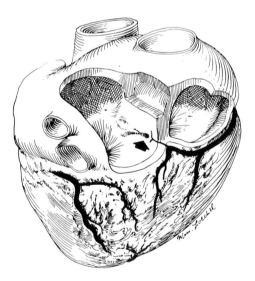

Fig. 1-8. Arterial supply to diaphragmatic surface of human heart as it occurs in approximately 90% of instances. (From James TN: Anatomy of the coronary arteries, New York, 1961, Hoeber Medical Division, Harper & Row, Publishers.)

valve. The fibers of the AV node are arranged in an interlacing pattern, functioning as a triage for atrial impulses and as a delay station in AV conduction. Delay is an important function since it allows time for atrial contraction to be effective in filling and stretching the ventricles. A diagrammatical representation of the ultrastructure of the AV node and bundle of His is presented in Fig. 1-10. Although the currents seem to be dispersed when entering the nodal area *(N)*, they emerge in the bundle of His *(H)* in a unified wave front.

As the AV node begins to penetrate the central fibrous body (the central core of fibrous tissue dividing atria and ventricles), its cells become more and more longitudinally oriented until they become the parallel pathways of the bundle of His and, as such, descend along the posterior border of the membranous ventricular septum.

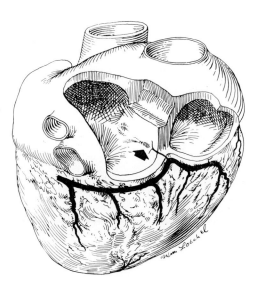

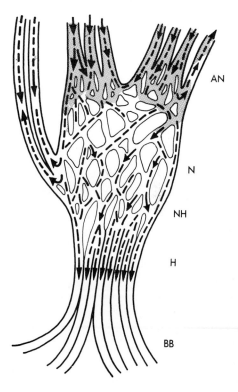

Fig. 1-9. Arterial supply to diaphragmatic surface of human heart as it occurs in approximately 10% of instances. (From James TN: Anatomy of the coronary arteries, New York, 1961, Hoeber Medical Division, Harper & Row, Publishers.)

Fig. 1-10. AV node and bundle of His. *AN,* atrionodal; *N,* nodal area; *NH,* nodal-His; *H,* bundle of His; *BB,* bundle branches. (From Sherf L and James TN: Am J Cardiol 29:529, 1972.)

Branching portion of the bundle of His

At approximately 6 weeks the bundle branches in the embryonic heart can be seen cascading down both sides of the septum with ramifications into the trabeculated pouches.[1] At 18 weeks the left bundle branch (LBB) is recognizable as a fanlike structure and the right bundle branch (RBB) as cordlike. [1]

   Left bundle branch. The main LBB lies on the left side of the ventricular septum, beginning at the level of the commissure formed by the aortic cusps and extending for approximately 1 to 2 cm before it divides. Here the bundle of His gives off a "fine stream"[20] of fibers (which have been described by James[21] as "a virtual sheet") that forms a large posterior radiation and a smaller anterior one. A third midseptal radiation was noted by Demoulin and Kulbertus[22,23] in 33 out of 49 normal hearts (type I, Fig. 1-11). This lesser-known fascicle was readily identified by

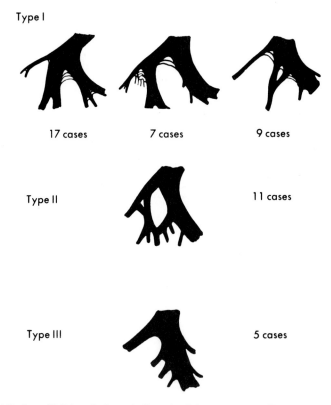

Fig. 1-11. Distribution of left bundle branch fibers in 49 human hearts. (From Kulbertus HE and Demoulin J. In Wellens HJJ, Lie KI, and Janse MJ, editors: The conduction system of the heart, Hingham, Mass, 1976, Martinus Nijhoff, Publishers.)

these investigators and was found to originate either from the common left bundle or from the anterior or posterior fascicle. In the remaining 16 cases the septum was supplied by radiations from the posterior fascicle or by combined radiations from both the anterior and the posterior fascicles. The findings of these investigators are illustrated in Fig. 1-11.

They observed the following:

1. There are three main interconnecting fascicles in the left ventricle rather than two. One supplies the anterior (superior) wall, another the posterior (inferior) wall, and a third the midseptum.
2. The electrocardiographic (ECG) pattern of left anterior hemiblock reflects LBB disease but is hardly ever confined solely to the anterior fascicle.

It is interesting to compare the drawings of these investigators with that in 1906 by Tawara,[24] who also depicted *three* fascicles in the left ventricle (Fig. 1-12), a concept supported by other investigators.[5,23,25,26]

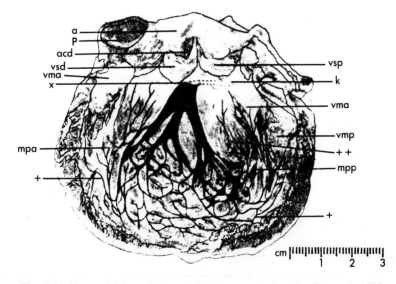

Fig. 1-12. Human left bundle branch anatomy as depicted by Tawara in 1906.

Right bundle branch. The RBB proceeds along the septal band to the moderator band, where it divides and fans out into the right ventricular wall. It is subendocardial at its origin and again before it fans out. The middle portion travels deeper within the muscle. The mature RBB is illustrated in Fig. 1-13.

The difference in size between the right and left bundle branches is striking and explains why the right bundle can be compromised by a lesser lesion than the larger LBB can. This fact may account for the frequent clinical innocence of right bundle branch block (RBBB).

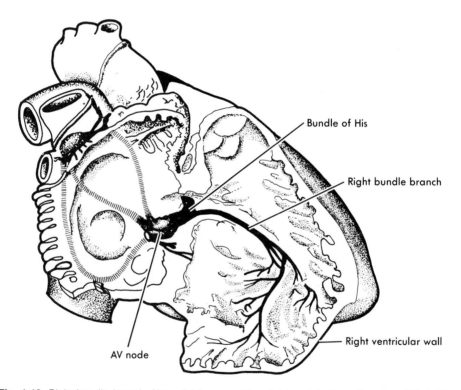

Fig. 1-13. Right bundle branch. Note division supplying right ventricular wall and septal division. (From Marriott HJL: Workshop in electrocardiography, Oldsmar, Fla, 1972, Tampa Tracings.)

REFERENCES

1. Anderson RH and others: The development of the cardiac specialized tissue. In Wellens HJJ, Lie KI, and Janse MJ, editors: The conduction system of the heart, Philadelphia, 1976, Lea & Febiger.
2. Retzer R: Some results of recent investigations on the mammalian heart, Anat Rec 2:149, 1908.
3. Patten BM: The development of the sinoventricular conduction system, Univ Mich Med Bull 22:1, 1956.
4. Truex RC: The sinoatrial node and its connections with the atrial tissues. In Wellens HJJ, Lie KI, and Janse MJ, editors: The conduction system of the heart, Philadelphia, 1976, Lea & Febiger.
5. Anderson RH and Becker AE: Gross anatomy and microscopy of the conducting system. In Mandel WJ, editor: Cardiac arrhythmias; their mechanisms, diagnosis and management, ed 2, Philadelphia, 1987, JB Lippincott Co.
6. Chuyacqui BJ: Uber die Ausbreitungsbundel des Simisknoten. Eine kritische Analyse der wichtigsten Arbeiten, Virchow's Arch, A Path Anat 335:179, 1972.
7. Spach MS and others: Excitation sequences of the atrial septum and A-V node in isolated hearts of the dog and the rabbit, Circ Res 29:156, 1971.
8. Spach MS and others: Electrical potential distribution surrounding the atria during depolarization and repolarization in the dog, Circ Res 24:857, 1969.
9. Sherf L and James TN: Fine structure of cells and their histologic organization within internodal pathways of the heart; clinical and electrocardiographic implications, Am J Cardiol 44:345, 1979.
10. Hoffman BF: Fine structure of internodal pathways, Am J Cardiol 44:387, 1979 (editorial).
11. Wenckebach KF: Beitrage zur Kenntnis der menschlichen Herztatigkeit, Arch Anat Physiol (Physiol Abth) 297, 1906.
12. Thorel C: Vorlaufige Mitteilung uber eine besondere Muskel-verbindung zwischen der Cava superior und den Hisschen Bundein, Munch Med Wschr 56:2159, 1906.
13. Bericht uber die Verhandlungen der XIV Tagung der deutchen pathologischen Gesellschaft in Erlangen, vom 4-6, Zentralbl Allg Pathol 21:433, April 1910.
14. Aschoff L: Referat uber die Herzstorungen in ihren Beziehungen zu den Spezifischen, Muskelsystem in Herzens, Verh Dtsch Ges Pathol 14:3, 1910.
15. Mönckeberg JG: Beitrage zur normalen und pathologischen Anatomie des Herzens, Verh Dtsch Ges Pathol 14:64, 1910.
16. Bachmann G: The inter-auricular time interval, Am J Physiol 41:309, 1916.
17. James TN: The connecting pathways between the sinus node and the AV node and between the right and left atrium in the human heart, Am Heart J 66:498, 1963.
18. Paes de Carvalho A: Cellular electrophysiology of the atrial specialized tissues. In Paes de Carvalho A, de Mello WC, and Hoffman BF, editors: Specialized tissues of the heart, Amsterdam, 1961, Elsevier North-Holland, Inc.
19. Walls EW: The development of the specialized conducting tissue of the human heart, J Anat 81:93, 1947.
20. Anderson RH and others: The atrioventricular junctional area of the human heart—a morphological study of the atrioventricular node and bundle, Eur J Cardiol 3:11, 1975.
21. James TN: Anatomy of the conduction system of the heart. In Hurst JW, editor: The heart, ed 4, New York, 1978, McGraw-Hill Book Co.
22. Demoulin JC and Kulbertus HE: Histopathological examination of concept of left hemiblock, Br Heart J 34:809, 1972.
23. Kulbertus HE and Demoulin J: Pathological basis of concept of left hemiblock. In Wellens HJJ, Lie KI, and Janse MJ, editors: The conduction system of the heart, Philadelphia, 1976, Lea & Febiger.
24. Tawara S: Das Reitzleitungssystem des Saugetierherzens, Jena Gustav Fischer, 1906.
25. Rossi L: Histopathology of the conducting system, G Ital Cardiol 2:484, 1972.
26. Uhley HN: The quadrifascicular nature of the peripheral conduction system. In Dreifus LS and Liboff W, editors: Cardiac arrhythmias, New York, 1973, Grune & Stratton, Inc.

CHAPTER 2

Sinus node and His bundle electrograms

Normal cardiac activation is initiated in the sinus node where pacemaker cells discharge at regular intervals and at a rate dependent on autonomic influences and the hemodynamic needs of the body.

The action potential generated in the sinus node is conducted to the atrial myocardium and from there across the AV node, bundle of His, and bundle branches into the ventricles. Specialized perinodal fibers connecting the sinus node and the atrium have been identified in the rabbit but not in humans. It is believed that conduction is facilitated between the sinus node and the atrial myocardium either by these specialized connecting fibers or simply because of the anatomical orientation of the atrial myocardial fibers.[1]

Propagation of current through the myocardium is dependent on the cable properties of myocardium. When the membrane potential changes in one segment of fiber, neighboring segments are affected so that they also depolarize and in turn act as an excitatory stimulus to the adjacent tissue. The current flows through the myocardium longitudinally along the length of the fibers. If for any reason the current is not strong enough or if the cells themselves have been functionally impaired, the velocity of the depolarization wave may slow considerably, or the wave may stop altogether.

Silent zones on surface ECG

The discharge of the sinus node is a silent event in that the magnitude of the electrical activity generated is too small to be picked up by the surface ECG; indeed, it was not recorded directly at all until 1978.[2-4]

The electrical activity generated during depolarization of the AV node and bundle of His is, like the sinus discharge, not strong enough to be recorded on the surface ECG. However, the PR interval offers a time frame for these events that is not available for the sinus node discharge and conduction through the sinus node to the atrial musculature.

Initial activation of the AV node occurs only 0.03 or 0.04 second after the beginning of the P wave, with the bundle of His and bundle branches activated during the PR segment.

Fig. 2-1 illustrates electrical events in the heart and relates them to what is actually seen on the surface ECG. Note that the discharge of the sinus node occurs before the onset of the P wave and that there is a measurable conduction time between sinus node discharge and the depolarization of atrial myocardium as signaled by the P wave.

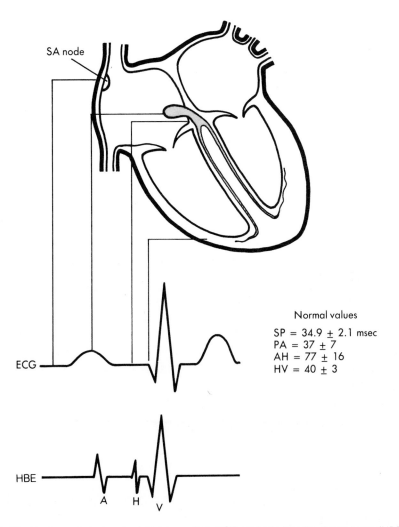

Normal values
SP = 34.9 ± 2.1 msec
PA = 37 ± 7
AH = 77 ± 16
HV = 40 ± 3

Fig. 2-1. Electrical events in heart related to surface ECG and His bundle electrogram *(HBE)*. Approximate relationship of sinus node discharge is also related to surface ECG. *SP,* SA conduction time; *PA,* intra-atrial conduction time; *AH,* AV nodal conduction time; *HV,* His-Purkinje conduction time.

Sinus node electrogram

Direct recording of the electrical discharge of the human sinus node was not available until, at Columbia University in 1978, the electrical potentials of the sinus node in the canine heart were successfully recorded.[2] In 1979 and 1980, the same team developed a technique for direct recording of the electrical potentials from the human sinus node.[3-5]

SA conduction time

During the above-mentioned experiments conduction time between the sinus node and the atrial myocardium (SA conduction time) was measured from the deflection on the SA nodal electrogram, attributed to SA nodal electrical activity, to the beginning of the P wave of the ECG in the bipolar records or to the beginning of the high right atrial electrogram in the unipolar records.

In 15 patients without SA nodal dysfunction, SA conduction time was 34.9 ± 2.1 msec. Accurate measurement of SA conduction time permits differentiation between normal and abnormal SA nodal function.

Clinically an understanding of SA conduction time illuminates the mechanism involved in type I and type II SA block and the difference between SA block and sinus arrest. We discuss these disorders in detail in Chapter 8.

The sinus node electrogram may also prove useful in cardiac surgery as an aid to avoiding damage to the sinus node. It may also provide a better method for differentiating normal from abnormal SA nodes.

His bundle electrogram

The electrical activity in the bundle of His was first recorded in 1960 in Europe[6] and in 1969 in the United States.[7]

The development of the catheter technique for recording His bundle electrograms (HBEs) has enabled the clinician to define the level of conduction delay within the AV junction and to establish the difference between type I and type II AV block.

HBE deflections

The deflections seen in the HBE and illustrated in Fig. 2-1 are as follows:

The A wave: The first deflection represents atrial activation and is called the A wave. This deflection represents low right atrial activation since the recording lead is either the bipolar His bundle lead or a low atrial lead.

The H deflection: This deflection follows the A wave and represents His bundle electrical activity as recorded by a catheter lying at the base of the tricuspid valve, close to the His bundle.

The V deflection: The last deflection on the His bundle electrogram represents ventricular activation and is concurrent with the QRS complex on the surface ECG.

HBE intervals and normal values

The HBE divides the PR interval into three components defined by the PA, AH, and HV intervals.

PA interval. This interval is an approximate measurement of intra-atrial conduction time from the area around the sinus node to the low right atrium. It is measured from the onset of the P wave on the standard ECG or from the atrial deflection of a high right atrial electrogram to the A wave on the HBE. The normal range is 25 to 45 msec (37 ± 7).

AH interval. This interval represents AV nodal conduction time. It is measured from the A wave on the HBE to the earliest onset of the His bundle potential. The normal range is 50 to 120 msec (77 ± 16).

HV interval. This interval represents the conduction time through the His-Purkinje system (from the bundle of His to the distal Purkinje fibers). The normal range is 35 to 45 msec (40 ± 3).

Sequence of activation through the conduction system

Fig. 2-2 relates the sequence of activation through the conduction system to the ECG. Note that the sinus node is activated before the P wave is inscribed and that the AV node is initially activated well before atrial depolarization is completed.

Activation of most of the His-Purkinje system naturally precedes activation of the working myocardium as represented by the QRS complex; the QRS therefore begins after most of the conduction system is already depolarized. An appreciation of this sequence helps one to grasp the concept of concealed conduction in the bundle branches as discussed in Chapter 17.

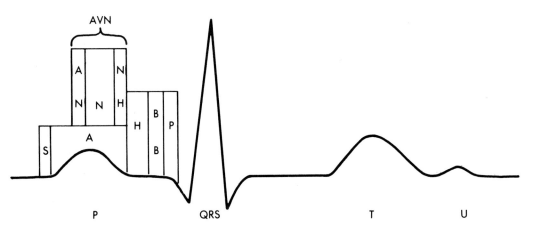

Fig. 2-2. Sequence of activation through conduction system related to surface ECG. Note that QRS begins only after most of conduction system has already been activated. *S,* SA conduction; *A,* atria; *AVN,* atrioventricular node; *AN,* atrionodal; *N,* nodal (central); *NH,* nodal-His; *H,* His bundle; *BB,* bundle branches; *P,* Purkinje fibers.

Noninvasive His bundle electrogram

In 1973 it was first demonstrated that the electrical activity arising from the His-Purkinje system could be recorded from the body surface.[8-10] Technical problems limited the success of these and further studies.[11-25] In 1981 Flowers and her group[26] developed a new system that records on a beat-to-beat basis but has a portability problem.

Indications for His bundle recordings

The extrapolation of data obtained from His bundle electrograms over the past decade has actually lessened the clinical need to use this technique.

In most cases of AV block the routine ECG and the clinical setting will provide enough information to deduce correctly the site of block. Even when the site of block cannot be deduced such as when the AV block is associated with a wide QRS complex, an HBE would be necessary only in the asymptomatic patient since the symptomatic patient should receive a pacemaker no matter at what level the block, and the treatment for the asymptomatic patient would depend on whether the pathology was in the AV node (type I) or in the His-Purkinje system (usually type II).

Even a diagnosis of concealed junctional extrasystoles, although not definitive, can generally be made from long continuous tracings.

In the realm of research His bundle electrograms will most certainly continue to contribute to the flow of information about reentrant phenomena, the mechanisms and actions of drugs, and the mechanisms of complex arrhythmias.

REFERENCES

1. Jordan JL and Mandel WJ: Disorders of sinus function. In Mandel WJ, editor: Cardiac arrhythmias; their mechanisms, diagnosis, and management, Philadelphia, 1980, JB Lippincott Co.
2. Cramer M and others: Electrograms from the canine sinoatrial pacemaker recorded in vitro and in situ, Am J Cardiol 42:939, 1978.
3. Reiffel J and others: Human sinus node electrograms: transvenous catheter recorded technique and normal sinoatrial conduction times in adults, Circulation 60:238, 1979 (abstract).
4. Hariman RJ and others: Method for recording electrical activity of the sinoatrial node and automatic atrial foci during cardiac catheterization in human subjects, Am J Cardiol 45:775, 1980.
5. Hariman RJ and others: Methods for recording electrograms of the sinoatrial node during cardiac surgery in man, Circulation 61:1024, 1980.
6. Giraud G and others: Variations de potentiel liées à l'activité du système de conduction auriculo-ventriculaire chez l'homme (enregistrement electrocardiographic endocavitaire), Arch Mal Coeur 53:757, 1960.
7. Scherlag BJ and others: Catheter technique for recording His bundle activity in man, Circulation 39:13, 1969.
8. Berbari EJ and others: Non-invasive technique for detection of electrical activity during the P-R segment, Circulation 48:1005, 1973.
9. Flowers NC and others: Surface recording of electrical activity from the His bundle area. Presented at the Annual Meeting of the Cardiac Electrophysiologic Group, Atlantic City, April, 1973.
10. Flowers NC and Horan LG: His bundle and bundle branch recordings from the body surface, Circulation 48:102, 1973.
11. Flowers NC and others: Surface recording of electrical activity from the region of the bundle of His, Am J Cardiol 33:384, 1974.
12. Flowers NC and others: Surface recordings of low-level internal signals. In Miller HA and Harrison DC, editors: Biomedical electrode technology: theory and practice, New York, 1974, Academic Press, Inc.
13. Berbari EJ and others: Extracardiac recordings of His-Purkinje activity during conduction disorders and junctional rhythms, Circulation 51:802, 1975.
14. Berbari EJ and others: The His-Purkinje electrocardiogram in man. An initial assessment of its uses and limitations, Circulation 54:219, 1976.
15. Stopczyk MJ and others: Surface recording of electrical heart activity during the P-R segment in man by a computer averaging technique. In Proceedings of the World Congress of Cardiology, p 162, 1974 (abstract).

16. Hishimoto Y and Sawayama T: Non-invasive recording of His bundle potential in man: simplified method, Br Heart J 37:635, 1975.

17. Furness A and others: The feasibility of detecting His-bundle activity from the body surface, Cardiovasc Res 9:390, 1975.

18. Takeda H and others: Noninvasive recording of His-Purkinje activity in patients with complete atrioventricular block: clinical application of an "automated descrimination circuit," Circulation 60:421, 1979.

19. Van Den Akker TJ and others: Real time method for noninvasive recording of His bundle activity of the electrocardiogram, Comput Biomed Res 9:559, 1976.

20. Sano T: Electrical activity of His bundle, Jpn Circ J 40:209, 1976.

21. Honda M and others: Clinical studies on noninvasive investigation of the His bundle electrogram. In Proceedings of the 5th International Symposium of Cardiac Pacing, p 19, 1977.

22. Hombach V, Behrenbeck DW, and Hilger HH: Osophagosternale and ösophagoapikale Ableitungen zur Registrierung von Oberflächen-His-Potentialen, Z Kardiol 66:565, 1977.

23. Denis JG and Cywinski JK: The use of microprocessor for noninvasive recordings of electrical activity from the conduction system of the heart. In Proceedings of the 29th Annual Conference of Engineers in Medicine and Biology, vol 18, p 187, 1976.

24. Ishijima M: Statistically compensated averaging method for noninvasive recording of His-Purkinje activity. In Proceedings of the 14th Rocky Mountain Bioengineering Symposium, Biomed Sci Instrum 14:129, 1978.

25. Vincent R and others: Noninvasive recording of electrical activity in the PR segment in man, Br Heart J 40:124, 1978.

26. Flowers NC and others: Surface recording of His-Purkinje activity on an every-beat basis without digital averaging, Circulation 63:948, 1981.

CHAPTER 3

Cellular electrophysiology

Historical highlights

In 1949 Hodgkin and Katz[1] demonstrated that a rapid influx of sodium into the cell (reflected by phase 0 of the action potential) was responsible for the depolarization of squid nerve cells and that this sudden increase in sodium permeability determined the amplitude and rate of rise of phase 0. Three years later Hodgkin and Huxley,[2] through the use of voltage-clamp technique, determined that this sudden, rapid inward flow of sodium was followed by an outward flow of potassium, which caused the repolarization phase of the action potential. The voltage clamp made it possible to set transmembrane voltage at selected values and then study ionic currents relative to time and voltage. Thus it became possible to describe depolarization and repolarization in terms of equations that show how the underlying membrane currents of sodium and potassium ions vary with transmembrane voltage and time. In the years that followed, sodium and potassium were assumed to be the only ions involved in the cardiac action potential,[3] although by this time it was well known that the initial rapid phase of depolarization was followed by a slower phase of depolarization.[4]

In 1966 Neidergerke and Orkand,[5] working with intracellular microelectrodes inserted into strips of frog heart muscle, demonstrated that there was an apparent sodium-calcium competition during depolarization. In that same year Hagiwara and Nakajima[6] demonstrated that there were two inward currents, one carried by sodium, which was responsible for the initial rise of the action potential, and one carried by calcium, which caused the plateau phase of the action potential. It was subsequently established that the initial depolarization, caused by the rapid inward sodium current, actually triggers the change in membrane permeability that gives rise to the second slow inward current, carried mainly by calcium.

Current flow in the heart: its cable properties

The normal cardiac cycle has its origin in the sinus node in which an impulse is regularly generated at a rate consistent with the needs of the body. This impulse then propagates through the atria, AV node, His-Purkinje system, and ventricular myocardium in a predictable and orderly fashion. A strand of cardiac muscle is like an electrical cable in that a current flows from a localized pacing area in the heart to adjacent cells, passing easily and rapidly because low-resistance gap junctions in the regions of the intercalated disks separate the end-to-end borders of the myocardial cells (Fig. 3-1). These disks, however, are not present between certain transitional cells of the proximal AV node, contributing to the normally slow conduction through the node.[7]

The generation and propagation of the impulse depends on the gradient of electrical potential that exists across the cell membrane when the cell is at rest (the resting membrane potential). When the membrane potential reaches threshold, a rapid sequence of changes in the transmembrane potential takes place. The electrical cycle of muscle cells is called an action potential.

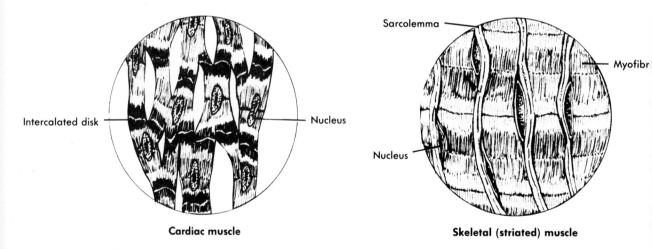

Cardiac muscle   **Skeletal (striated) muscle**

Fig. 3-1. Comparison of myocardial and skeletal tissue. Note distinctive way cardiac cells branch and intercalated disks separate their connecting ends. (From Conover, M: Understanding electrocardiography, ed 5, St. Louis, 1988, The CV Mosby Co.)

Normal cellular electrophysiology

The integrity of the cell is dependent on an intact resting membrane potential, which in turn is dependent on the sodium pump and sodium-potassium ATPase, sodium-potassium exchange, sodium concentration gradient, sodium-calcium exchange, and potassium concentration gradient, in addition to normal electrolyte balance and absence of certain drugs.

RESTING MEMBRANE POTENTIAL. The resting membrane potential is the electrical potential gradient that exists across cell membranes during electrical diastole (phase 4 of the action potential). When a microelectrode penetrates the membrane of a healthy cardiac cell, it records a negative potential with respect to a reference electrode outside the cell in the extracellular fluid. Everywhere in the normal heart, except in the AV and SA nodes and on the atrial surfaces of the two AV valves, this potential is approximately -90 mV.[8]

The normal resting membrane potential of -90 mV in myocardial cells is maintained mainly by the electrogenic negativity produced by (1) the sodium-potassium exchange pump and (2) the flow of potassium out of the cell down its concentration gradient. The resting membrane potential determines conduction velocity and the ability of the cell to respond to a stimulus.

SODIUM PUMP AND SODIUM-POTASSIUM ATPase. The sodium pump is an ion transport system in the cardiac sarcolemma. Its main function is to generate large sodium (Na^+) and potassium (K^+) gradients across the cell membrane by transporting Na^+ out of the cell in exchange for K^+. Energy for the pumping of Na^+ out of and K^+ into the cell is derived from the hydrolysis of adenosine triphosphate (ATP) by sodium-potassium ATPase. The rate at which ATP is hydrolyzed is increased by Na^+ and/or by K^+ (more so by the two together). However, before this energy can be used for the sodium pump, ATP must form a complex with magnesium (Mg^{++}). Thus the ATPase reaction requires various substrates, including Na^+, K^+, ATP, and Mg^{++}.[9]

SODIUM-POTASSIUM EXCHANGE. The active transport of Na^+ out of the cell in exchange for K^+ is depicted on the right side of the cell in Fig. 3-2. The binding sites for the cations of sodium-potassium ATPase are on either side of the membrane. The binding site for Na^+ is on the inside and for K^+ is on the outside of the sarcolemma. Sodium ions are transported to the outside of the cell from binding sites on the inside in exchange for K^+ bound to sites on the outside of the cell membrane. For every three Na^+ that are transported out of the cell, only two K^+ are brought in, causing generation of a current. Thus the sodium pump generates a net positive charge that moves out of the cell, contributing to the normal negative intracellular resting potential of -90 mV by approximately 10 mV.

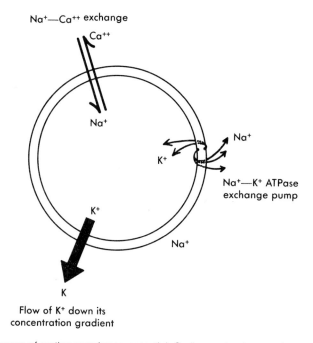

Fig. 3-2. Maintenance of resting membrane potential. Sodium-potassium exchange pump extrudes three sodium ions for every two postassium ions, generating a net negative flow of 10 mV; flow of potassium out of cell down its concentration gradient generates approximately 80 mV, accounting for most of the -90 mV resting membrane potential. Energy created by the sodium gradient removes calcium from the cell (sodium-calcium exchange). (From Conover M: Understanding electrocardiography, ed 5, St. Louis, 1988, The CV Mosby Co.)

SODIUM CONCENTRATION GRADIENT. The large Na^+ concentration gradient created by the Na^+ pump determines cardiac electrophysiological properties because it permits the fast inward current during rapid depolarization. Once the fast sodium channels are open, this gradient causes Na^+ to rush into the cell, reversing its polarity. The Na^+ gradient also provides a reserve of osmotic energy that is used to transport other ions across the membrane; the sodium-calcium exchange is an example of this transportation.

SODIUM-CALCIUM EXCHANGE. The sodium pump takes part in the regulation of myocardial contractility by creating a Na^+ concentration gradient that provides the energy to remove calcium (Ca^{++}) from the cell against an electrochemical gradient. If the sodium gradient is reduced, there is less energy for this work, and calcium ions accumulate inside the cell, explaining the inotropic effect of digitalis, which inhibits the sodium pump and causes intracellular sodium and therefore calcium to accumulate, resulting in a stronger contraction.[9]

POTASSIUM CONCENTRATION GRADIENT. The electrogenic effect of the sodium-potassium exchange pump itself accounts for only approximately 10 mV of the resting membrane potential. The remainder of the resting membrane potential is achieved because of the large concentration gradient of K^+ across the membrane (approximately 40:1) established by the sodium-potassium exchange pump. Since the cell membrane is highly permeable to K^+, this ion flows out of the cell down its concentration gradient (see Fig. 3-2). More K^+ leaves the cell than Na^+ enters, creating an electrogenic current of approximately -80 mV. The electrochemical gradient thus generated by the sodium pump and the flow of K^+ down its concentration gradient cannot be neutralized by a flow of Na^+ into the cell because the membrane is far less permeable to Na^+ than it is to K^+ and because of the sodium pump. This pump clears the cytosol of even small amounts of Na^+ that remain after rapid depolarization and returns the K^+ that remain after repolarization to the cytosol from the extracellular fluid.

If the concentration gradient of K^+ is smaller than normal (for example, because of a loss of K^+ from the cell such as occurs with ischemia), then the exodus of K^+ from the cell is less and so is the resting membrane potential. A less negative resting membrane potential causes a decrease in conduction velocity and encourages arrhythmias.

SUMMARY OF FUNCTIONS OF SODIUM PUMP. In summary, the functions of the sodium pump are as follows:

1. Creation of the Na^+ gradient across the cell membrane, which in turn provides the electrochemical gradient for rapid depolarization
2. Generation of the osmotic energy to rid the cell of Ca^{++} by means of the sodium-calcium exchange
3. Maintenence of the resting membrane potential, thus assuring optimal conduction
4. Regulation of myocardial contractility by providing osmotic energy for the active transport of Ca^{++} out of the cell
5. Extrusion of Na^+ from the cell after rapid depolarization
6. Restoration of K^+ to the cell after repolarization
7. Creation of a net outward positive current through an unequal exchange with K^+, contributing to the resting membrane potential
8. Creation of a K^+ concentration gradient, which generates a net outward positive current, contributing to the resting membrane potential

Membrane channels

Membrane channels are depicted by Rosen and Wit[10] in Fig. 3-3. They are specific for certain ions and functions, and they open in response to a certain voltage—their threshold potential. They are composed of a channel protein, selectivity filter, and gating proteins. The channel protein (nonstippled area) separates the portal itself from the lipid bilayer of the cell membrane (stippled area). The selectivity filter

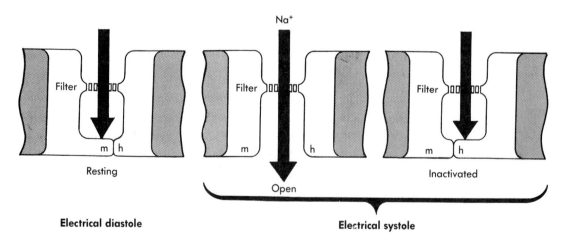

Fig. 3-3. States of the fast sodium *(Na⁺)* channel during different phases of the action potential. Resting state is that seen during phase 4 of the transmembrane potential; open state correlates with phase 0, and inactivated state correlates with phase 2 and part of phase 3. *(m* and *h,* Gating proteins.) (From Rosen MR and Wit AL: Am J Cardiol 59[11]:10E, 1987.)

guards the channel and is ion-specific, being situated near the channel's outer surface and having a diameter specific for certain ions. For example, the selectivity filter for the fast channel is specific for Na^+, although hydrogen (H^+) may also pass through.[11]

The gating proteins, designated by Hodgkin and Huxley[12] as "m" and "h" (see Fig. 3-3), function to provide resting, open, and inactivated states. In the resting state (electrical diastole), the *m* protein is in a closed position. It will move to an open position when threshold potential (-70 mV for the fast channels and -30 mV for the slow channels) is reached. Sodium enters through fast channels, and both Ca^{++} and Na^+ enter through slow channels. During rapid depolarization the *h* protein inactivates the fast channel by moving to a closed position. As the cell repolarizes and returns to its resting state, the *m* protein again takes over the closed position. The movement of these gating proteins to open and closed positions is determined by transmembrane voltage and by the length of time that the cell has maintained that voltage. Fig. 3-3 illustrates a membrane channel during the electrical cardiac cycle.

The slow Ca^{++} channels operate in the same way as the fast Na^+ channels except that the threshold potential of the two differ, with that of the slow channels -30 to -40 mV (as opposed to -70 mV for the fast channels). Also, the slow channels stay open longer than those of the fast Na^+ channels, rendering the myocardium refractory for a longer time. Because of a slow inward current of positive ions (Ca^{++} and Na^+) into the cell through the slow Ca^{++} channels, rapid repolarization is delayed, and the refractory period is prolonged. Cells with only slow Ca^{++} channels have a resting potential of -60 mV.

Electrical cardiac cycle and action potential

The action potential is divided into five phases, which constitute a rapid sequence of changes in electrical potential across the cell membrane during depolarization and repolarization. Phase 4 constitutes electrical diastole, and phases 0 to 3 constitute electrical systole.

Study of the action potential is possible with use of a glass capillary microelectrode inserted into a single cardiac fiber. This impalement does not result in significant cell injury because the microelectrode tip is so small (<1 μm). Thus the normal electrophysiological properties of the fiber can be studied. The flow of ions across the cell membrane can be identified by using voltage clamp techniques. The graph in Fig. 3-4 reflects the voltage across the cell membrane as recorded by the microelectrode at the moment of impalement of the cell and during the electrical cardiac cycle (electrical diastole and electrical systole) in both nonpacemaker and pacemaker cells. Note the difference in phase 4 (electrical diastole) between the pacemaker cell and the nonpacemaker cell; the nonpacemaker cell waits for a stimulus from outside (Fig. 3-4, *A*), whereas the pacemaker cell is able to reach threshold potential on its own (Fig. 3-4, *B*).

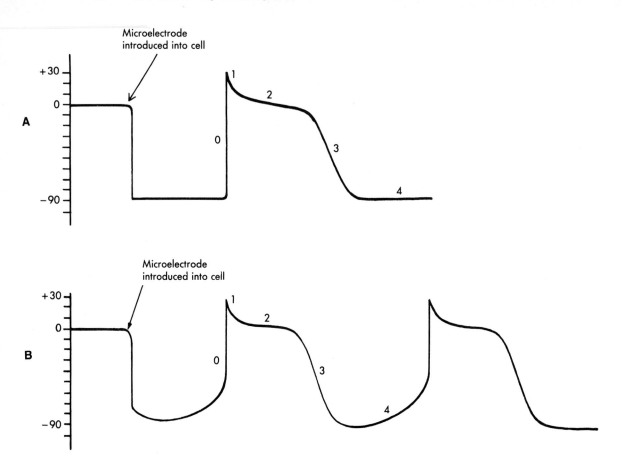

Fig. 3-4. Action potentials of **A,** a myocardial fiber and, **B,** a pacemaker fiber. Arrow indicates point at which microelectrode was introduced into cell. Note graph suddenly dips to −90 mV as it records resting membrane potential.

Phase 4

Phase 4 is the time between two consecutive action potentials, or electrical diastole—the resting stage of the cardiac cell. At the end of phase 3 and the beginning of phase 4, the cell has been completely repolarized, achieving its maximal resting membrane potential. Note in Fig. 3-4 that the membrane potential is negative to −90 mV when phase 4 begins. Normally, nonpacemaker cells steadily maintain this membrane potential until they are driven to threshold potential by the current from the sinus node; in pacemaker cells phase 4 rises slowly. During phase 4, the pacemaker cell is either driven to threshold by an outside stimulus or it slowly depolarizes until threshold potential is reached (see Fig. 3-4, *B,* phase 4 depolarization).

Phase 4 depolarization

Depolarization is the reduction of the resting membrane potential to a less negative value; phase 4 depolarization is sometimes called *slow diastolic depolarization*. It is a normal process in pacemaker cells, although it may be abnormal if accelerated. In pacemaker cells the resting membrane potential is slowly reduced (becomes less negative) during phase 4 until threshold potential is reached or until the cell is suddenly driven to threshold potential by an outside current before it can reach that point on its own. The slow depolarization of the cell during phase 4 was formerly thought the result of a slow diastolic buildup of intracellular K^+ coupled with an inward Na^+ current, but recent studies[13-16] have shown that diastolic depolarization may instead be caused by a slow diastolic build-up of Na^+ influx, as illustrated in Fig. 3-5.

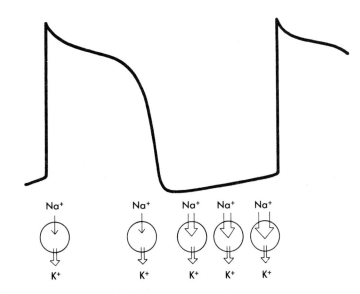

Fig. 3-5. Pacemaker current. During phase 4 in pacemaker cells, a slow buildup of intracellular positive ions occurs (slow diastolic depolarization) as a result of an increasing amount of Na^+ entering the cell until the cell reaches threshold potential and depolarizes rapidly. (From Conover M: Understanding electrocardiography, ed 5, St. Louis, 1988, The CV Mosby Co.)

Threshold potential

The threshold potential is the voltage to which the cell must be reduced before a reversal in potential can occur. Normally, the sinus node cells are the only ones to achieve threshold potential without outside help; they do so by slow diastolic depolarization. In the remainder of the heart, the cells are driven to threshold potential by the current emanating from the sinus node. The threshold potential of the cells in the healthy heart ranges from −70 mV to −80 mV, except for the SA and AV nodes, in which it is approximately −40 mV. When these membrane potentials are reached, the cell rapidly reverses its potential (rapid depolarization or phase 0).

Phase 0 depolarization

Phase 0 is the sharp, tall upstroke of the action potential—the phase of rapid depolarization; it occurs when the membrane is suddenly brought to threshold potential (−70 mV) and the activation gates of the fast sodium channels open to allow the sudden rush of sodium into the cell. The rate of rise of phase 0 (Vmax) is determined both by the number of available sodium ions and by the number of fast sodium channels, which are in turn related to the negativity of the membrane in its resting state.

During phase 0 of the fast response action potential, a second inward current is initiated at approximately −30 to −40 mV. This current is probably carried by both calcium and sodium, and its upstroke velocity and the velocity at which it propagates are much slower than those of the fast response; hence the term "slow response" action potential is used for cells that do not have fast sodium channels. Phase 0 is immediately followed by repolarization.

Repolarization

Repolarization is the restoration of the cell to its maximal diastolic potential, a process that begins immediately after rapid depolarization (phase 0) when the sodium influx is abruptly terminated because the fast sodium channels close (the slow calcium channels stay open until the onset of phase 3). Repolarization is divided into three phases.

PHASE 1. Phase 1 is the rapid brief beginning of repolarization immediately following phase 0. It results because the fast sodium channels close abruptly and because of a transient outward potassium current. Phase 1 ends in the plateau of the action potential.

PHASE 2. Phase 2 is maintained by the influx of positive ions (Ca^{++} and Na^{+}) into the cell through the slow calcium channels. It is the plateau phase of the action potential; this phase is relatively long in myocardial cells compared to skeletal muscle cells. Fig. 3-6 illustrates the effect of this slower current on the fast-response action potential graph. The slower calcium current is represented by a heavy line. This inward calcium current that is initiated during phase 0 of the action potential has three main functions:

1. Prolongation of refractoriness. It maintains the cell in a prolonged depolarized state, allowing time for one muscle contraction to be completed before another is initiated.
2. Delivery of calcium, which is essential to electromechanical coupling, to the inside of the cell.
3. Stimulation of the sarcoplasmic reticulum. This stimulation causes the release of the intracellular stores of calcium that also take part in the contraction process.

During phase 2, inward and outward currents are balanced as chloride and calcium ions flow in and potassium ions flow out, and there is an outward net positive flow caused by the sodium pump, all of which tends to maintain a positive level of membrane potential.[17]

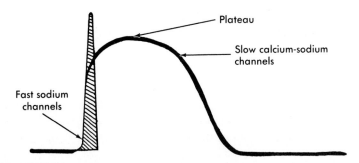

Fig. 3-6. Differing effects of fast sodium channels and slow calcium-sodium channels on action potential. Flow of sodium through fast sodium channels initiates the action potential, and then these channels close *(shaded area)*. Flow of current through slow calcium channels is responsible for the plateau and duration of action potential. (From Conover M: Understanding electrocardiography, ed 5, St. Louis, 1988, The CV Mosby Co.)

PHASE 3. Phase 3 is the rapid repolarization phase. It is initiated by the closing of the slow calcium channels. During phase 3, the exodus of potassium from the cell increases, and the sodium pump restores the cell to its maximal diastolic negativity. When the cell has repolarized to −30 mV, some of the slow calcium channels are ready for another stimulus; by −70 mV some of the fast sodium channels are also ready to respond to another stimulus. However, these responses are poor and may not be propagated. Optimal response occurs at the end of phase 3 when the cell has attained its maximal diastolic potential.

Membrane channels related to the action potential

Fig. 3-7 illustrates the typical action potential of a ventricular myocardial cell as related to the fast sodium and slow calcium membrane channels, both of which are operative during the fast response action potential. Note that the fast sodium channels close almost as soon as they open, producing phase 0 and initiating phase 1, but that the slow calcium channels are open longer, creating the long phase 2 (plateau) and providing the heart with a longer refractory period than that of skeletal muscle. The closing of the slow calcium channels initiates the rapid repolarization phase (phase 3).

Types of action potentials

There are three types of action potentials—fast response, depressed fast response, and slow response (Fig. 3-8), depending on the cell's location in the heart and its diseased state. As the membrane potential is reduced, fewer fast sodium channels are available (depressed fast response action potential) until finally none are available (slow response action potential). A fast response action potential is recorded from a cell that has fast sodium channels available at the onset of depolarization (atrial and ventricular myocardial cells and the cells of the His-Purkinje system); the more negative a cell is during its resting state, the more fast sodium channels that are available. A slow response action potential is recorded from cells that have only slow calcium channels available at the onset of depolarization; normally such cells are found in the sinus and AV nodes and on the atrial surface of the AV valves. In diseased states, slow response action potentials may be recorded from elsewhere as may be action potentials that still possess fast (but fewer than normal) sodium channels, i.e., the depressed fast response action potential. Such an action potential is never normal.

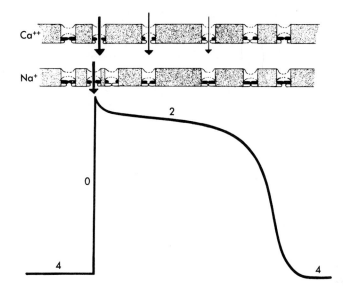

Fig. 3-7. Phases of action potential correlated with mechanism of fast sodium channels and slow calcium channels. Activation gates *(dark bar)* of both channels are closed during electrical diastole *(phase 4)* and both open at their own particular threshold potential during phase 0. (From Conover M: Understanding electrocardiography, ed 5, St. Louis, 1988, The CV Mosby Co.)

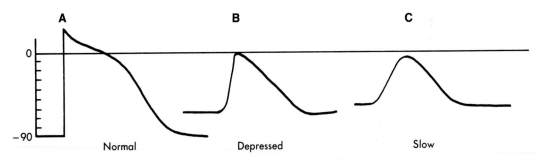

Fig. 3-8. The three types of action potential. **A,** Fast response action potential is found everywhere in the normal heart except, notably, in the two nodes. **B,** Depressed fast response is never normal. **C,** Slow response is found normally in the two nodes and abnormally elsewhere. (From Conover M: Understanding electrocardiography, ed 5, St. Louis, 1988, The CV Mosby Co.)

Refractory periods

Refractoriness is the inability of a cell or fiber to respond normally to a stimulus because it has been too recently activated by a previous stimulus. The *refractory period* is the interval during which the cell or fiber remains unresponsive (effective refractory period) or responds inadequately (relative refractory period) to a second stimulus as recorded by electrodes some distance from the stimulating electrode. Fig. 3-9 illustrates the effective and relative refractory periods. During the *effective refractory period (ERP)*, from phase 0 to −60 mV in phase 3, no stimulus can evoke a propagated response; during the *relative refractory period (RRP)*, that time in phase 3 from −60 mV to −85 mV, a propagated response can result from a strong stimulus.[18] For example, the ERP of the AV node is that interval during which it is impossible for a stimulus to activate and penetrate the node; in its RRP the stimulus can penetrate the node if it is strong enough, but its conduction velocity through the node is impaired.

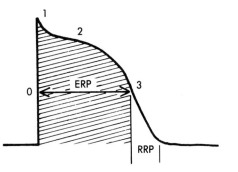

Fig. 3-9. The two parts of refractory period. Effective refractory period *(ERP)* extends from phase 0 to approximately −60 mV in phase 3. Remainder of action potential is relative refractory period *(RRP)*. (From Conover M: Understanding electrocardiography, ed 5, St. Louis, 1988, The CV Mosby Co.)

Cellular physiology. The refractory period itself is determined by the level of the transmembrane potential, which in turn is regulated by the availability of the voltage-dependent fast sodium channels. After phase 0 of the action potential, the fast sodium channels are inactivated and cannot be reactivated until the membrane potential has achieved at least −70 mV (during phase 3 of the action potential). During this time the membrane cannot respond with a propagated action potential to even a strong stimulus. When the membrane achieves −70 mV, the fast sodium channels become partially activated; and as the recovery of excitability proceeds, a strong stimulus may elicit a propagated response (relative refractory period). Such a response is characterized by slow conduction.

Cardiac action potential compared to other action potentials

The cardiac action potential has a much longer duration than that of skeletal muscle, nervous tissue, and smooth muscle because the heart must perform as a pump, with adequate time to fill and with a contraction that propels the chamber contents with the same force each beat. Whereas skeletal muscle may be stimulated rapidly and repetitively, cardiac muscle needs time to relax. Moreover, the vigor of contraction in skeletal muscle can be altered by changing the number of muscle bundles activated; however, cardiac muscle must be activated in precisely the same sequence each beat, and the spread of the impulse must be uniform if arrhythmias are to be avoided.

The cardiac action potential differs markedly from that of skeletal muscle, but even among cardiac action potentials there are characteristic differences. For example:

1. Pacemaker cells possess the property of automaticity; nonpacemaker cells do not. Phase 4 of the action potential reflects this property.

2. The cells of the two nodes (sinus and AV) depolarize because of the relatively slow inward current, which is mainly carried by calcium and probably some sodium, to produce what has been called a "slow response action potential."[8] In addition, the sinus node possesses the property of automaticity, and the AV node in the intact heart does not. All other cells (atrial and ventricular, pacemaker and nonpacemaker) normally depolarize because of the rapid inward sodium current, and that depolarization itself triggers the relatively slower inward calcium current, although under abnormal situations, these cells may be depolarized by the slow calcium current alone.

3. Within the ventricles, the duration of the action potential, and hence the refractory period, of the intraventricular conduction system becomes progressively longer from the beginning of the bundle branches to their endings and then gets progressively shorter again through the transitional cells to the ventricular muscle, resulting in a mechanism called "gating" (Fig. 3-10).[19]

Gating mechanism

The action potential duration increases progressively from the AV node to the distal Purkinje system, where it reaches its maximum; beyond this point its duration decreases.[19-21] This trend can be seen in Fig. 3-10. The region of maximal action potential duration, and therefore refractory period, is referred to as the "gate." For a premature stimulus to propagate through the entire conduction system, it must arrive at the Purkinje fibers (the gate) after the effective refractory period is complete. Thus the gate protects the ventricular myocardium from premature depolarizations arising proximal to the Purkinje fibers.

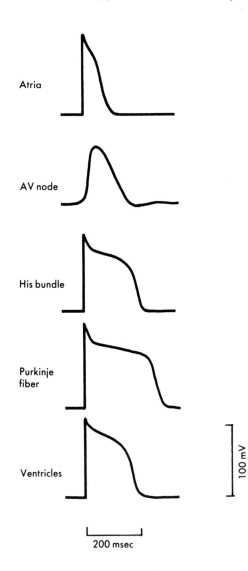

Atria

AV node

His bundle

Purkinje fiber

Ventricles

100 mV

200 msec

Fig. 3-10. Action potential configuration from different areas of the heart. Note that action potential gets longer and longer in duration until it reaches its maximal duration in Purkinje fibers and decreases in duration in ventricular myocardium. The result is a mechanism called "gating."

Supernormal period

"Supernormal" is the name given to the short portion of phase 3 just before the fiber returns to its resting potential (**x** in Fig. 3-11). It is so named because a weaker stimulus than is normally required can initiate a propagated action potential at that time. The explanation of this unexpected phenomenon is that the cell presumably has recovered enough that an adequate number of fast sodium channels are available and yet the membrane potential is closer to threshold potential than if the cell had achieved full repolarization. Thus the cell requires a smaller stimulus to bring it to threshold.[22] Supernormal excitability and conduction are discussed in Chapter 18.

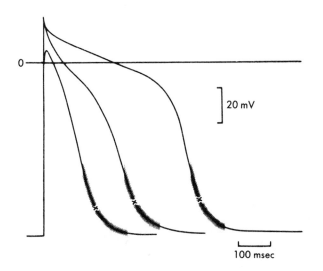

Fig. 3-11. Relationship between supernormal period and total refractory period (X indicates moment of maximal supernormality). Above are shown superimposed action potentials. Longest duration action potential was evoked at a basic cycle length of 800 msec. Shorter action potentials were successively evoked premature beats at cycle lengths of 460 msec and 251 msec. Shaded areas delineate the boundaries of the period of supernormal excitability. The Xs within the shaded area indicate the point of minimal current requirements. (From Spear JF and Moore EN: Circulation 50:144, 1974. By permission of the American Heart Association, Inc.)

Membrane potential related to conduction velocity

An important determinant of conduction velocity is the magnitude of the sodium influx during rapid depolarization. Other determinants are the level of the threshold potential, the electrical cable properties of the fibers, and the diameter and structure of the fiber.[23]

The magnitude of the fast sodium influx is reflected in the speed with which phase 0 rises and in the level of the positive overshoot (dV/dt).[24,25] The size of the sodium current is, in turn, dependent on the membrane potential at the time of stimulation. The more negative this potential, the greater the number of sodium channels available to allow sodium to rush into the cell will be and the faster and higher phase 0 will climb. When the membrane potential just before excitation is approximately −95 mV, conduction velocity is optimal.[26,27] When the membrane potential is less negative, −70 mV for example, some of the sodium channels will be unavailable because their inactivation gates remain closed, resulting in a smaller sodium current of depolarization. Phase 0 of the resulting action potential will, in turn, have a slower rate of rise and a smaller amplitude. This action potential might be an inadequate stimulus for neighboring cells in its conduction path so that the amplitude of phase 0 of the action potential diminishes progressively as the impulse propagates. Such a sequence has been termed "decremental conduction."[4,28] The relationship between the membrane potential at the time of stimulation and the maximal rate of depolarization of the action potential reflects a property known as *membrane responsiveness*.

Fig. 3-12 illustrates the action potentials elicited when stimuli are applied during phase 3. Note that as the stimulus is applied at a more negative level, phase 0 of the resulting action potential becomes steeper and taller. The first two stimuli re-

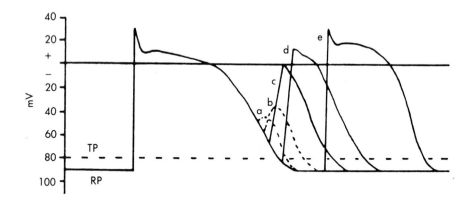

Fig. 3-12. Normal action potential and responses *(a-e)* elicited by stimuli applied at various stages of repolarization. Amplitude and upstroke velocity of such responses are related to level of membrane potential from which they arise. Earliest responses *(a and b)* are slow response action potentials, which arise from low levels of membrane potential; they do not propagate. Response *c* represents earliest propagated action potential (depressed fast response), but it propagates slowly because of its low upstroke velocity and low amplitude. Response *d* is elicited just before complete repolarization, and its rate of rise and amplitude are greater than those of *c* because it arises from a higher membrane potential. However, it still propagates more slowly than normal. Response *e* is elicited after complete repolarization and, therefore, has a normal rate of depolarization and amplitude and so propagates rapidly. *TP,* threshold potential; *RP,* resting potential. (From Singer DH and Ten Eick RE: Prog Cardiovasc Dis 11:488, 1969.)

sult in slow response action potentials with no fast sodium channels involved. Stimulus "c" and "d" result in depressed fast response action potentials. Finally, when a stimulus is delivered at maximal diastolic depolarization, the action potential has a steep phase 0 with a positive overshoot of approximately 30 mV and the possibility for optimal conduction velocity.

Normal automaticity

Automaticity is the capability of a cell to depolarize spontaneously, reach threshold potential, and initiate a propagated action potential. It is accomplished during phase 4 (diastole) through a slow buildup of positive ions inside the cell (thus the terms "slow diastolic depolarization," "spontaneous diastolic depolarization," or "phase 4 depolarization").

In healthy hearts only the cells of the sinus node reach threshold potential without an outside stimulus, although cells in other areas are capable of automaticity and are referred to as subsidiary or latent pacemakers. Those potential pacemaking areas are the cells of the His-Purkinje system. The atrial surface of the mitral and tricuspid valves also possess pacemaker cells; the clinical importance is not known. The two types of altered automaticity (enhanced normal and abnormal) are discussed in Chapter 4.

The rate of the slow diastolic depolarization decreases from the sinus node down to the Purkinje fibers (Fig. 3-13) so that the sinus node depolarizes fastest during electrical diastole and reaches threshold potential before latent pacemaker cells have time to do so. A current speeds from the sinus node through the rest of the heart, driving all of the subordinate pacemaker cells to threshold potential before they can reach that point themselves.

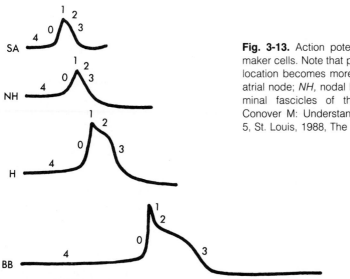

Fig. 3-13. Action potentials of four types of pacemaker cells. Note that phase 4 becomes flatter as the location becomes more distal in the heart. *SA*, sinoatrial node; *NH*, nodal His; *H*, bundle of His; *BB*, terminal fascicles of the bundle branches. (From Conover M: Understanding electrocardiography, ed 5, St. Louis, 1988, The CV Mosby Co.)

Overdrive suppression

Overdrive suppression is the inhibitory effect of a faster pacemaker on a slower one. This suppression, along with the successful race to threshold potential exhibited by the SA node, normally assures the node of its role as the dominant pacemaker of the heart and makes it more difficult for a subsidiary pacemaker to emerge and compete with the SA node. An example of overdrive suppression is seen in sudden complete AV block when the rate of the escape beats from the junctional focus is sluggish at first but eventually settles at a rate that is a little faster. Overdrive suppression of the SA node generally refers to the inhibitory effect of a period of driven activity (by use of an electrical stimulus) on the automatic activity of the SA node,[28] but is a well-known phenomenon even after a single atrial extrasystole.[29,30]

Mechanism. The mechanism of overdrive suppression is hyperpolarization. The effect of an outside stimulus on a pacemaker cell is enhancement of the activity of the sodium-potassium exchange pump. When a pacemaker cell is driven at a rate faster than its self-stimulated rate, there is an accumulation of intracellular Na^+, which in turn acts as a stimulus for the sodium pump. The faster the pacemaker cell fires, the harder the sodium pump works, rendering the driven cells more negative than normal (hyperpolarized).[13,14,31] When the stimulation is stopped, these hyperpolarized cells take longer to reach threshold than had they not been hyperpolarized, resulting in the brief period of quiescence called overdrive suppression.

The automatic firing of all pacemaker cells is controlled primarily by the autonomic nervous system; sympathetic stimulation inhibits the effects of overdrive suppression by causing steepening of phase 4 depolarization in pacemaker cells.[11] Changes in cell environment (K^+, pH, partial pressure of oxygen [Po_2], and Ca^{++}) also have a secondary effect on the rate of automatic fibers.

During sinus bradycardia the rate-dependent suppression of the subsidiary pacemakers is reduced. They can thus become active pacemakers without much delay if the SA node slows sufficiently or fails. This action is in contrast to the effects of a sudden suppression of the SA node or events after the sudden development of complete heart block. In such cases it will take several seconds for the overdrive suppression to subside and the escape pacemaker to assume its intrinsic rate. Thus, although vagal stimulation inhibits the atria, the resulting bradycardia secondarily removes an inhibition from the ventricles and may allow escape beats to appear more promptly.

Fig. 3-14 gives examples of the overdrive suppression exerted on the SA node by an atrial extrasystole. In Fig. 3-14, *A*, the lengthening of the cycle after the premature atrial beat is a manifestation of normal overdrive suppression; but in Fig. 3-14, *B*, the exaggerated slowing after the atrial premature beats is clearly indicative of abnormal SA nodal function.

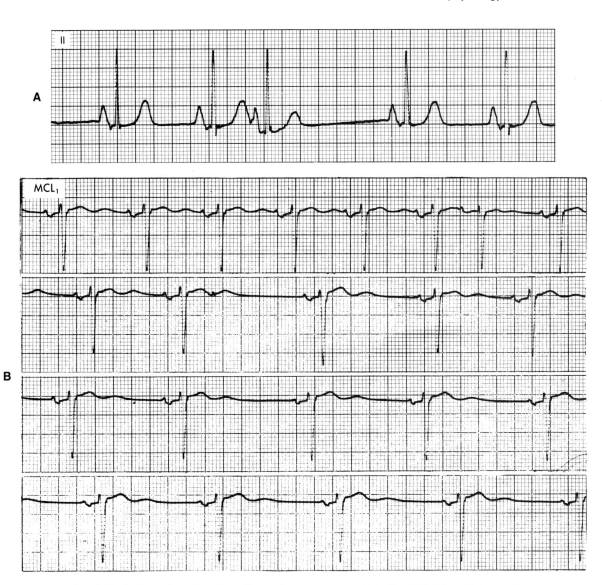

Fig. 3-14. A, Normal manifestation of overdrive suppression. Note that P'-P interval is longer than P-P interval that precedes it. Instead of resetting the SA node, the atrial premature beat has suppressed it. **B,** Abnormal response by sinus node to overdrive suppression by two atrial premature beats.

Action potential of the two nodes

Fig. 3-15 demonstrates the action potential from the dominant SA nodal pacemaker as recorded in 1965 by Sano and Yamagishi.[32] The resting potential of the SA and AV nodes is approximately −60 mV, and the threshold potential is approximately −30 mV. Thus there are no fast sodium channels in the two nodes. Because of this lack and because of the anatomical structure of AV nodal cells, conduction velocity slows through their fibers, a property well suited to the primary function of the AV node.

Sherf and James[7] found the action potentials of the proximal AV node are located anterior to the coronary sinus and just above the tricuspid valve in the canine heart. Diastolic depolarization (automaticity) was found in 82% of the proximal AV nodal cells and in 100% of the distal ones. Conduction velocity through the AV node becomes progressively slower as the impulse proceeds toward the distal portion of the node. When the sinus node is depressed, Urthaler and others[33,34] have shown that there are two pacemaker centers in the canine heart. The main center is probably located in the NH region (junction of the AV node and His bundle). Thus the AV node has two functions: (1) slowing AV conduction velocity to allow time for ventricular filling, and (2) serving as the principal alternate pacemaker of the heart.

If portions of the AV node have an action potential like that of the sinus node, including diastolic depolarization, why does the AV node not compete with the sinus node? Practically speaking, it is unthinkable that it would do so since this action would result in chaos. The question becomes even more intriguing in the light of 1980 and 1982 studies[35,36] of the rabbit heart that demonstrated rapid AV nodal automaticity when the AV node was severed from its atrial connections. Wit and Rosen[14] have proposed that, in the intact animal, AV nodal automaticity is suppressed not only by overdrive suppression but also by a background current flowing between nodal and atrial tissue in a retrograde direction (from the lower membrane potential of the node to the higher one of the atria).

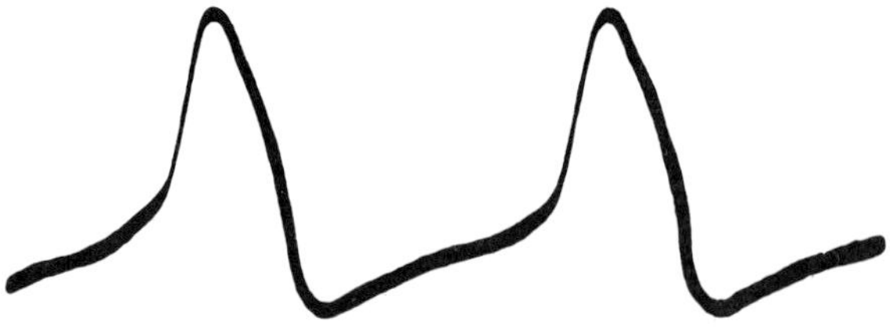

Fig. 3-15. Sinus node action potential. (Modified from Sano T and Yamagishi S: Circ Res 16:423, 1965.)

Automaticity versus excitability

All normal myocardial cells are excitable; that is, they are all capable of giving rise to an action potential when driven by an adequate stimulus. However, only the specialized cells (pacemaker cells) can reach threshold potential without an outside stimulus. These cells possess the property of automaticity. This distinction is illustrated in Fig. 3-16.

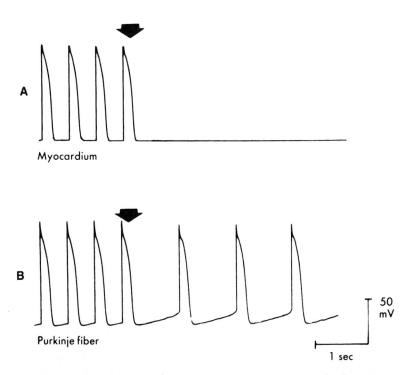

Fig. 3-16. Excitability and automaticity. Fibers in **A** and **B** are being driven by an extracellular electrode. Both types of cells are excitable. At the arrows the stimulus is discontinued. Myocardial fiber, **A,** will not begin to fire again until the stimulus is reinstated, but Purkinje fiber, **B,** can depolarize spontaneously during phase 4 until threshold potential is attained and an action potential is initiated (automaticity). (From Rosen MR and others: Cardiac arrhythmias in the neonate, infant, and child, New York, 1977, Appleton-Century-Crofts.)

Action potential related to the electrocardiogram

Fig. 3-17 relates the action potential to the electrocardiogram (ECG). Whenever there is a difference in electrical potential between fibers within the heart, a current will flow; such is the case during the QRS and the T wave. It is the difference in potential between the first and last cells to depolarize that causes displacement of the ECG stylus from the isoelectric line to produce the QRS complex. Thus abnormalities in depolarization are reflected in the QRS complex, and those abnormalities in repolarization are reflected in the ST segment, the T wave, and the QT interval. During phase 2 of the action potential there is little difference in potential between the first and last fibers to depolarize. Thus no current flows, and the ECG has an isoelectric ST segment. During rapid repolarization (phase 3) there is again a difference in potential, which produces the T wave.

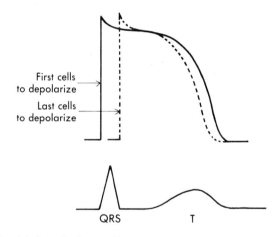

Fig. 3-17. Action potentials from the first and last cells to depolarize related to the ECG. Because of difference in potential between the first and last cells to depolarize, the QRS is inscribed. ST segment results when there is no difference in potential and is therefore isoelectric. T wave reflects the difference in potential during phase 3. (Modified from Surawicz B and Saito S: Am J Cardiol 41:943, 1978.)

Summary

Current flow in the heart is facilitated by the unique structure of the myocardial cells and the negativity of the membrane potentials. This negativity and the availability of fast sodium channels are maintained by the electrogenic sodium pump and sodium-potassium ATPase. The electrical cardiac cycle consists of electrical diastole (phase 4) and electrical systole (phases 0-3). During phase 4, pacemaker cells are slowly depolarized, but the sinus node reaches threshold potential first, causing rapid (phase 0) depolarization followed by repolarization (phases 1-3). Phase 0 results when the fast sodium channels open at their threshold potential (-90 mV); the slow calcium channels also open during this phase at their threshold potential (approximately -30 mV) and are responsible for the plateau stage (phase 2) of the action potential.

REFERENCES

1. Hodgkin AL and Katz B: Ionic currents underlying activity in the giant axon of the squid, J Physiol 108:37, 1949.
2. Hodgkin AL and Huxley AF: A quantitative description of membrane current and its application to conduction and excitation in nerve, J Physiol 117:500, 1952.
3. Noble D: A modification of the Hodgkin-Huxley equations to Purkinje-fibre action and pacemaker potentials, J Physiol 160:317, 1962.
4. Hoffman BF and Cranefield PF: Electrophysiology of the heart, New York, 1960, McGraw-Hill Book Co.
5. Neidergerke R and Orkand RK: The dependence of the action potential of the frog's heart on the external and intracellular sodium concentration, J Physiol 84:312, 1966.
6. Hagiwara S and Nakajima S: Differences in Na and Ca spikes as examined by application of tetrodotoxin, procainamide and manganese ions, J Gen Physiol 49:793, 1966.
7. Sherf L, James TN, and Woods WT: Function of the atrioventricular node considered on the basis of observed histology and fine structure, J Am Coll Cardiol 5:770, 1985.
8. Cranefield PF: The conduction of the cardiac impulse, Mount Kisco, NY, 1975, Futura Publishing Co.
9. Katz AM: Effects of digitalis on cell biochemistry: sodium pump inhibition, J Am Coll Cardiol 5:16A, 1985.
10. Rosen MR and Wit AL: Arrhythmogenic actions of antiarrhythmic drugs, Am J Cardiol 59:10E, 1987.
11. Hille B: Ionic channels of excitable membranes. Sunderland, Mass, 1984, Sinauer Assoc.
12. Hodgkin AL and Huxley AF: A quantitative description of membrane current and its application to conduction excitation in nerve, J Physiol 117:500, 1952.
13. Wit AL: Cellular electrophysiologic mechanisms of cardiac arrhythmias, Ann NY Acad Sci 432:1, 1986.
14. Wit AL and Rosen MR: Cellular electrophysiology of cardiac arrhythmias. In Josephson ME and Wellens HJJ, editors: Tachycardias: mechanisms, diagnosis, treatment, Philadelphia, 1984, Lea & Febiger.
15. Yanagihara K and Irisawa H: Potassium current during the pacemaker depolarization in rabbit sinoatrial node cell, Pflugers Arch 388:255, 1980.
16. Noma A and others: Slow current systems in the AV node in the rabbit heart, Nature 285:228, 1980.
17. Gadsby DC and Wit AL: Electrophysiologic characteristics of cardiac cells and the genesis of cardiac arrhythmias. In Wilkerson RD, editor: Cardiac pharmacology, New York, 1981, Academic Press, Inc.
18. Surawicz B: Contributions of cellular electrophysiology to the understanding of the electrocardiogram, 1987, unpublished.

19. Myerburg RJ: The gating mechanism in the distal AV conducting system, Circulation 43:955, 1971.

20. Myerburg RJ, Stewart JW, and Hoffman BF: Electrophysiological properties of the canine peripheral AV conducting system, Circ Res 26:361, 1970.

21. Myerburg RJ and others: Electrophysiology of endocardial intraventricular conduction: the role and function of the specialized conducting system. In Wellens HJJ, Lie KI, and Janse MJ, editors: The conduction system of the heart, Philadelphia, 1976, Lea & Febiger.

22. Spear JF, and Moore EN: Supernormal excitability and conduction. In Wellens HJJ, Lie KI, and Janse MJ, editors: The conduction system of the heart: structure, function and clinical implications, Philadelphia, 1976, Lea & Febiger.

23. Cranefield PF and Hoffman BF: Conduction of the cardiac impulse. II. Summation and inhibition, Circ Res 28:220, 1971.

24. Weidmann S: The effect of the cardiac membrane potential on the rapid availability of the sodium-carrying system, J Physiol 127:213, 1955.

25. Jack JJB, Noble D, and Tsien RW: Electric current flow in excitable cells, Oxford, 1975, Clarendon Press.

26. Draper MH and Weidmann S: Cardiac resting and action potentials recorded with an intracellular electrode, J Physiol 115:74, 1951.

27. Vassalle M: The relationship among cardiac pacemakers: overdrive suppression, Circ Res 41:269, 1977.

28. Erlanger J: Further studies on the physiology of heart block. The effects of extra systoles upon the dog's heart and upon strips of terrapin's ventricle in the various stages of block, Am J Physiol 16:160, 1906.

29. Katz LN and Pick A: Clinical electrocardiography. I. The arrhythmias, Philadelphia, 1956, Lea & Febiger.

30. Paulay MKL, Varghese PJ, and Damato AN: Atrial rhythms in response to an early atrial premature depolarization in man, Am Heart J 85:323, 1973.

31. Vassalle M: Electrogenic suppression of automaticity in sheep and dog Purkinje fibers, Circ Res 27:361, 1970.

32. Sano T and Yamagishi S: Spread of excitation from the sinus node, Circ Res 16:423, 1965.

33. Urthaler F and others: Mathematical relationship between automaticity of the sinus node and the AV junction, Am Heart J 86:189, 1973.

34. Urthaler F and others: Electrophysiological and mathematical characteristics of the escape rhythm during complete AV block, Cardiovasc Res 8:173, 1979.

35. Wit AL and Cranefield PF: Mechanisms of impulse initiation in the atrioventricular junction and the effects of acetylstrophanthidin, Am J Cardiol 49:921, 1982 (abstract).

36. Kokubun S and others: The spontaneous action potential of rabbit atrioventricular node cells, Jap J Physiol 30:529, 1980.

CHAPTER 4

Altered automaticity and triggered activity

Abnormal impulse formation, along with abnormal impulse conduction, is the basis of all cardiac arrhythmias.[1,2] Abnormalities of impulse formation include altered automaticity and triggered activity. Abnormalities of impulse conduction involve mechanisms such as unidirectional block, bidirectional block, functional and anatomical reentry, and reflection. These mechanisms are secondary to disease processes such as ischemia, electrolyte derangements, autonomic nervous system abnormalities, and vagotonia and anatomical abnormalities such as accessory pathways or may actually be induced by the very drugs that are used to treat the arrhythmias.

Normal automaticity is a characteristic of the sinus node at low diastolic membrane potentials (−60 mV) and of Purkinje fibers at high diastolic membrane potentials (−90 mV). The rate of normal automaticity in Purkinje fibers is 30 to 40 beats/min.

Altered automaticity, whether emanating from fibers with high or low membrane potentials, occurs de novo; it needs only phase 4 depolarization to initiate it. Triggered activity cannot occur de novo; it must be initiated by an afterdepolarization (early or delayed), which, as its name implies, needs a prior action potential to initiate it.[3] An arrhythmia caused by a reentry mechanism also cannot initiate itself; like the afterdepolarization, it requires a preceding action potential for its generation; unlike the afterdepolarization, it is dependent on abnormal conduction rather than focal oscillations in the membrane potential. This chapter is concerned with altered automaticity and triggered activity; abnormalities of impulse conduction such as reentry are covered in subsequent chapters.

Altered automaticity

Altered automaticity may be caused either by enhanced normal automaticity in Purkinje fibers with a high membrane potential or by abnormal automaticity in severely depressed Purkinje or myocardial tissue. Because enhanced-normal automaticity involves cells that retain a normal resting membrane potential and abnormal automaticity involves cells with markedly reduced membrane potentials, altered automaticity may occur across a broad range of membrane potentials, from approximately −90 to −50 mV in Purkinje cells and at membrane potentials of less than −60 mV in most myocardial cells.

ENHANCED NORMAL AUTOMATICITY. Enhanced normal automaticity is an acceleration (steepening) of phase 4 depolarization in pacemaker cells and is a cause of arrhythmias in Purkinje fibers with high membrane potentials; in such cases, automaticity is readily suppressed by overdrive pacing.[4] In fact, if the membrane potential is decreased (becomes less negative), the response to overdrive pacing is blunted and ultimately does not occur.[5] Ectopic beats or rhythms result when the cell reaches threshold potential prematurely.

Enhancement of normal automaticity is secondary to excess catecholamines and can result in an increase of firing rate in Purkinje fibers to approximately 100 beats/min and rarely to a faster rate. This mechanism is illustrated in Fig. 4-1, in which the normal Purkinje cell action potential is depicted by a solid line. Note that the action potential with enhanced-normal automaticity is normal in every aspect except for the steepening of phase 4 depolarization. The cells involved are not necessarily ischemic and have normal or slightly depressed resting membrane potentials and fast-response action potentials.

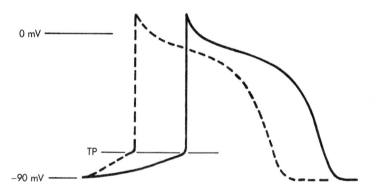

Fig. 4-1. Enhanced normal automaticity *(dashed line)*. This mechanism occurs in fibers with high membrane potentials (−70 to −90 mV). *TP*, threshold potential.

ABNORMAL AUTOMATICITY. Abnormal automaticity occurs in fibers with low levels of membrane potential (usually less than approximately −60 mV). This is true not only for the specialized conducting fibers of the Purkinje system but also for myocardial fibers, which normally do not possess the property of automaticity.[6,7] At such low membrane potentials the action potential is dependent more on calcium (Ca^{++}) than it is on sodium (Na^+). The rhythms are spontaneous, persistent, do not respond to lidocaine, are difficult if not impossible to overdrive, and may actually slightly increase their rate in response to overdrive stimulation.[5]

In the past it was suggested that all abnormal automatic rhythms resulted from steepening of phase 4 depolarization in pacemaker cells. It is now known that automaticity may occur in other than pacemaker cells. This abnormal situation is caused by the loss of fast sodium channels and the presence of a pacemaker current that differs from the normal one. Thus atrial and ventricular cells that are so depressed that they have lost their fast sodium channels and have slow response action potentials are capable of generating automatic beats. Such an abnormal action potential is illustrated in Fig. 4-2, *B*, and is compared with normal and enhanced normal automaticity in Fig. 4-2, *A*.

The reduction in membrane potential responsible for abnormal automaticity may occur in Purkinje fibers during the first 24 hours after an infarction and is the most frequent cause of ventricular tachycardia during that period.[8] The ventricular tachycardia would be persistent and unresponsive to lidocaine. Abnormal automaticity may also be the result of ischemia, hypocalcemia, cardiomyopathy, increased extracellular or decreased intracellular potassium, and increased sodium permeability or decreased potassium permeability. Such rhythms are difficult if not impossi-

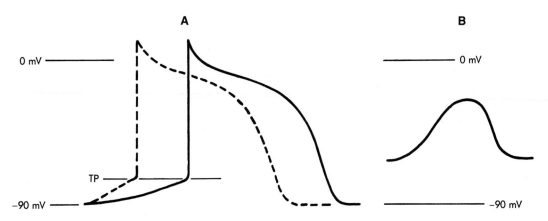

Fig. 4-2. A, Enhanced normal automaticity *(dashed line)* and, **B,** abnormal automaticity.

ble to subdue by overdrive pacing.[9,10] Thus they may emerge in the presence of an adequate sinus rhythm such as in the case of an accelerated idioventricular rhythm. The sinus node easily suppresses normal His-Purkinje cells, even during rather marked sinus bradycardia. However, this suppression may not be possible when cells of the His-Purkinje system or of the atrial or ventricular myocardium are severely depressed and act as automatic foci.[11,12]

ENHANCED NORMAL AUTOMATICITY VERSUS ABNORMAL AUTOMATICITY

Clinical setting. Often the clinical setting and the behavior of the tachycardia or the accelerated rhythm suggest the mechanism. For example, in patients with an acute myocardial infarction in whom there are sure to be severely depressed myocardial cells with membrane potentials below approximately -60 mV, ventricular tachycardia is usually caused by abnormal automaticity; it will not respond to lidocaine and cannot be suppressed by overdrive pacing. Conversely, in a patient with a complete AV block with an idioventricular rhythm, the mechanism of the ventricular rhythm is more likely to be enhanced-normal automaticity, and care must be taken not to administer lidocaine, which would suppress the lifesaving ventricular focus.

Antiarrhythmic drugs. Enhanced-normal automaticity (high potential) is suppressed by class I antiarrhythmics. Abnormal automaticity (low potential) can be further suppressed and therefore blocked from producing arrhythmias by calcium channel blockers (verapamil and nifedipine) and by acetylcholine and ethmozin.[13] Lidocaine does not suppress arrhythmias resulting from abnormal automaticity since the cells involved have slow calcium channel action potentials,[14] and lidocaine blocks fast sodium channels in cells that are only slightly depressed.

Overdrive suppression. The parallel relationship of membrane potential with the possibility of overdrive suppression is one characteristic that distinguishes automaticity at a high membrane potential (enhanced-normal automaticity) from that at a lower level (abnormal automaticity); as the one decreases, so does the other, and overdrive suppression becomes less and less possible. Overdrive suppression is not possible in depressed fibers because they are unable to hyperpolarize like fibers with high membrane potentials.

Overdrive suppression is dependent on the creation of a state of hyperpolarization. This suppression takes place in a series of steps: (1) the rapid pacing causes an increased influx of Na^+ into the cells through the fast Na^+ channels; (2) the increase in intracellular Na^+ is in turn a stimulus to the sodium-potassium ATPase pump, which relentlessly empties the cell of Na^+ and eventually renders it more negative than normal (hyperpolarization); and (3) when the rapid stimulus ceases, the cells begin phase 4 depolarization from their supernegative status, from which it takes longer to reach threshold potential.

Depressed cells, on the other hand, cannot achieve the state of hyperpolariza-

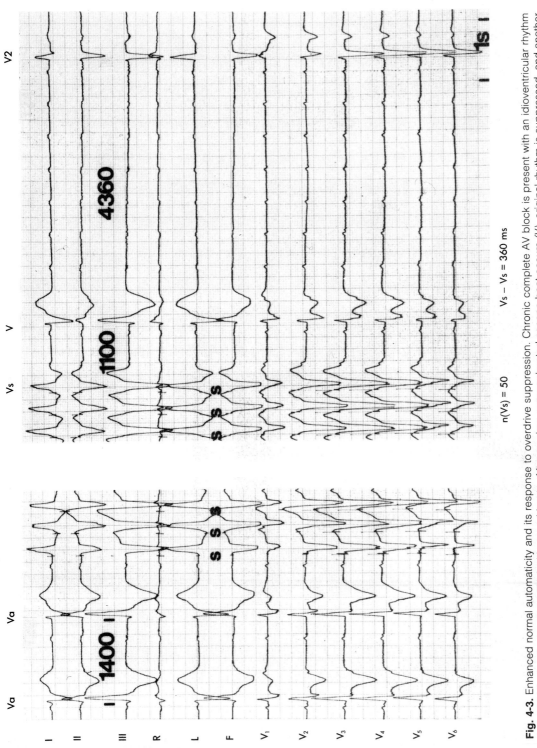

Fig. 4-3. Enhanced normal automaticity and its response to overdrive suppression. Chronic complete AV block is present with an idioventricular rhythm (Va). This rhythm is overdriven (Vs) with paced beats. After pacing, an accelerated escape beat occurs (V), original rhythm is suppressed, and another focus emerges (V2). (From Gorgels APM and others: The clinical relevance of abnormal automaticity and triggered activity. In Brugada P and Wellens HJJ: Cardiac arrhythmias: where to go from here? Mt Kisco, NY, 1987, Futura Publishing Co, Inc.)

n(Vs) = 50   Vs – Vs = 360 ms

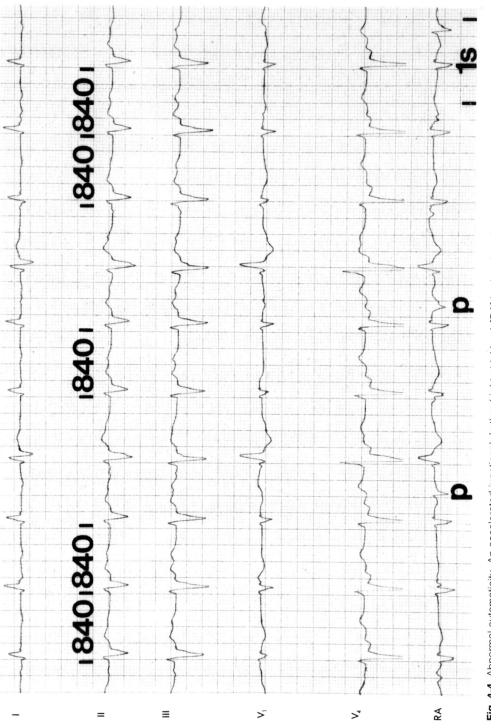

Fig. 4-4. Abnormal automaticity. An accelerated junctional rhythm (right atrial lead *[RA]* is also shown) is interrupted by ventricular captures that are conducted with right bundle branch block (RBBB). (From Gorgels APM and others: The clinical relevance of abnormal automaticity and triggered activity. In Brugada P and Wellens HJJ: Cardiac arrhythmias: where to go from here? Mt Kisco, NY, 1987, Futura Publishing Co, Inc.)

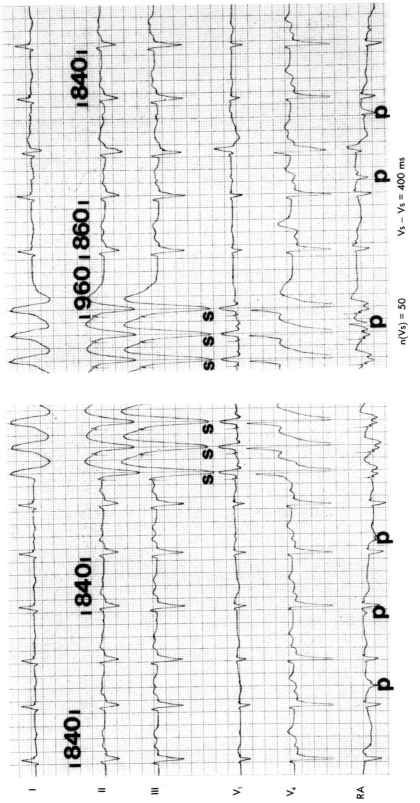
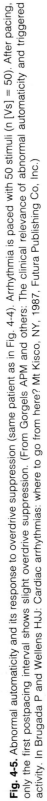

Fig. 4-5. Abnormal automaticity and its response to overdrive suppression (same patient as in Fig. 4-4). Arrhythmia is paced with 50 stimuli (n [Vs] = 50). After pacing, only the first postpacing interval shows slight overdrive suppression. (From Gorgels APM and others: The clinical relevance of abnormal automaticity and triggered activity. In Brugada P and Wellens HJJ: Cardiac arrhythmias: where to go from here? Mt Kisco, NY, 1987, Futura Publishing Co, Inc.)

tion because they have no fast Na$^+$ channels to help build the above series of events. They are not depolarized by fast Na$^+$ currents but by slow calcium currents.

Figs. 4-3, 4-4, and 4-5 are tracings from Brugada and Wellens' laboratories[14] that illustrate the use of overdrive suppression to confirm the arrhythmogenic mechanisms. The patient whose ECG is in Fig. 4-3 has complete AV block and an idioventricular rhythm of 42/min, which is overdriven. A long pause follows, and an idioventricular rhythm from a different focus takes over. Thus the mechanism of the first automatic focus was normal automaticity because it was suppressed by overdrive stimuli. Figs. 4-4 and 4-5 are from the same patient and show an arrhythmia compatible with abnormal automaticity. The patient had an old myocardial infarction and was in severe heart failure with an accelerated junctional rhythm at a rate of 75/min (see Fig. 4-4). Overdrive pacing (see Fig. 4-5) did not suppress the junctional rhythm, and neither did lidocaine.[14] Thus the mechanism of this arrhythmia was abnormal automaticity caused by severely depressed cells in the AV junction.

Triggered activity

Triggered activity is rhythmic activity that results from the attainment of threshold potential by an afterdepolarization. In electrophysiological studies, the rate of the triggered rhythm tends to increase as the drive rate increases.[15]

Afterdepolarizations are oscillations in the membrane potential that are induced and strongly influenced by the preceding cardiac rhythm.[4,16-21] They are not the same as altered automaticity in either of its forms, nor are they sustained by a reentry circuit; they are the result of a second depolarization that occurs either after full repolarization (delayed afterdepolarization) or during the final stage of repolarization (early afterdepolarization).

DELAYED AFTERDEPOLARIZATIONS. Delayed afterdepolarizations are oscillations in transmembrane potential that follow full repolarization of the membrane; that is, they occur after phase 3 of the action potential.[22] They are dependent on the preceding action potential for their initiation. A delayed afterdepolarization is shown in Fig. 4-6, A *(open arrow)*. Note that since this afterdepolarization has not reached threshold potential, an extra beat is not initiated. In Fig. 4-6, B *(solid arrow)*, the afterdepolarization reaches threshold potential and produces tachycardia. In electrophysiological studies,[23] an increase in the stimulus rate causes the amplitude of the delayed afterdepolarization to increase (bringing it to threshold potential) and shortens the coupling interval that links it to the preceding action potential. Clinically, achievement of threshold potential results in triggered activity in the form of an ectopic atrial, junctional, or ventricular tachycardia or in ventricular bigeminy.

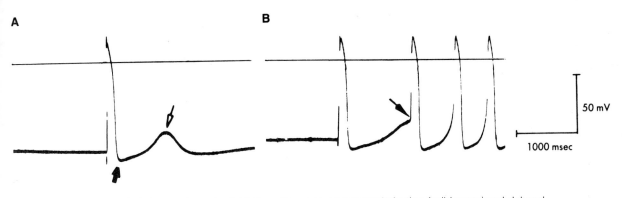

Fig. 4-6. A, Driven action potential followed by delayed hyperpolarization *(solid arrow)* and delayed afterdepolarization *(open arrow)*. **B,** Driven action potential followed by delayed afterdepolarization that reaches threshold and nondriven action potential *(arrow)* that arises from the peak of the afterdepolarization. (From Wit AL and others. In Narula OS, editor: Cardiac arrhythmias: electrophysiology, diagnosis, and management, Baltimore, 1979, The Williams & Wilkins Co.)

Clinical implications. Triggered activity secondary to delayed afterdepolarizations may occur in the following clinical settings: hypokalemia, hypercalcemia, hypomagnesemia, digitalis toxicity, diuretic use, ischemia and reperfusion, increased sympathetic tone, increased wall tension, and heart failure.[14]

Mechanisms and suppression. Delayed afterdepolarizations occur because of an increase in intracellular calcium concentration, which in turn results in a transient inward sodium current. This sodium current causes the delayed afterdepolarization. Intracellular calcium overload occurs because of the following:

1. Inhibition of the sodium-potassium ATPase pump by digitalis glycosides.[24,25] Hypokalemia and hypomagnesemia also inhibit the sodium-potassium ATPase pump and are suspects in the production of triggered activity apart from their well-known role in producing QT prolongation and torsades de pointes.[26]

   The typical arrhythmias of digitalis toxicity are atrial tachycardia with 2:1 block,[27] ventricular bigeminy,[28] accelerated idiojunctional rhythm,[29] fascicular tachycardia, and bidirectional ventricular tachycardia.[23,30-36] These arrhythmias are illustrated and further discussed in Chapter 5.

   Digitalis inhibits the sodium-potassium ATPase pump because it competes with potassium for a binding site on the membrane; when it replaces the potassium, the pump is inhibited at that site. This process can be suppressed by (1) accelerating the pump with potassium supplements,[37] (2) suppressing the triggered activity with magnesium[38] or doxorubicin,[39] or (3) hyperpolarizing the cell membrane with cholinomimetic drugs.[40]

2. Calcium overload in myocardial tissue during the reperfusion phase after coronary artery occlusion[41,42] and thrombolytic therapy. This mechanism probably produces the accelerated idioventricular rhythm typical of this clinical setting.[14] Calcium overload can be inhibited by calcium entry blockers.[43-45]

3. Catecholamine-induced calcium overload[46-49] (the resulting triggered activity that results can be inhibited by beta-blocking drugs). Other suppressants of triggered activity are diphenylhydantoin,[14] aprindine,[50] and caffeine.[51,52]

WARNING: When using drugs to treat digitalis toxicity, a temporary pacemaker should first be inserted[14] because digitalis, in addition to causing triggered activity, suppresses phase 4 in Purkinje cells and in the sinus node and causes different degrees of SA and AV block. Thus, when the antiarrhythmic abolishes the triggered activity, cardiac arrest may result. Also to be avoided is beta stimulation (e.g., by anxiety, exercise, sympathicomimetic drugs)[14] because shortening the cycle length and catecholamines aggravate the situation by causing delayed afterdepolarizations to heighten and reach threshold potential.

EARLY AFTERDEPOLARIZATIONS. Early afterdepolarizations are oscillations in transmembrane potential that occur before the completion of phase 3 repolarization.[4,18,19] Fig. 4-7 compares them with delayed afterdepolarizations. The two mechanisms differ in that the early afterdepolarization is more inclined to trigger an arrhythmia in a patient with bradycardia, whereas the delayed afterdepolarization is amplified by a shortening of the cycle length. Early afterdepolarizations terminate with overdrive suppression as long as the resting membrane potential remains high. Their termination is often associated with hyperpolarization, a factor that negates the transmembrane current responsible for the early afterdepolarization.[18]

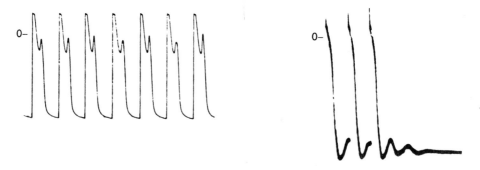
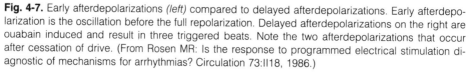

Fig. 4-7. Early afterdepolarizations *(left)* compared to delayed afterdepolarizations. Early afterdepolarization is the oscillation before the full repolarization. Delayed afterdepolarizations on the right are ouabain induced and result in three triggered beats. Note the two afterdepolarizations that occur after cessation of drive. (From Rosen MR: Is the response to programmed electrical stimulation diagnostic of mechanisms for arrhythmias? Circulation 73:II18, 1986.)

Clinical implications. Early afterdepolarizations in fibers with high membrane potentials have been implicated as a mechanism of tachycardias secondary to prolonged QT intervals (torsades de pointes).[53-55] The clinical implications of early afterdepolarizations in fibers with low membrane potentials is not known.[14]

Early afterdepolarizations versus abnormal automaticity. Clinically, it is impossible to distinguish between arrhythmias caused by early afterdepolarizations and those caused by abnormal automaticity. Both actually share the same mechanism—automaticity resulting from stimulation at a low membrane potential, although in one it is primary and in the other it is secondary. It is the primary mechanism in abnormal automaticity since the low potential carries with it an abnormal pacemaker current, which produces the abnormal automaticity. In triggered activity caused by early afterdepolarization, it is the secondary mechanism since the primary mechanism is the afterdepolarization, which occurs when the membrane has a low potential.

Early afterdepolarizations versus enhanced normal automaticity. The arrhythmia caused by triggered activity induced by early afterdepolarizations has in common with enhanced normal automaticity the propensity to emerge at slower rates; in addition, both may be suppressed by overdrive pacing. They differ in their initial performance in that arrhythmias resulting from enhanced normal automaticity tend to have a warm-up period before a steady rate is reached, whereas those arrhythmias triggered by early afterdepolarizations settle into a stable rate after approximately the third beat. Fig. 4-8 is an example of triggered activity caused by early afterdepolarizations; its onset is regular, i.e., no warm-up.

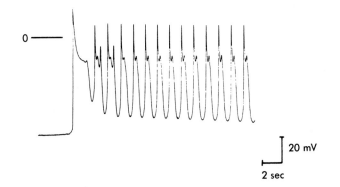

0 ———

20 mV

2 sec

Fig. 4-8. Triggered activity caused by early afterdepolarizations. Note that from the onset the rhythm is quite regular, requiring no period of warm-up. (From Damiano BP and Rosen MR: Effects of pacing on triggered activity induced by early afterdepolarizations, Circulation 69:1013, 1984.)

Summary

Arrhythmias caused by abnormal impulse formation are classified as either altered automaticity or triggered activity. Altered automaticity is either enhanced normal or abnormal automaticity and may occur over a broad range of resting membrane potentials from -90 to -50 mV. The membrane potential determines the type of altered automaticity.

Among the fibers that have high membrane potentials, only Purkinje fibers are capable of automaticity, enhanced normal automaticity, or abnormal automaticity. Enhanced normal automaticity can be caused in Purkinje fibers by catecholamines, in which case the rate may accelerate from its normal 30 to 40 beats/min to approximately 100 beats/min. Conversely, all myocardial cells, both Purkinje cells and working cells, are capable of abnormal automaticity if their membrane potential is depressed enough so that there are no fast sodium channels available. Abnormal automaticity is caused by a reduction in the membrane potential and the presence of a pacemaker current that is different from normal. Some clinical settings for abnormal automaticity are infarction, ischemia, and electrolyte derangements. Both enhanced normal and abnormal automaticity occur de novo.

Triggered activity does not occur de novo; it results when threshold potential is reached by oscillations during (early afterdepolarization) or immediately after (delayed afterdepolarization) the action potential. Early afterdepolarizations are oscillations in the membrane potential before full repolarization and may be secondary to prolonged repolarization (long QT interval). Delayed afterdepolarizations are caused by intracellular calcium overload, which may in turn be the result of digitalis toxicity, reperfusion, or catecholamines.

Although it is not yet possible to differentiate clinically with certainty between these four arrhythmogenic mechanisms, in many cases we can apply our present knowledge to the clinical setting, consider the etiology and behavior of the arrhythmia, and make the proper therapeutic choice. We can now at least bring to the bedside the certain knowledge that not all arrhythmias will respond to one certain antiarrhythmic drug and that some will need very specific pharmacological intervention or no intervention at all.

REFERENCES

1. Cranefield PF, Wit AL, and Hoffman BF: Genesis of cardiac arrhythmias, Circulation 47:190, 1973.
2. Hoffman BF and Cranefield PF: The physiological basis of cardiac arrhythmias, Am J Med 37:670, 1964.
3. Rosen MR: Is the response to programmed electrical stimulation diagnostic of mechanisms for arrhythmias? Circulation 73:II18, 1986.
4. Vassalle M: The relationship among cardiac pacemakers: overdrive suppression, Circ Res 41:269, 1977.
5. Dangman K and Hoffman BF: Studies on overdrive stimulation of canine cardiac Purkinje fibers: maximal diastolic potential as a determinant of the response, J Am Coll Cardiol 2:1183, 1983.
6. Imanishi S and Surawicz B: Automatic activity in depolarized guinea pig ventricular myocar-

dium: characteristics and mechanisms, Circ Res 39:751, 1976.

7. Katzung BG and Morgenstern JA: Effects of extracellular potassium on ventricular automaticity; and evidence for a pacemaker current in mammalian ventricular myocardium, Circ Res 40:105, 1977.

8. Marec HL and others: An evaluation of automaticity and triggered activity in the canine heart 1 to 4 days after myocardial infarction, Circulation 71:1224, 1985.

9. Cranefield PF: Action potentials, afterpotentials and arrhythmias, Circ Res 41:415, 1977.

10. Wit AL: Cellular electrophysiologic mechanisms of cardiac arrhythmias, Ann NY Acad Sci 432:1, 1986.

11. Dangman KH and Hoffman BF: Studies on overdrive stimulation of canine cardiac Purkinje fibers: maximum diastolic potential as a determinant of the response, J Am Coll Cardiol 2:1183, 1983.

12. Hoffman BF and Rosen MR: Cellular mechanisms for cardiac arrhythmias, Circ Res 49:1, 1981.

13. Hoffman BF: Disturbances of cardiac electrogenesis. In Rosenbaum MB and Elizari MV, editors: Frontiers of cardiac electrophysiology, development in cardiovascular medicine, Boston, 1983, Martinus Nijhoff, Publishers.

14. Gorgels APM and others: The clinical relevance of abnormal automaticity and triggered activity. In Brugada P and Wellens HJJ: Cardiac arrhythmias: where to go from here? Mt Kisco, NY, 1987, Futura Publishing Co, Inc.

15. Moak JP and Rosen MR: Induction and termination of triggered activity by pacing in isolated canine Purkinje fibers, Circulation 69:149, 1984.

16. Johnson NJ and Rosen MR: The distinction between triggered activity and other cardiac arrhythmias. In Brugada P and Wellens HJJ: Cardiac arrhythmias: where to go from here? Mt Kisco, NY, 1987, Futura Publishing Co, Inc.

17. Rosen MR and others: Mechanics of digitalis toxicity. Effects of ouabain on phase 4 of canine Purkinje fiber transmembrane potentials, Circulation 47:681, 1973.

18. Rosen MR and others: Correlation between effects of ouabain on the canine electrocardiogram and transmembrane potentials of isolated Purkinje fibers, Circulation 47:65, 1973.

19. Ferrier GR: The effects of tension on acetylstrophanthidin-induced transient depolarizations and aftercontractions in canine myocardial and Purkinje tissue, Circ Res 38:156, 1976.

20. Cranefield PF: The conduction of the cardiac impulse: the slow response and cardiac arrhythmias, Mt Kisco, New York, 1975, Futura Publishing Co, Inc.

21. Cranefield PF: Does spontaneous activity arise from phase 4 depolarization or from triggering? In Bonke FIM, editor: The sinus node: structure, function and clinical relevance, The Hague, 1978, Martinus Nijhoff, Publishers.

22. Rosen MR: Cellular electrophysiology of digitalis toxicity, J Am Coll Cardiol 5:22A, 1985.

23. Rosen MR and Reder RF: Does triggered activity have a role in the genesis of cardiac arrhythmias, Ann Intern Med 94:794, 1981.

24. Schatzmann HJ: Herzglykoside als Hemmstofe fuer den aktiven Kaliumund Natriumtransport durch die Erhthrocytenmenbran, Helv Physiol Pharmacol Acta 11:346, 1953.

25. Skou JC: The influence of some cations on an adenosine triphosphatase from peripheral nerves, Biochim Biophys Acta 23:394, 1957.

26. Coumel P and others: Torsade de pointes. In Josephson ME and Wellens HJJ, editors: Tachycardias, mechanisms, diagnosis, treatment, Philadelphia, 1984, Lea and Febiger.

27. Wellens HJJ: The electrocardiogram in digitalis intoxication. In Yu PN and Goodwin JF, editors: Progress in cardiology, Philadelphia, 1976, Lea & Febiger.

28. Kieval RS and others: Triggered activity as a cause of bigeminy, J Am Coll Cardiol 8:644, 1986.

29. Rosen MR and others: Can accelerated atrioventricular junctional escape rhythms be explained by delayed afterdepolarizations? Am J Cardiol 45:1272, 1980.

30. Ferrier GR: Digitalis arrhythmias: role of oscillatory afterpotentials, Prog Cardiovasc Dis 19:459, 1977.

31. Hoffman BF and Rosen MR: Cellular mechanisms for cardiac arrhythmias, Circ Res 49:1, 1981.

32. Wit AL and others: Triggered activity. In Zipes DP, Bailey JC, and Elharrar V, editors: The slow inward current and cardiac arrhythmias, The Hague, 1980, Martinus Nijhoff, Publishers.

33. Zipes DP and others: Accelerated cardiac escape rhythms caused by ouabain intoxication, Am J Cardiol 32:2489, 1974.

34. Zipes DP and others: Atrial induction of ventricular tachycardia: reentry versus triggered automaticity, Am J Cardiol 44:1, 1979.

35. Whalen DA and others: Effect of a transient period of ischemia on myocardial cells. I. Effects on cell volume regulation, Am J Pathol 74:381, 1974.

36. Gorgels APM and others: Extrastimulus related shortening of the first post-pacing interval in digitalis-induced ventricular tachycardia, J Am Coll Cardiol 1:840, 1983.

37. Wallick DW and others: Effects of ouabain and vagal stimulation on heart rate in dog, Cardiovasc Res 18:75, 1984.

38. Specter MJ and others: Studies on magnesium's mechanism of action in digitalis induced arrhythmias, Circulation 52:1001, 1975.

39. Le Marec H and others: The effects of doxorubicin on ventricular tachycardia, Circulation 74:881, 1986.

40. Cranefield P: Triggered arrhythmias. In Rosenbaum MB and Elizari MV, editors: Frontiers of cardiac electrophysiology, Boston, 1975, Martinus Nijhoff, Publishers.

41. Wellens HJJ: The electrocardiogram 80 years after Einthoven, J Am Coll Cardiol 7:484, 1986.

42. Ferrier GR and others: Possible mechanisms of ventricular arrhythmias elicited by ischemia followed by reperfusion, Circ Res 56:184, 1985.

43. Rosen M and Danilo P: Effects of tetrodotoxin, lidocaine, verapamil and AHRE-2666 on ouabain induced delayed afterdepolarizations in canine Purkinje fibers, Circ Res 46:117, 1980.

44. Gough WB and others: Effects of nifedipine on triggered activity in 1-day-old myocardial infarction in dogs, Am J Cardiol 53:303, 1983.

45. Klevans LR and Kelly RJ: Effect of autonomic neural blockade on verapamil-induced suppression of the accelerated ventricular escape beat in ouabain-treated dogs, J Pharmacol Exp Ther 206:259, 1978.

46. Wit AL and others: Electrogenic sodium extrusion can stop triggered activity in the canine coronary sinus, Circ Res 49:1029, 1981.

47. Valenzuela F and Vasalle M: Interaction between overdrive excitation and overdrive suppression in canine Purkinje fibers, Cardiovasc Res 17:608, 1983.

48. Vasalle M and others: The effect of adrenergic enhancement on overdrive excitation, J Electrocardiol 9:335, 1976.

49. Lerman BB and others: Adenosine-sensitive ventricular tachycardia: evidence suggesting cyclic AMP-mediated triggered activity, Circulation 74:881, 1986.

50. Wellens HJJ and others: New studies on triggered activity. In Harrison DC, editor: Cardiac arrhythmias: a decade of progress, Boston, 1981, GK Hall Medical Publishers.

51. Di Gennaro M and others: Abolition of digitalis tachyarrhythmias by caffeine, Am J Physiol 244:H215, 1983.

52. Di Gennaro M and others: On the mechanism by which caffeine abolishes the fast rhythms induced by cardiotonic steroids, J Mol Cell Cardiol 16:851, 1984.

53. Brachmann J and others: Bradycardia dependent triggered activity: relevance to drug induced multiform ventricular tachycardia, Circulation 68:846, 1983.

54. Brugada P and Wellens HJJ: Early afterdepolarizations: role in conduction block, prolonged repolarization dependent reexcitation, and tachyarrhythmias in the human heart, PACE 8:889, 1985.

55. Franz MR: Long-term recording of monophasic action potentials from human endocardium, Am J Cardiol 51:1629, 1983.

CHAPTER 5

Digitalis dysrhythmias

↑ in delayed afterpotential

Digitalis intoxication should be ruled out in any patient with arrhythmias who is taking the drug, especially in those patients who have myocardial ischemia. In concentrations that have no effect on normal Purkinje fibers, digitalis can enhance arrhythmias in ischemic Purkinje fibers by increasing the magnitude of delayed afterdepolarizations and causing triggered activity, the most probable mechanism for the abnormal impulse formation in digitalis toxicity. Digitalis also causes AV block and suppresses phase 4 depolarization in normal pacemaker cells.[1-20]

Mortality in undiagnosed digitalis toxicity

The mortality rate after the misinterpretation of digitalis dysrhythmias was published by Dreifus.[13] In the patients studied, when atrial tachycardia with block went unrecognized and digitalis was continued, 100% (7:7) died; when the drug was stopped, there was a 6% mortality rate (1:16). When junctional tachycardia was not recognized as a digitalis dysrhythmia, 81% died (25:31); and when the diagnosis was made and the drug stopped, the mortality rate was 16% (7:43).

Cellular basis for positive inotropy

↑ intracellular Na + ↑ Ca²⁺

Digitalis competes with potassium (K^+) for a binding site on the cell membrane, interfering with the sodium-potassium ATPase pump.[7,8] This competition impairs sodium (Na^+) efflux and results in an accumulation of intracellular Na^+, which in turn influences the sodium-calcium exchange, causing a net gain in intracellular calcium (Ca^{++}). These known facts support the hypothesis that the inhibition of the sodium pump explains the ability of digitalis to increase myocardial contractility.[7,8,21]

Cellular basis for digitalis dysrhythmias

The increase in intracellular Ca^{++} caused by digitalis is in turn followed by a transient inward Na^+ current. As illustrated in Fig. 5-1 (solid line), this transient current occurs after full repolarization, causing a *delayed afterdepolarization*.[8,22-24] If this afterdepolarization does not reach threshold potential, it cannot cause ectopic beats or rhythms on the surface electrocardiogram (ECG). Shortening the cycle length and/or increasing catecholamines may cause the delayed afterdepolarization to heighten and reach threshold potential, in which case a propagated action potential results. This action potential is called a triggered beat since it does not result from either type of altered automaticity but is dependent on the preceding beat. An abnormal rhythm is then perpetuated (triggered activity) because each triggered beat is followed by its own afterdepolarization, which is guaranteed to reach threshold potential because of the short cycle preceding it. The rhythm finally terminates itself when the enhanced activity of the sodium pump produces hyperpolarization, with the sodium pump itself stimulated by the increase in intracellular Na^+ secondary to the rapid rate. Triggered activity is also illustrated in Fig. 5-1 (dashed line).

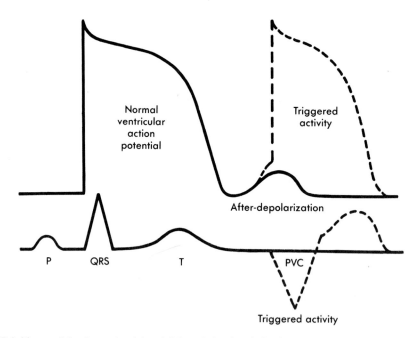

Fig. 5-1. Myocardial action potential and delayed afterdepolarization as it relates to the surface electrocardiogram (ECG). Dashed lines represent the sequence of events that result when an afterdepolarization reaches threshold potential. (From Conover M: Understanding electrocardiography, ed 5, St. Louis, 1988, The CV Mosby Co.)

Digitalis and potassium

Maintenance of the serum K^+ levels within the physiological range is the goal during digitalis therapy because both hypokalemia of <3 to 4 mM and hyperkalemia of >5 mM exacerbate digitalis dysrhythmias.[8] This exacerbation is because of the following:

1. Digitalis and K^+ vie for binding sites on the membrane; thus the inhibitory effects of digitalis on the sodium pump are partially reversed when extracellular K^+ concentration is elevated.[8,25]
2. Hypokalemia is an arrhythmogenic mechanism on its own, setting the stage for abnormal automaticity and slow conduction. When digitalis is administered to the hypokalemic patient, arrhythmogenesis is compounded because the binding of digitalis to its receptor site on the membrane is facilitated by the lack of K^+, promoting the development of delayed afterdepolarizations and triggered activity.
3. An elevation in extracellular K^+ to more than approximately 5 mM has the same end result as does hypokalemia. Although the extra K^+ in the extracellular compartment reduces the binding of digitalis to the cellular membrane, it also accelerates repolarization and lowers the resting membrane potential, slowing or blocking conduction.[8,26]

Drugs that interact with digoxin

Digitalis dysrhythmias may result from adding other drugs to the patient's regimen. Quinidine and amiodarone markedly increase the steady state serum digoxin levels, as do certain calcium channel blockers, especially verapamil.[27]

Quinidine. When quinidine is added to digoxin therapy, the dose of digoxin should be decreased by approximately 50%. When quinidine is given to patients receiving digoxin, the serum digoxin concentration increases because of a reduction in the volume of digoxin distribution and a decrease in renal and nonrenal clearance of digoxin. The implication is that quinidine interferes with digoxin tissue binding.[28,29]

Amiodarone. In one study, there was a mean increase in plasma digoxin concentration of 70% when amiodarone (600 mg/day) was administered along with the digoxin. This result is caused in part by a decrease in renal and nonrenal clearance of digoxin and in part by an increase in half-life.[27,30]

Verapamil. Both renal and nonrenal clearance of digoxin decreases when digoxin and verapamil are combined. This effect develops gradually during the first few days and reaches a steady state within 7 days.[31]

Diltiazem. A 22% increase in steady state plasma digoxin concentration occurs when diltiazem (180 mg/day) is added to digoxin.[32]

Drugs that apparently do not affect digoxin concentration are procainamide, disopyramide, mexiletine, flecainide, ethmozine, and nifedipine.

ECG recognition of digitalis dysrhythmias

Digitalis dysrhythmias can be divided into two categories based on excitant and suppressant effects. The excitant effects are probably caused by afterdepolarizations that reach threshold potential and produce triggered activity[5,15,17]; the suppressant effects are caused by depression of phase 4 depolarization in pacemaker cells and by prolonged AV conduction. Both extrasystoles and blocks occur in chronic users of digitalis, whereas AV block is the predominant problem in the acute setting (e.g., accidental or intentional overdose).

Certain digitalis dysrhythmias can be identified by specific features on the surface ECG. These features were pointed out as early as 1974[14] and 1976[15] and have been reiterated and expanded over the years.[16-20] Two such arrhythmias encountered in patients taking digitalis are easily identified by their typical features—atrial tachycardia with block and fascicular ventricular tachycardia. Other typical digitalis arrhythmias are ventricular bigeminy,[33] accelerated idiojunctional rhythm,[34] and bidirectional ventricular tachycardia.[35-42] With patients on digitalis, any new arrhythmia or change from one type of arrhythmia to another should be suspected of being digitalis induced.[17] Accidental or suicidal acute overdosage with digitalis tend to cause profound AV block, whereas tachycardias are more common with chronic users.

Arrhythmias that are rarely, if ever, caused by digitalis are atrial fibrillation, atrial flutter, parasystole, type II second degree AV block, and chaotic atrial tachycardia.[17]

ATRIAL TACHYCARDIA WITH BLOCK. Atrial tachycardia caused by digitalis toxicity is the result of triggered activity and is often associated with AV block, not only secondary to the rapid atrial rate, but also to the lengthening of the AV nodal refractory period. The ECG is typical[15-17]:

1. The atrial rate is 130 to 250 beats/min.
2. AV conduction is usually 2:1 but sometimes manifests Wenckebach periods. When digitalis is discontinued, transient 1:1 conduction may appear before the rhythm converts to sinus rhythm.
3. At times (60%)[15] there is ventriculophasic behavior of PP intervals; i.e., the PP interval embracing the R wave is shorter than the PP interval without an R wave. In some cases this behavior is so marked that it may resemble bigeminal nonconducted atrial premature beats (PACs). The mechanism of ventriculophasic changes in PP intervals is the same as that seen in complete heart block. Peak sympathetic activity occurs just before the upstroke of the aortic pressure (shortly after the onset of the QRS), causing the atrial cycle to shorten. Sympathetic activity then decreases sharply, and vagal tone increases, causing the next atrial cycle to lengthen.[17,43,44]

4. The shape of the P waves is identical or almost so to the sinus P waves. When this shape is also associated with 2:1 block and ventriculophasic changes in PP intervals, the diagnosis of digitalis toxicity becomes more certain.

Fig. 5-2, *A*, is an example of atrial tachycardia with 2:1 block in a patient with digitalis toxicity. Note that the P waves resemble sinus P waves (Fig. 5-2, *B*) and that the PP interval without the R wave is longer than the PP interval that includes an R wave.

A

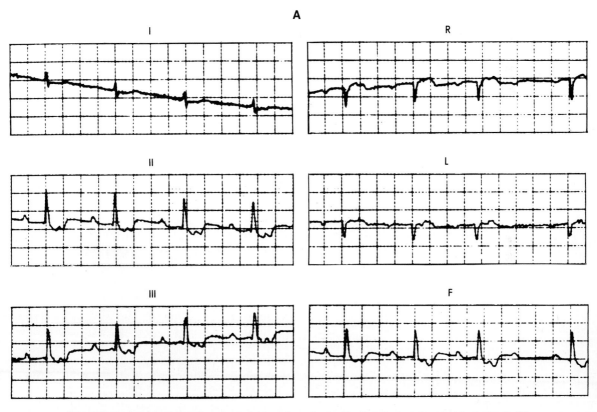

Fig. 5-2. A, Atrial tachycardia with 2:1 block in patient with digitalis toxicity. Ventriculophasic PP intervals are present. (**A** and **B** from Vanagt EJ and Wellens HJJ: The electrocardiogram in digitalis intoxication. In Wellens HJJ and Kulbertus HE, editors: What's new in electrocardiography? The Hague, 1981, Martinus Nijhoff Publishers.)   *Continued.*

B

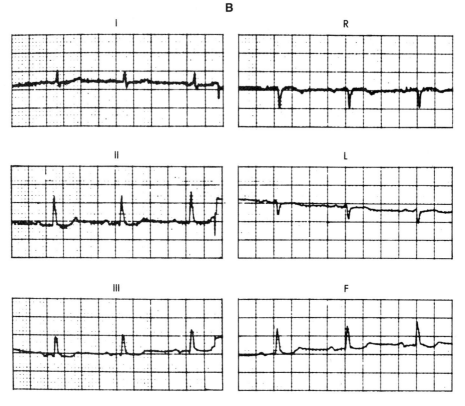

Fig. 5-2, cont'd. B, Digitalis has been discontinued and sinus rhythm restored; note similarity in P wave configuration during atrial tachycardia and sinus rhythm.

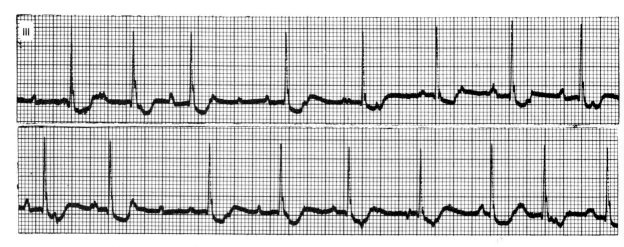

Fig. 5-3. Atrial tachycardia with block (strips are continuous). Note variable P wave morphology, irregular atrial rhythm, changing AV conduction ratio, and sagging ST segments.

Fig. 5-3 shows atrial tachycardia with various shaped P' waves and variable conduction ratio. The sagging ST segments are characteristic of digitalis effect.

Fig. 5-4 illustrates profound AV block seen in a patient with acute digitalis toxicity—in this case, in one who had attempted suicide.

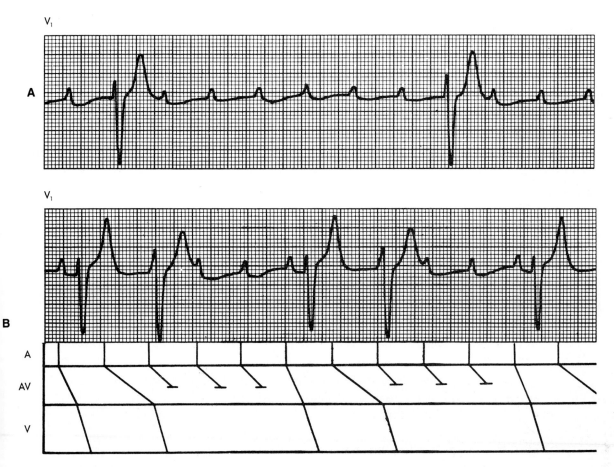

Fig. 5-4. Profound AV block in patient with acute digitalis toxicity (attempted suicide). **A,** Conduction ratio is 7:1. **B,** Situation has improved with conduction ratio of 5:2. (From Conover M: Cardiac arrhythmias, St. Louis, 1974, The CV Mosby Co.)

Fig. 5-5 illustrates results of acute digitalis toxicity from accidental overdose. The patient was mistakenly given 2 mg of digoxin intravenously, with disturbing results.

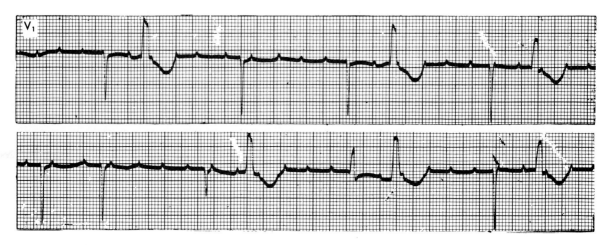

Fig. 5-5. Atrial tachycardia with 4:1 block and ventricular ectopic beats in patient with acute digitalis toxicity (accidental overdose).

FASCICULAR VENTRICULAR TACHYCARDIA. In digitalis toxicity, ventricular arrhythmias are thought to originate in one of the fascicles of the left bundle branch, producing a pattern that resembles incomplete right bundle branch block (RBBB) with right or left axis deviation. In the fascicular ventricular tachycardia that occurs with digitalis toxicity, the following are typical:

1. The QRS is narrower than usual (0.12 to 0.14 sec).
2. The pattern is that of incomplete RBBB.
3. The rate is usually 90 to 160 beats/min.
4. The axis is abnormal. A focus in the anterosuperior fascicle produces right axis deviation, and a focus in the posteroinferior fascicle produces left axis deviation.

Competition for the pacing role may also exist among the Purkinje fibers, causing the QRS configuration during the tachycardia to be inconstant.[15-18] This fact can be noted in Fig. 5-6, in which the shape of the QRS changes with the different sites of impulse formation in the left ventricular Purkinje system.

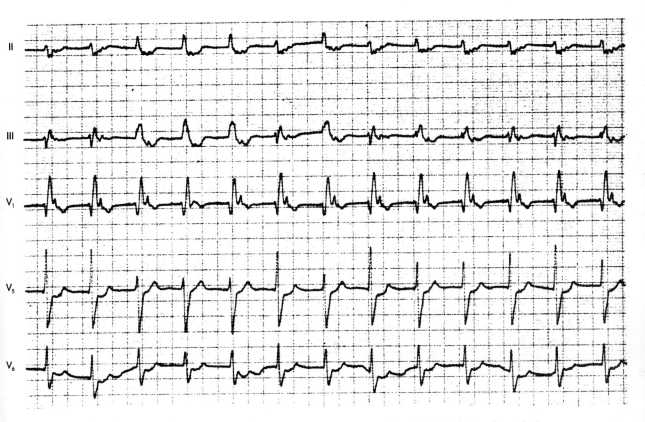

Fig. 5-6. Accelerated fascicular ventricular rhythm—an example of digitalis-induced ventricular rhythm, with impulse formation at different sites in the left ventricular Purkinje system. Characteristically, the QRS width is 0.12 to 0.14 sec. One-to-one ventriculoatrial conduction is present. (From Vanagt EJ and Wellens HJJ: The electrocardiogram in digitalis intoxication. In Wellens HJJ and Kulbertus HE, editors: What's new in electrocardiography? The Hague, 1981, Martinus Nijhoff Publishers.)

In the past it was not uncommon for the accelerated fascicular or ventricular rhythms common to digitalis overdosage to be misdiagnosed as preexcitation with conduction over Mahaim fibers. However, research has shown that, with digitalis toxicity, these rhythms probably have their origin in one of the fascicles of the left bundle branch just distal to the His bundle.[45-48] Fig. 5-7 shows fascicular tachycardia seen in atrial fibrillation. It has typical morphology (incomplete RBBB) and typical rate (140 beats/min).

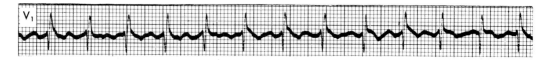

Fig. 5-7. Atrial fibrillation with typical fascicular tachycardia seen in digitalis toxicity; note the incomplete right bundle branch block and the rate of 140/min.

Fig. 5-8 is from a 50-year-old woman with an acute inferior infarction in whom sinus tachycardia developed at a rate of 130 beats/min. She was given 0.75 mg of digoxin intravenously, and the dose was repeated 1 hour later. During the subsequent several hours many manifestations of digitalis intoxication appeared, including severe vomiting and the cardiotoxic effects illustrated in Fig. 5-8. The initial manifestations of toxicity are seen in Fig. 5-8, *A,* in which there is significant AV block and a junctional escape rhythm of 50 beats/min; the last beat is a conducted one. As the toxicity progresses, a fascicular rhythm emerges (Fig. 5-8, *B).* The incomplete RBBB pattern typical of this rhythm is thought caused by triggered activity. In Fig. 5-8, *C,* when two fascicular beats are closely linked, there is a pause, and the junctional escape rhythm takes over. In Fig. 5-8, *D,* there are two junctional escape beats; the rest are conducted. The profound AV block and suppression of phase 4 in His-Purkinje fibers, caused by digitalis, are manifested in Fig. 5-8 *E,* when the fascicular rhythm fails. Fig. 5-8, *E,* illustrates the need for the insertion of a temporary pacemaker when digitalis toxicity is being treated; if the afterpotentials are abolished before normal AV conduction and normal automaticity are restored, the result may be profound bradycardia or cardiac standstill. By the same token, beta stimulation (including anxiety, exercise, sympathicomimetic drugs) and cholinolytic drugs (atropine) should be avoided.[5,17]

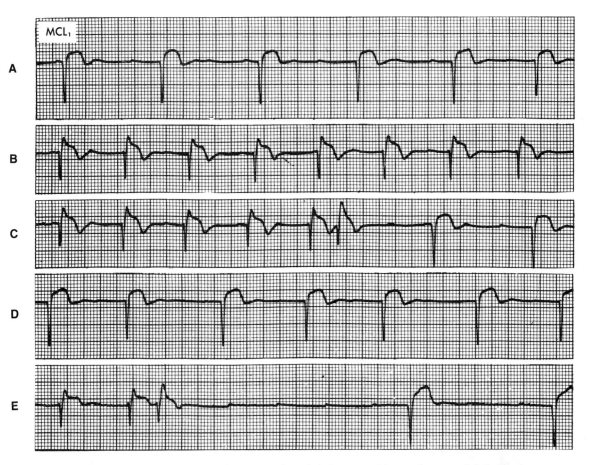

Fig. 5-8. Strips are not continuous but were selected during several hours of severe digitalis intoxication in a patient with acute inferior infarction who received 1.5 mg of digoxin intravenously in 1 hour. **A,** Sinus tachycardia (rate, 135 beats/min) with significant AV block and junctional escape rhythm (rate, 50 beats/min). **B,** Fascicular rhythm. Note typical incomplete right bundle branch block pattern. **C,** Cessation of fascicular rhythm after two closely linked beats; junctional escape rhythm follows. **D,** AV Wenckebach period with junctional escape. **E,** When fascicular rhythm fails again, so does the junctional escape, another manifestation of digitalis toxicity. There is now complete heart block.

BIDIRECTIONAL VENTRICULAR TACHYCARDIA. This term is purely descriptive and does not imply a mechanism. Although the axis changes have been thought in the past to be caused by alternating conduction over the anterior and posterior fascicles,[49] recent His bundle studies support the mechanisms of either dual ventricular foci or one focus with alternating routes.[17,50-52] Fig. 5-9 illustrates the characteristic digitalis-induced bidirectional ventricular tachycardia with RBBB configuration and alternating right and left axis deviation. Fig. 5-10 is less typical with its left bundle branch block (LBBB) configuration.

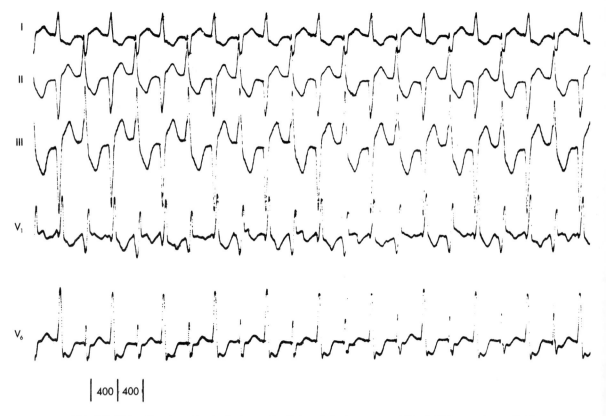

Fig. 5-9. Bidirectional ventricular tachycardia. Note relatively narrow width of QRS complexes (0.12 sec), right bundle branch block configuration, and alternating left and right axis deviation. (From Vanagt EJ and Wellens HJJ: The electrocardiogram in digitalis intoxication. In Wellens HJJ and Kulbertus HE, editors: What's new in electrocardiography? The Hague, 1981, Martinus Nijhoff Publishers.)

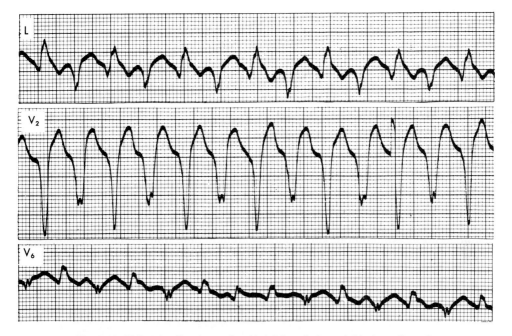

Fig. 5-10. Bidirectional tachycardia with left bundle branch block configuration.

VENTRICULAR BIGEMINY. Ventricular extrasystoles are the most frequent cardiac manifestation of digitalis overdosage except in children, in whom supraventricular ectopics are more common. However, ventricular arrhythmias are in no sense diagnostic of digitalis intoxication, being common in both health and disease of any kind, with ventricular bigeminy most commonly seen in patients with coronary artery disease.[17] Furthermore, digitalis is often an effective drug for reducing or eliminating ventricular extrasystoles that are not caused by the drug.[53,54]

Ventricular bigeminy has long been regarded as a common manifestation of digitalis toxicity[55-57] and has been shown as the result of afterdepolarizations and triggered activity (see Chapter 4).[33] Because Purkinje fibers compete for the pacing role, the ventricular ectopic beats often have different configurations, even though the coupling interval is fixed.

Fig. 5-11 is from a patient with atrial fibrillation and severe digitalis intoxication. There is at least high-grade and probably complete AV block, with resultant escaping idiojunctional rhythm at the slow rate of approximately 40 beats/min. Note the two different shapes of the junctional escape beats. Impulse formation from two or even three sites in the AV junction has been observed after digitalis excess.[58-61] There is ventricular bigeminy, and, as is often the case, the extrasystolic complexes vary in shape ("multiform" or "variform").[53,62] Scherf and Schott[53] claim that the ventricular ectopic beats of a digitalis-induced bigeminy always show variation in morphology if long enough strips are taken. A nondysrhythmic sign diagnostic of digitalis intoxication is also seen in this tracing—sagging ST segments in leads in which the QRS is predominantly negative.[63]

Sometimes the bigeminy caused by digitalis is intermittently concealed; bigeminal runs may be seen, and all interectopic intervals contain only odd numbers of sinus beats.[64] Fig. 5-12 is an example of concealed ventricular bigeminy in which two runs of bigeminy are seen and the number of sinus beats intervening between consecutive ectopic beats is always an odd number—1, 3, 5, 7, etc.

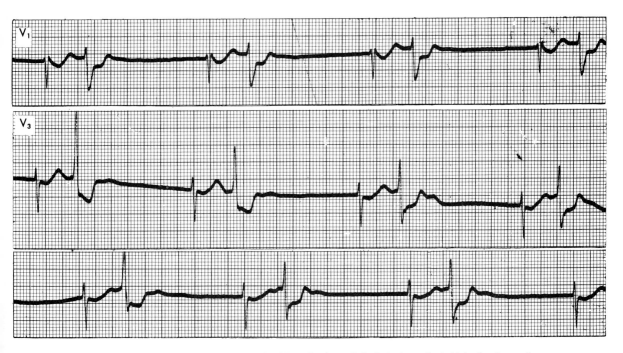

Fig. 5-11. Atrial fibrillation with ventricular bigeminy in a digitalis-toxic patient. Note fixed coupling intervals and three different configurations of the ventricular premature beats. Junctional escape beats also change in configuration.

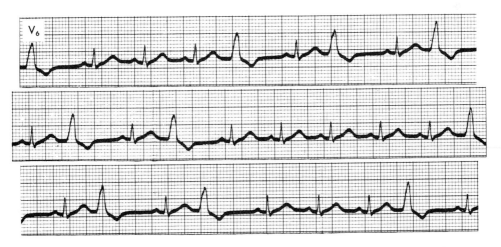

Fig. 5-12. Concealed ventricular bigeminy—a short sample of a much longer strip in which the number of sinus beats intervening between consecutive ectopics was always an odd number. Tendency to bigeminy is apparent in this sample, in which the intervening sinus beats consecutively number 3, 1, 1, 1, 1, 5, 1, 1, 3.

ACCELERATED IDIOJUNCTIONAL RHYTHM AND JUNCTIONAL TACHYCARDIA.
Digitalis in toxic doses not only impairs AV conduction through the AV node, but it also depresses phase 4 in His-Purkinje cells and causes afterdepolarizations and triggered activity. The junctional rhythms that result have a gradual onset and are manifested when they attain a rate greater than that of the sinus node, usually approximately 70 beats/min. From a rate of 60 to 100 beats/min, the arrhythmia is called "accelerated idiojunctional rhythm"—"idio" because there is often retrograde block and AV dissociation. When the rate is greater than 100 beats/min, the term "idiojunctional tachycardia" is used, although the mechanism remains the same. The rate commonly does not exceed 140 beats/min.[17,65] Because of its gradual onset, this tachycardia was termed "nonparoxysmal" by Pick and Dominguez.[65]

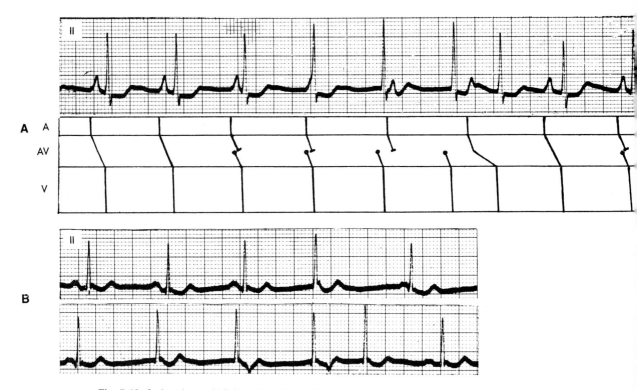

Fig. 5-13. A, Accelerated idiojunctional rhythm (rate, 78 beats/min) in digitalis toxicity usurps control from a sinus rhythm (rate, 70 to 75 beats/min). Seventh beat is a ventricular capture conducted with prolonged PR interval. **B,** Accelerated junctional rhythm resulting from digitalis overdosage. In second strip there is retrograde conduction to the atria.

Fig. 5-13, *A,* is a tracing from a 12-year-old girl who required a mitral commissurotomy. After successful surgery her digitalis dosage was not reduced, and signs of intoxication soon developed in the form of the accelerated idiojunctional rhythm seen in this tracing. Note the AV dissociation in the same tracing.

Fig. 5-13, *B,* illustrates a case of accelerated junctional rhythm resulting from digitalis overdosage. In this case there is retrograde conduction to the atria (second strip). The patient was a young woman with a rheumatic heart who was 1-day postpartum. By mistake, she received an extra dose of digoxin (0.5 mg) intravenously and began to show this irregular junctional rhythm.

VENTRICULAR TACHYCARDIA. Fig. 5-14 is the tracing from a patient who was being relentlessly nudged toward his death by repeated intravenous doses of digoxin. Hypokalemia and/or hypomagnesemia may also have been factors. Fascicular ventricular tachycardia is present (note the RBBB pattern). When the cycle lengthens to 0.90 sec in the bottom strip, ventricular tachycardia resembling torsade de pointes follows. Torsade de pointes is often, although not always, associated with a long QT interval and is precipitated by lengthening of the cycle. The mechanism of the morphology of torsade de pointes is not known, although the long QT interval is associated with oscillations before repolarization is completed (early afterdepolarization).[66-68] This concept is discussed more completely in Chapter 4.

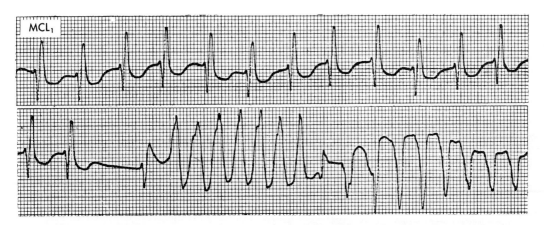

Fig. 5-14. Fascicular ventricular tachycardia that is somewhat irregular. There is a long QT interval, and after a pause in the second strip, what apparently is torsade de pointes ensues.

DOUBLE TACHYCARDIA. Digitalis toxicity is the most common cause of "double tachycardia,"[69] the simultaneous existence of two rapidly firing but independent foci. Figs. 5-15 and 5-16 illustrate simultaneous atrial and junctional tachycardia. In Fig. 5-15 both rhythms have the same rate, producing an isorhythmic AV dissociation. Notice that the P waves are always in the same place relative to the R wave but that they are too close to conduct across the AV node. In Fig. 5-16 the slight shortening of some of the cycles is probably the result of conduction of the atrial impulse into the ventricles (ventricular capture).

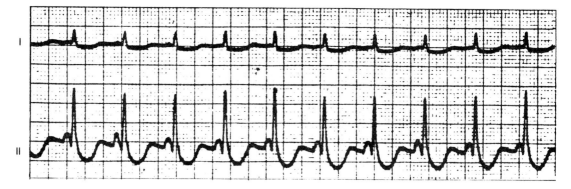

Fig. 5-15. Double tachycardia—atrial tachycardia and junctional tachycardia with isorhythmic AV dissociation. (Courtesy of William P Nelson, MD, Tampa, Fla.)

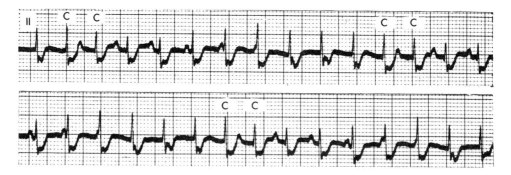

Fig. 5-16. Strips are continuous. Simultaneous but independent atrial tachycardia (rate, 172 beats/min) and junctional tachycardia (rate, 154 beats/min). Pairs of captured beats *(C)* are recognized by the slight shortening of the ventricular cycles.

SINUS BRADYCARDIA AND SA WENCKEBACH PERIOD. Digitalis suppresses not only impulse formation in the SA node but conduction out of the node as well. Fig. 5-17 shows both sinus bradycardia and a simultaneous 5:4 SA Wenckebach period. The loss of every fifth P wave causes this mild sinus bradycardia to be more profound. The SA Wenckebach period exists when conduction from the sinus node to atrial tissue gets longer and longer until finally an impulse is not conducted at all, and the period begins again. In the classical SA Wenckebach period, the PP intervals get progressively shorter, and the pause is less than twice the shortest cycle. The PR remains constant unless there is a concurrent AV Wenckebach period.

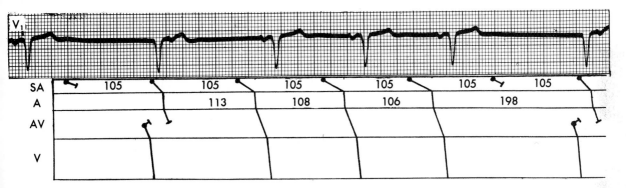

Fig. 5-17. SA Wenckebach period. Second and last beats are junctional escape beats (see laddergram.) Wenckebach-type conduction from sinus node to atrial tissue is inferred from progressive shortening of PP interval.

AV WENCKEBACH PERIOD. Digitalis exerts its suppressant effects on AV nodal conduction and on normal automaticity. It lengthens the refractory period of AV nodal tissue and depresses phase 4 depolarization in pacemaker cells. The AV nodal block occurs at two levels, producing both entrance and exit block. The upper level of block occurs between atrial tissue and the site of impulse formation in the AV junction (entrance block); the lower level of block occurs between the site of impulse formation and the ventricles (exit block).[17] Fig. 5-18 is an example of 6:5 type I AV block (Wenckebach period) caused by digitalis.

ATRIAL FIBRILLATION WITH ACCELERATED IDIOJUNCTIONAL RHYTHM AND WENCKEBACH EXIT BLOCK. Fig. 5-19 is from a patient with atrial fibrillation, true posterior infarction, and digitalis intoxication. In lead V_2 there are 5:4 and 4:3 Wenckebach periods; in lead V_4 there is the more common 3:2 ratio, producing bigeminal grouping. Note in the laddergram that the junctional focus is firing regularly and conduction time from the junctional focus to the ventricles lengthens and then fails. A higher degree of exit block from a subsidiary pacemaker could cause severe bradycardia but is thought rare in digitalis intoxication.[70]

Fig. 5-20 illustrates atrial fibrillation, with some degree of AV block and an accelerated idiojunctional rhythm, the combination of which has caused complete AV dissociation.

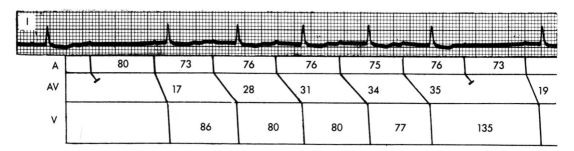

Fig. 5-18. Second degree AV block, type I. This typical Wenckebach period shows progressive lengthening of PR interval until sixth beat is dropped (6:5 AV block).

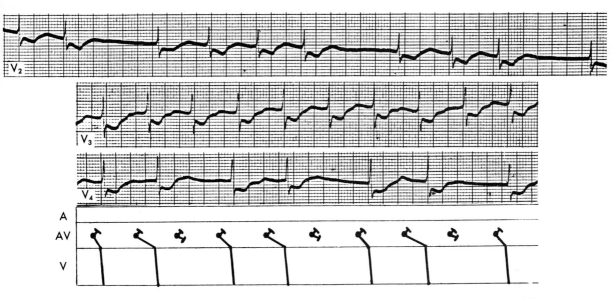

Fig. 5-19. Atrial fibrillation with accelerated junctional rhythm and Wenckebach exit block. Lead V₃ shows accelerated junctional rhythm, with a rate of 98 beats/min resulting from digitalis toxicity. Leads V₂ and V₄ have same accelerated rhythm but with Wenckebach exit block, causing group beating.

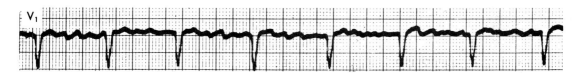

Fig. 5-20. Atrial fibrillation with AV block and accelerated idiojunctional rhythm, producing AV dissociation.

ACCELERATED IDIOVENTRICULAR RHYTHM. Fig. 5-21 is from a 10-year-old boy who, after mitral valve surgery, was mistakenly maintained on a double dose of digitalis. He manifested an accelerated idioventricular (probably fascicular) rhythm dissociated from his sinus rhythm, with ventricular bigeminy. There is also some degree of block since the atrial impulses in lead I land beyond the T wave and yet are not conducted. Four days later, after discontinuance of the digitalis, the rhythm reverted to sinus, uncomplicated except for residual first-degree AV block.

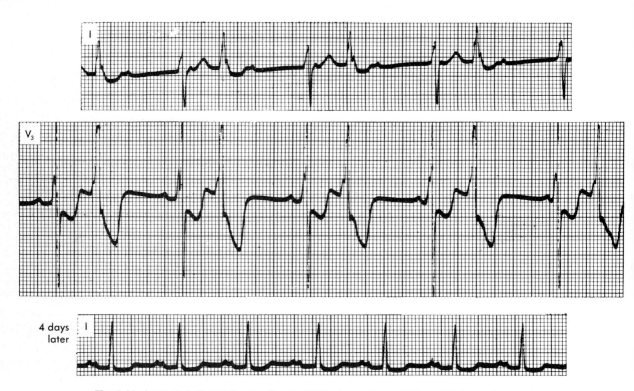

Fig. 5-21. Acute digitalis toxicity, resulting in AV block, accelerated idioventricular rhythm, and ventricular bigeminy and reverting to sinus rhythm with first degree AV block after 4 days.

SINUS BRADYCARDIA AND JUNCTIONAL TACHYCARDIA. Fig. 5-22 illustrates a threefold effect of digitalis toxicity: sinus bradycardia, junctional tachycardia, and a minor degree of AV block.[71]

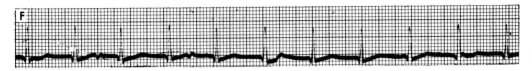

Fig. 5-22. Digitalis toxic trio: sinus bradycardia, accelerated idiojunctional rhythm, and some degree of AV block.

Summary

Digitalis intoxication causes (1) AV block because of its vagomimetic effect; (2) abnormal impulse formation, which is often typical and is caused by delayed afterdepolarizations causing triggered activity; and (3) suppression of normal escape pacemakers because of a depression of phase 4 depolarization. Certain digitalis arrhythmias can be identified by very specific features on the surface ECG. Two of these arrhythmias are atrial tachycardia with block and fascicular ventricular tachycardia. Other typical digitalis dysrhythmias are ventricular bigeminy, accelerated idiojunctional rhythm, and bidirectional ventricular tachycardia. Any new arrhythmia or change from one type of arrhythmia to another in patients on digitalis should be suspected of being digitalis induced.

REFERENCES

1. Hariman RJ and others: Enhancement of triggered activity in ischemic Purkinje fibers by ouabain: a mechanism of increased susceptibility to digitalis toxicity in myocardial infarction, J Am Coll Cardiol 5:672, 1985.
2. Lynch JJ and others: Facilitation of lethal ventricular arrhythmias by therapeutic digoxin in conscious post infarction dogs, Am Heart J 111:883, 1986.
3. Aronson RS and Gelles JM: The effect of ouabain, dinitrophenol and lithium on the pacemaker current in sheep Purkinje fibers, Circ Res 40:517, 1977.
4. Wittenberg SM and others: Acceleration of ventricular pacemakers by transient increase in heart rate in dogs during ouabain administration, Circ Res 30:167, 1972.
5. Gorgels APM and others: The clinical relevance of abnormal automaticity and triggered activity. In Brugada P and Wellens HJJ, editors: Cardiac arrhythmias: where to go from here? Mt Kisco, NY, 1987, Futura Publishing Co, Inc.
6. Johnson NJ and Rosen MR: The distinction between triggered activity and other cardiac arrhythmias. In Brugada P and Wellens HJJ, editors: Cardiac arrhythmias: where to go from here? Mt Kisco, NY, 1987, Futura Publishing Co, Inc.
7. Katz AM: Effects of digitalis on cell biochemistry: sodium pump inhibition, J Am Coll Cardiol 5:16A, 1985.
8. Rosen MR: Cellular electrophysiology of digitalis toxicity, J Am Coll Cardiol 5:22A, 1985.

9. Rosen MR and others: Correlation between effects of ouabain on the canine electrocardiogram and transmembrane potentials of isolated Purkinje fibers, Circulation 47:65, 1973.

10. Ferrier GR and others: A cellular mechanism for the generation of ventricular arrhythmias by acetylstrophanthidin, Circ Res 32:600, 1973.

11. Davis LD: Effect of changes in cycle length of diastolic depolarization produced by ouabain in canine Purkinje fiber, Circ Res 32:206, 1973.

12. Rosen MR and Danilo Jr P: Digitalis-induced delayed afterdepolarizations. In Zipes DP, Bailey JC, and Elharrar V, editors: The slow inward current and cardiac arrhythmias, The Hague, 1980, Martinus Nijhoff Publishers.

13. Dreifus LS and others: Digitalis intolerance, Geriatrics 18:494, 1963.

14. Zipes DP and others: Accelerated cardiac escape rhythms caused by ouabain intoxication, Am J Cardiol 33:248, 1974.

15. Wellens HJJ: The electrocardiogram in digitalis intoxication. In Yu PN and Goodwin JF, editors: Progress in cardiology, Philadelphia, 1976, Lea & Febiger.

16. Wellens HJJ: The electrocardiogram 80 years after Einthoven, J Am Coll Cardiol 7:484, 1986.

17. Vanagt EJ and Wellens HJJ: The electrocardiogram in digitalis intoxication. In Wellens HJJ and Kulbertus HE, editors: What's new in electrocardiography? The Hague, 1981, Martinus Nijhoff Publishers.

18. Gorgels APM and others: Extrastimulus related shortening of the first post-pacing interval in digitalis-induced ventricular tachycardia, J Am Coll Cardiol 1:840, 1983.

19. Rosen MR and Reder RF: Does triggered activity have a role in the genesis of cardiac arrhythmias? Ann Intern Med 94:794, 1981.

20. Rosen MR and others: Can accelerated atrioventricular junctional escape rhythms be explained by delayed afterdepolarizations? Am J Cardiol 45:1272, 1980.

21. Fozzard HA and Sheets MF: Cellular mechanism of action of cardiac glycosides, J Am Coll Cardiol 5:10A, 1985.

22. Tsien RW and others: Cellular and subcellular mechanisms of cardiac pacemaker oscillation, J Exp Biol 81:205, 1979.

23. Kass RS and others: Role of calcium ions in transient inward current and aftercontractions induced by strophanthidin in cardiac Purkinje fibers, J Physiol 281:187, 1978.

24. Lederer WJ and Tsien RW: Transient inward current underlying arrhythmogenic effects of cardiotonic steroids in Purkinje fibers, J Physiol 263:73, 1976.

25. Lee KS and Klaus W: The subcellular basis for the mechanism of inotropic action of cardiac glycosides, Pharmacol Rev 23:193, 1971.

26. Fisch C: Relation of electrolyte disturbances to cardiac arrhythmias, Circulation 47:408, 1973.

27. Marcus FI: Pharmacokinetic interactions between digoxin and other drugs, J Am Coll Cardiol 5:82A, 1985.

28. Leahey Jr EB and others: Quinidine-digoxin interaction. Time course and pharmacokinetics, Am J Cardiol 48:1141, 1981.

29. Warner NJ and others: Tissue digoxin concentrations and digoxin effect during the quinidine-digoxin interaction, J Am Coll Cardiol 5:680, 1985.

30. Moysey JO and others: Amiodarone increases plasma digoxin concentrations, Br Med J 282:272, 1981.

31. Klein HO and others: The influence of verapamil on serum digoxin concentration, Circulation 65:998, 1982.

32. Yoshida A and others: Effect of diltiazem on plasma level and urinary excretion of digoxin in healthy subjects, Clin Pharmacol Ther 35:681, 1984.

33. Kieval RS and others: Triggered activity as a cause of bigeminy, J Am Coll Cardiol 8:644, 1986.

34. Rosen MR and others: Can accelerated atrioventricular junctional escape rhythms be explained by delayed afterdepolarizations? Am J Cardiol 45:1272, 1980.

35. Rosen MR and Reder RF: Does triggered activity have a role in the genesis of cardiac arrhythmias, Ann Intern Med 94:794, 1981.

36. Ferrier GR: Digitalis arrhythmias: role of oscillatory afterpotentials, Prog Cardiovasc Dis 19:459, 1977.

37. Hoffman BF and Rosen MR: Cellular mechanisms for cardiac arrhythmias, Circ Res 49:1, 1981.

38. Wit AL and others: Triggered activity. In Zipes DP, Bailey JC, and Elharrar V, editors: The slow inward current and cardiac arrhythmias, The Hague, 1980, Martinus Nijhoff, Publisher.

39. Zipes DP and others: Accelerated cardiac escape rhythms caused by ouabain intoxication, Am J Cardiol 32:248, 1974.

40. Zipes DP and others: Atrial induction of ventricular tachycardia: reentry versus triggered automaticity, Am J Cardiol 44:1, 1979.

41. Whalen DA and others: Effect of a transient period of ischemia on myocardial cells. I. Effects on cell volume regulation, Am J Pathol 74:381, 1974.

42. Gorgels APM and others: Extrastimulus related shortening of the first post-pacing interval in digitalis-induced ventricular tachycardia, J Am Coll Cardiol 1:840, 1983.

43. Roth IR and Kish B: Mechanisms of irregular sinus rhythm in auriculo-ventricular heart block, Am Heart J 36:257, 1948.

44. Rosenbaum MB and Lepeschkin E: Effects of ventricular systole on auricular rhythm in auriculo-ventricular block, Circulation 11:240, 1955.

45. Massumi RA: Aberrancy of junctional escape beats: evidence for origin in the left bundle branch, Am J Cardiol 29:351, 1972.

46. Cohen HC and others: Ventricular tachycardia with narrow QRS complexes (left posterior fascicular tachycardia), Circulation 45:1035, 1972.

47. Rosenbaum M: Classification of ventricular extrasystoles according to form, J Electrocardiogr 2:289, 1969.

48. Rosenbaum M and others: The mechanism of narrow ventricular ectopic beats. In Sandoe E, Flensted-Jensen E, and Olesen KH, editors: Symposium on cardiac arrhythmias, Sweden, 1970, AB Astra.

49. Rosenbaum MB and others: The mechanism of bidirectional tachycardia, Am Heart J 78:4, 1969.

50. Cohen HC and others: Ventricular tachycardia with narrow QRS complexes (left posterior fascicular tachycardia), Circulation 45:1035, 1972.

51. Cohen SI and others: Infra-His bundle origin of bidirectional tachycardia, Circulation 47:1260, 1973.

52. Morris SN and Zipes DP: His bundle electrocardiography during bidirectional tachycardia, Circulation 48:32, 1973.

53. Scherf D and Schott A: Extrasystoles and allied arrhythmias, ed 2, London, 1973, William Heinemann Medical Books, Ltd.

54. Lown B and others: Effect of a digitalis drug on ventricular premature beats, N Engl J Med 296:301, 1977.

55. Sagal EL and Wolff L: Digitalis bigeminy: analysis of 50 cases, N Engl J Med 240:676, 1949.

56. Schrager MW: Digitalis intoxication, AMA Arch Intern Med 100:881, 1957.

57. Von Capeller D and others: Digitalis intoxication: clinical report of 148 cases, Ann Intern Med 50:869, 1959.

58. Chung K and others: Double AV nodal rhythm, Jpn Heart J 5:171, 1964.

59. Chung EK: Unusual form of digitalis induced triple AV nodal rhythm, Am Heart J 79:250, 1970.

60. Jonas S and Richman SM: Double nodal rhythm with A-V dissociation, Am Heart J 60:811, 1960.

61. Castellanos Jr A and Lemberg J: The relationship between digitalis and atrioventricular nodal tachycardia with block, Am Heart J 66:605, 1963.

62. Friedberg CK and Donoso E: Arrhythmias and conduction disturbances due to digitalis, Prog Cardiovasc Dis 2:408, 1959.

63. Lepeschkin E: Modern electrocardiography, Baltimore, 1951, The Williams & Wilkins Co.

64. Schamroth L and Marriott HJL: Concealed ventricular extrasystoles, Circulation 27:1043, 1963.

65. Pick A and Dominguez P: Nonparoxysmal A-V nodal tachycardia, Circulation 16:1022, 1957.

66. Brachmann J and others: Bradycardia dependent triggered activity: relevance to drug induced multiform ventricular tachycardia, Circulation 68:846, 1983.

67. Brugada P and Wellens HJJ: Early afterdepolarizations: role in conduction block, prolonged repolarization dependent reexcitation, and tachyarrhythmias in the human heart, PACE 8:889, 1985.

68. Franz MR: Long-term recording of monophasic action potentials from human endocardium, Am J Cardiol 51:1629, 1983.

69. Castellanos and others: Digitalis-induced arrhythmias: recognition and therapy, Cardiovasc Clin 1:108, 1969.

70. Pick A and Langendorf R: Recent advances in the differential diagnosis of A-V junctional arrhythmias, Am Heart J 76:553, 1968.

71. Kastor JA: Digitalis intoxication in patients with atrial fibrillation, Circulation 47:888, 1973.

CHAPTER 6

The reentry mechanism

"Reentry" is well named: it implies that an impulse, after activating a segment of tissue once, returns and activates it again. The impulse cannot double back on its tracks and retrace its steps since tissue in its wake is refractory; there must be a separate return pathway. It must not return too soon or the just-activated tissue will still be refractory. Therefore prerequisites for reentry include a second approach to the involved segment (which implies the existence of a circuit) and slow enough conduction to give surrounding tissue time to repolarize.

However, there is a third requirement as well: there must be unequal responsiveness in two segments of the dual circuitous path; otherwise, the spreading impulse would synchronously activate all in its path, and there would be no opportunity for it to turn back and reactivate the tissue it had previously depolarized. This third requirement is often described as "unidirectional block"; and, of course, this block would and does favor reentry. However, unidirectional block—implying that conduction is possible in only one direction—is essential only when the block is permanent. When the block is transient (because of refractoriness), the difference in the refractory periods of two limbs of the circuit suffices.

In Fig. 6-1 the segment of tissue, X, is initially activated from left to right *(continuous line)*. If the impulse finds that path Y is still refractory after path Z has recovered from a previous activation, the impulse will traverse Z but will be unable to enter Y. If, however, Y has recovered by the time the impulse approaches its other end, the impulse will be able to activate it from right to left; and if, in turn, the impulse has traveled slowly enough that X or Z has had time to recover, the impulse will reenter X and/or Z to initiate a single reentry (reciprocal, echo) beat or a run of reciprocating tachycardia.

Reentry may be either random (e.g., in fibrillation), or it may be ordered (a fixed pathway). When the circuit involved is tiny such as in the AV node or a distal

Purkinje circuit, the phenomenon is *"microreentry."* When the circuit takes a longer pathway as in the circus movement tachycardia of Wolff-Parkinson-White (WPW) syndrome or the ventricular tachycardia using the divisions of the left bundle branch (LBB), the term *"macroreentry"* is appropriate.

The requirements for reentry can be summarized as follows:

1. An available circuit
2. Unequal responsiveness in two segments of the circuit
3. Slow conduction

Because one of the factors favoring reentry is delayed conduction, rhythms that depend on reentry for their development or perpetuation are disorders of conduction rather than of impulse formation. In fact, the existence of conduction delay may be the decisive clue to the fact that the underlying mechanism is reentry.

Among the disturbances of rhythm known to be caused by reentry are the following:

1. Some extrasystoles (usually bigeminal or trigeminal)
2. Some ventricular tachycardias
3. Paroxysmal supraventricular tachycardias (AV nodal reentry; AV reentry using the AV node and an accessory pathway; SA nodal reentry; and intra-atrial reentry)

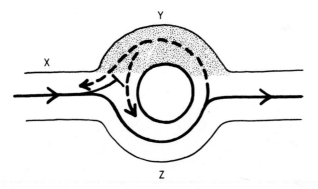

Fig. 6-1. Reentry. The segment of tissue *(X)* is initially activated from left to right *(continuous line)*. One path *(Y)* is still refractory, and the impulse cannot enter. The other path *(Z)* has recovered partially, and the impulse travels slowly through it, by which time the Y path has recovered. The impulse then travels retrogradely in Y to reenter X and Z.

Historical background

Reentry was mentioned as early as 1887[1]; but first proof of its existence was adduced by Mayer in 1906[2] and 1908[3] through his work with jellyfish, an animal that also provided early researchers with an understanding of the concepts of cardiac rhythmicity, pacemaker function, and conduction block.[4-7]

   The concepts of reciprocating rhythms and reciprocal or "echo" beats arose from the experiments of Mines in 1913[8] and 1914,[9] using portions of the atria and ventricles of the frog and the electrical ray.

   The original jellyfish studies by Mayer are worth recounting here since the results of his experiments can be applied to atrial, ventricular, and Purkinje fibers in the human heart. Fig. 6-2 represents the subumbrella tissue of the jellyfish, which Mayer cut into a ring. Note in Fig. 6-2, A, that when the ring was stimulated at one point, the excitation waves traveled in opposite directions around the ring to meet and cancel each other. When pressure was applied (the shaded area in Fig. 6-2, B) on one side of the ring near the point of origin, the impulse was blocked there and traveled only in the opposite direction. When the impulse was on its one-way journey around the ring, the pressure was released, and the impulse was able to continue around and around (Fig. 6-2, C). The impulse continued to propagate because it traveled in only one direction and because the ring was long enough to allow the point of stimulation to recover before the impulse arrived from the opposite direction. In the human heart more than simply a long pathway is necessary since normal conduction velocity is so fast that it is unlikely that such a circuit could exist in

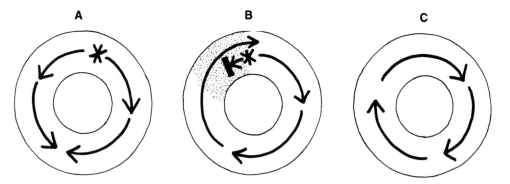

Fig. 6-2. Diagrammatic representation of the first studies by Mayer proving reentry. In **A,** the impulses travel from the stimulus in opposite directions around the ring to meet and cancel each other. In **B,** pressure has been applied at the shaded area in the ring, at which point the impulse is blocked and travels only in the opposite direction. Pressure is then removed, and the impulse continues, **C,** around and around on its one-way journey as long as refractory tissue is not encountered.

functional isolation.[10] In the following pages we discuss the additional requirement of *slow conduction*, as well as other mechanisms involved in reentry such as summation, inhibition, and reflection.

Slow conduction

As stated in Chapter 3, one of the determinants of conduction velocity is the level of the resting membrane potential at the time of stimulation. The more negative the resting membrane potential, the more sodium channels are available, and the quicker these channels open to allow sodium to rush into the cell. This mechanism has been referred to as the "fast response" action potential.[11] It occurs in fibers in which the resting membrane potential is optimal (-80 to -90 mV) and, in the Purkinje system, results in conduction velocity of 1 to 4 m/sec.[12,13] Depressed fast response and slow response action potentials may develop in the heart because of disease processes.[14,15] These action potentials may result in conduction that is slow enough to support a reentry circuit.

DEPRESSED FAST RESPONSE.[16] When the resting membrane potential is between -60 and -70 mV, only approximately half the fast sodium channels are available, and consequently, the upstroke velocity and amplitude of phase 0 of the action potential are less than normal, and conduction velocity decreases. Such an action potential is the result of both sodium and calcium influxes into the cell, which are slower and of less magnitude than at a more negative resting membrane potential.

SLOW RESPONSE.[17,18] When the resting membrane potential is less than -55 or -60 mV, the action potential is mainly the result of a relatively slow influx of calcium, along with some sodium, since the fast sodium channels are completely inactivated at approximately -50 mV.[12] A strong depolarizing current may initiate the slow upstroke velocity and low amplitude. This type of action potential results in slow conduction and may result in one-way conduction block[19]; or with further reduction of the resting membrane potential, the action potential no longer acts as a stimulus for the fibers ahead of it, and conduction is blocked in both directions.

In a sufficiently long segment with slow response action potentials and depressed fast response action potentials, conduction can proceed slowly enough to be still traveling when the normal tissue has completed its effective refractory period. This impulse can then reenter the newly repolarized normal tissue and produce an ectopic beat. Actually the slow response action potentials are conducted so slowly that the length of depressed tissue may be short indeed and still support a current until the surrounding tissue has recovered.

Fig. 6-3 illustrates and compares the normal fast response action potential with the depressed fast response and the slow response action potentials. Note that as the resting membrane potential decreases (becomes less negative), so do the upstroke velocities and heights of phase 0.

Within minutes after a coronary occlusion, the resulting anoxia produces continuous localized electrical activity, the action potential duration shortens, and the resting membrane potential decreases.[20-22] Thus the depressed fast response and the slow response are the rule in infarcted tissues.

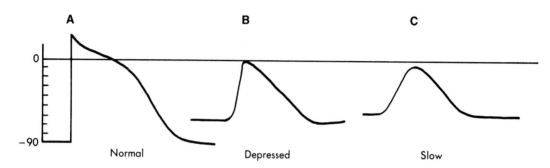

Fig. 6-3. Comparison of the normal fast response action potential, **A,** with the depressed fast response, **B,** and the slow response, **C,** action potentials.

Unidirectional block

Unidirectional block, as mentioned previously, is one of the conditions that favors reentry and may result from a lowered resting membrane potential.

When bundles of myocardial tissue (atrial, ventricular, or Purkinje) are stimulated at both ends, the impulse travels at almost equal velocities in both directions. If the resting membrane potential is so reduced that the upstroke velocity and amplitude of phase 0 are less (a depressed fast response), conduction is slower in both directions. If the resting membrane potential is reduced even further to produce a slow response action potential, conduction may proceed slowly in only one direction and not at all in the other.[12]

Summation

Summation has been mentioned by Cranefield[17] as a possible cause of one-way conduction block. It requires a particular arrangement of fibers: if two fibers converge to form one, it is possible that two impulses, both traveling toward the convergence, could meet and form a stronger current.

If the segment is depressed, then conduction may actually depend on this convergence and the resulting "summation," as illustrated in Fig. 6-4, A. Note that in 6-4, B, on the other hand, one of the impulses reaches the depressed area at the convergence before the other and is therefore unable to propagate through alone. In Fig. 6-4, C, the impulse is traveling in the opposite direction through the depressed area, and because it divides instead of uniting, block results.

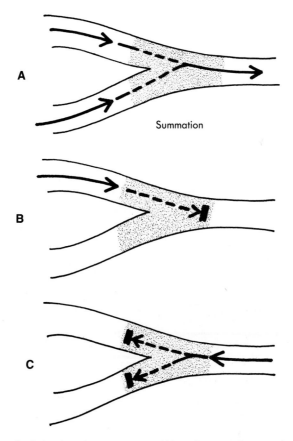

Fig. 6-4. Summation. In **A,** two impulses converge within a depressed area to form a current strong enough to emerge from the depressed area, whereas only one impulse entering the depressed area, **B,** would be blocked. In **C,** an impulse traveling in the opposite direction through the depressed area divides, instead of converging, and is blocked.

Inhibition

The term inhibition is used to describe the mechanism when one impulse, which is unable to travel through a depressed segment, reaches that segment first and leaves it refractory so that a stronger impulse entering the depressed segment through another fiber is blocked.

In Fig. 6-5 impulse 1 is able to travel through the depressed segment (Fig. 6-5, *A*), whereas impulse 2 is not (Fig. 6-5, *B*). However, if impulse 2 reaches the depressed segment first (Fig. 6-5, *C*), not only will it be blocked, but it will leave refractory tissue in the pathway of impulse 1 and thus block that impulse as well.

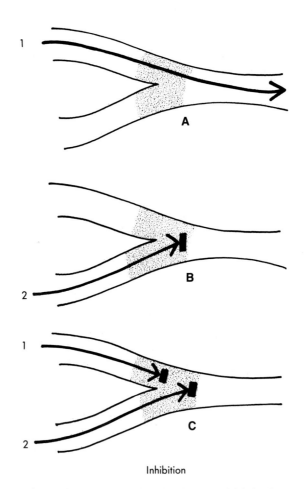

Inhibition

Fig. 6-5. Inhibition. In **A,** impulse 1 can negotiate the depressed *(shaded)* area; impulse 2, on the other hand, cannot. **B.** If this weaker impulse reaches the depressed area first, **C,** it will also block the stronger impulse *(1)*.

Reflection

Another form of reentry is produced through reflection in unbranching, parallel pathways of fibers that have depressed segments.[23,24] If the site of impulse origin has completed its effective refractory period by the time the reflected impulse returns to it, a premature beat will result. This mechanism is diagrammatically illustrated in Fig. 6-6; two adjacent depressed fibers are shown, with the upper fiber more severely depressed than the lower one. The originating wave front *(1)* is blocked in the severely depressed fiber *(2)* but proceeds slowly in the other fiber. At 3 the wave front returns through the severely depressed fiber to the area of its origin. If the normal myocardium has completed its effective refractory period by the time the impulse reaches the interface between normal and depressed tissue, it will be propagated through the normal myocardium to produce a premature complex.

Reflection may occur in Purkinje fibers or in myocardial tissue. In Purkinje fibers the reentry is caused by longitudinal dissociation[25]; in myocardial tissue reentry may occur between severely depressed segments through electrotonic propagation.[26-28]

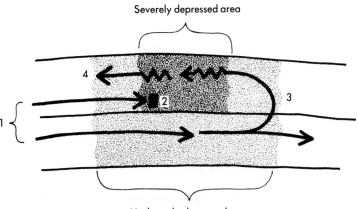

Fig. 6-6. Reflection. The impulse *(1)* is blocked in the severely depressed fiber *(2)* but proceeds slowly in the less depressed fiber to return in the opposite direction *(3)* through the severely depressed fiber to its origin *(4)*.

Summary

Reentry is the reactivation of tissue by a returning impulse. The mechanism requires an area of slow, one-way conduction to sustain it. Since slow conduction is a normal feature of the sinus and AV nodes, reentry through these structures can occur without the structures themselves being abnormal. For reentry to occur elsewhere in the heart, conduction slow enough to sustain the circuit is only achieved by depressed tissue, i.e., depressed fast response or slow response action potentials. Reentry can occur both in branching fibers and in parallel pathways (reflection). It is the sustaining mechanism in some cases of ventricular bigeminy or trigeminy, ventricular tachycardia, and paroxysmal supraventricular tachycardia (SA reentry, intra-atrial reentry, AV nodal reentry, or AV reentry using an accessory pathway and the AV node or two accessory pathways).

REFERENCES

1. McWilliams JA: Fibrillar contraction of the heart, J Physiol (Lond.) 8:296, 1887.
2. Mayer AG: Rhythmical pulsation in scyphomedusae, Carnegie Institution of Washington, Pub No 47, 1906.
3. Mayer AG: Rhythmical pulsation in scyphomedusae. II. In Papers from the Tortugas Laboratory of the Carnegie Institution of Washington, Pub No 102, Part 7, 1908.
4. Romanes GJ: Preliminary observations on the locomotor system of medusae, Philos Trans R Soc Lond 166:269, 1876.
5. Romanes GJ: Further observations on the locomotor system of medusae, Philos Trans R Soc Lond 167:659, 1877.
6. Romanes GJ: Concluding observations on the locomotor system of medusae, Philos Trans R Soc Lond 171:161, 1880.
7. Romanes GJ: Jelly-fish, star-fish, and sea-urchins: being a research on primitive nervous systems, London, 1885, Kegan Paul, Trench & Co.
8. Mines GR: On dynamic equilibrium in the heart, J Physiol (Lond.) 46:349, 1913.
9. Mines GR: On circulating excitations in heart muscles and their possible relation to tachycardia and fibrillation, Trans R Soc Can 8:43, 1914.
10. Cranefield PF and Hoffman BF: Reentry: slow conduction, summation, and inhibition, Circulation 44:309, 1971.
11. Cranefield PF, Wit AL, and Hoffman BF: Conduction of the cardiac impulse. III. Characteristics of very slow conduction, J Gen Physiol 59:227, 1972.
12. Gadsby DC and Wit AL: Normal and abnormal electrophysiology of cardiac cells. In Mandel WJ, editor: Cardiac arrhythmias; their mechanisms, diagnosis, and management, Philadelphia, 1980, JB Lippincott Co.
13. Rosen MR and Hordof AJ: Mechanisms of arrhythmias. In Roberts NK and Gelband H, editors: Cardiac arrhythmias in the neonate, infant, and child, New York, 1977, Appleton-Century-Crofts.
14. Hordof AJ and others: Electrophysiologic properties and response to pharmacologic agents of fibers from diseased human atria, Circulation 54:774, 1976.
15. Boyden PA and others: Effects of atrial dilatation on atrial cellular electrophysiology: studies on cats with spontaneous cardiomyopathy, Circulation 56 (suppl. III):48, 1977 (abstract).
16. Wit AL, Rosen MR, and Hoffman BF: Electrophysiology and pharmacology of cardiac arrhythmias. II. Relation of normal and abnormal electrical activity of cardiac fibers to the genesis of arrhythmias, Am Heart J 88:515, 1974.
17. Cranefield PF: The conduction of the cardiac impulse, Mt Kisco, NY, 1975, Futura Publishing Co.

18. Carmeliet EE and Vereecke J: Adrenaline and the plateau phase of the cardiac action potential, Pflugers Arch 313:303, 1969.
19. Cranefield PF, Wit AL, and Hoffman BF: The genesis of cardiac arrhythmias, Circulation 47:190, 1973.
20. Cranefield PF: Action potentials, afterpotentials, and arrhythmias, Circ Res 41:415, 1977.
21. MacLeod DP and Prasad K: Influence of glucose on the transmembrane action potential of papillary muscle, J Gen Physiol 53:792, 1969.
22. Han J: Ventricular ectopic activity in myocardial infarction. In Han J, editor: Cardiac arrhythmias: a symposium, Springfield, Ill, 1972, Charles C Thomas, Publisher.
23. Rosen MR: Is the response to programmed electrical stimulation diagnostic of mechanisms for arrhythmias? Circulation 73(suppl II):18, 1986.
24. Dangman KH and Hoffman BF: Studies on overdrive stimulation of canine cardiac Purkinje fibers: maximum diastolic potential as a determinant of the response, J Am Coll Cardiol 2:1183, 1983.
25. Wit AL, Hoffman BF, and Cranefield PF: Slow conduction and reentry in the ventricular conducting system. I. Return extrasystole in canine Purkinje fibers, Circ Res 30:1, 1972.
26. Antzelevitch C, Jalifé J, and Moe GK: Characteristics of reflection as a mechanism of reentrant arrhythmias and its relationship to parasystole, Circulation 61:182, 1980.
27. Jalifé J and Moe GK: Excitation, conduction and reflection of impulses in isolated bovine and canine cardiac Purkinje fibers, Circ Res 49:233, 1981.
28. Rozanski GJ, Jalifé J, and Moe GK: Reflected reentry in nonhomogeneous ventricular muscle as a mechanism of cardiac arrhythmias, Circulation 69:163, 1984.

CHAPTER 7

Intraventricular reentry

Although from time to time there has been vociferous opposition to the claim that reentry causes ventricular extrasystoles, tachycardia, and fibrillation, there is little doubt that reentry is one of the responsible mechanisms. Moreover, since 1971 evidence has rapidly accumulated that many ventricular tachycardias—following the example of supraventricular tachycardias—owe their existence to a reentry mechanism.

Reentry within terminal Purkinje fibers

In 1971[1] and 1972[2,3] reentrant activity was demonstrated in vitro in canine terminal Purkinje fibers with the use of microelectrodes. This type of reentry was described as early as 1906 by Mayer[4] and later by Schmitt and Erlanger,[5] Mines,[6] and Garrey.[7]

Fig. 7-1 is a diagrammatic representation of conduction through normal terminal Purkinje fibers. The impulse travels at the same speed through all segments of the fiber, thus eliminating any possibility for reentry. It is important that conduction velocity be uniform within one locality, although conduction velocities do differ from location to location in the myocardium, ranging from 0.5 to 5 m/sec in cardiac fibers other than those of the two nodes.

Fig. 7-2 represents conduction through a severely depressed segment of the terminal Purkinje network. The shaded area has a resting membrane potential of -55 to -60 mV. Thus depolarization in this area is accomplished by Na^+ and Ca^{++} currents passing through slow channels to produce a slow response action potential. The impulse *(1)* travels normally through the unaffected Purkinje twig *(2)* but is blocked at the border of the severely depressed segment *(3)*. Normal conduction, however, proceeds through the normal Purkinje network and on into the myocardium. When the propagated impulse arrives at the distal end of the severely depressed segment *(4)*, it may be blocked in this direction as well, or it may enter the depressed segment and propagate slowly. When it reaches the border of normal tissue, one of two things may happen: (1) it may be blocked because the normal tissue is still refractory, in which case no extrasystole occurs, or (2) it may reenter the newly repolarized normal segment and proceed into the myocardium to produce a premature beat.

Other mechanisms for reentry within the Purkinje fibers include summation and reflection, described in the previous chapter.

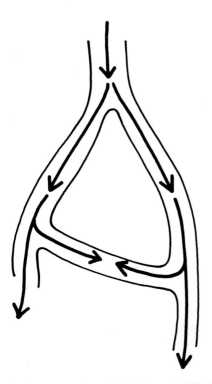

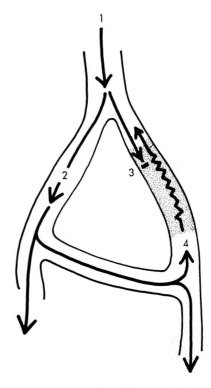

Fig. 7-1. Conduction through normal terminal Purkinje fibers. The conduction velocity is uniform.

Fig. 7-2. Conduction through severely depressed segment of terminal Purkinje fibers. The impulse *(1)* travels normally through normal tissue *(2)*, is blocked at the severely depressed tissue *(3)*, but returns, with delay, through this tissue from the opposite direction *(4)*.

Reentry through ischemic myocardial tissue

In 1977 El-Sherif and co-workers[8,9] demonstrated that the conduction disorders in ischemic myocardium closely simulated those in ischemic and depressed His-Purkinje tissue. Until this time all the models for reentry involved conductive tissue.

Fig. 7-3 is a diagrammatic representation of the conduction delays leading to re-entry in the canine myocardium 3 to 7 days after myocardial infarction. It shows a web of interconnecting, depressed, slowly conducting myocardial tissue (white paths) within a bed of more severely depressed nonconducting tissue (stippled areas) surrounded by normal myocardium. This model is consistent with the known pathology of ischemic zones, in which relatively viable myocardium is interspersed with areas of infarction.[10] The depressed tissue provides "electrical avenues" as opposed to the anatomical pathways of the His-Purkinje system.

In Fig. 7-3 there are several "doors" through which the initiating impulse may gain entrance into the depressed electrical pathways. However, at some entries propagation is blocked. Note the slow devious pathway taken by the impulse until it finds an exit into nonrefractory normal tissue. Reentry then takes place; and if the strength of the activating wave front is sufficient to excite the normal tissue, a premature beat results.

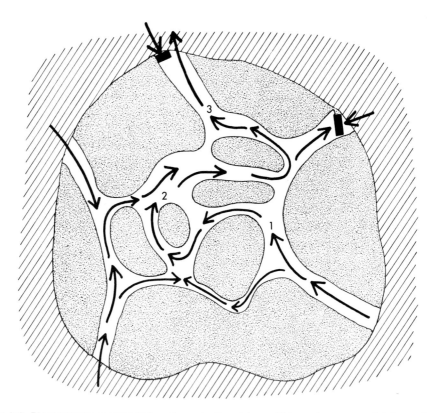

Fig. 7-3. Diagrammatic representation of conduction delays within canine myocardial tissue 3 to 7 days after an infarction. Anatomical electrical pathways are provided by a web of depressed conducting tissue *(white paths)* lying in a bed of severely depressed nonconducting tissue *(stippled areas)*. The impulse travels into the depressed area through some of the paths but is blocked from doing so in others. The slowly propagating impulse may then exit through the "doors" in which there was one-way block. (Modified from El-Sherif N and others: Circulation 55:686, 1977.)

The complex interconnections in the ischemic zone would seem to invite summation and inhibition, although so far these mechanisms have been demonstrated only for depressed Purkinje fibers and not for depressed ischemic myocardium.

Fig. 7-4 is a diagrammatic illustration of the conduction disorder in an infarcted zone leading to reentry. Displayed below it are the records obtained from that zone by a specially designed composite electrode and multiple bipolar electrodes.[8] The dashed rectangle outlines the area covered by these electrodes when placed on the left ventricular epicardial surface. This combination of electrodes recorded a continuous series of multiple asynchronous spikes, thus providing evidence for the link between an initiating complex and the subsequent premature one.

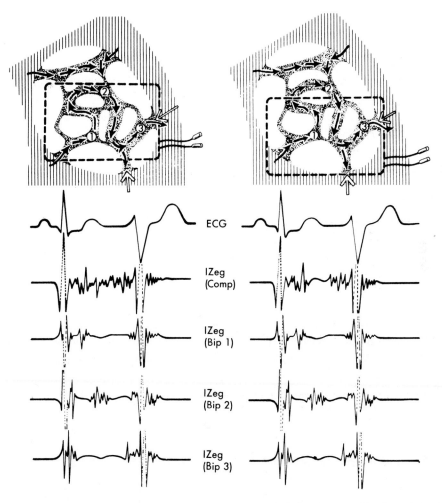

Fig. 7-4. Schematic representation of conduction disorder in infarction zone, leading to reentry. Tracings from top to bottom represent a standard ECG lead, a composite electrode recording (IZeg-*[Comp]*), and three close bipolar recordings (IZeg *[Bip, 1-3]*). (From El-Sherif, N and others: Circulation 55:686, 1977. By permission of the American Heart Association, Inc.)

Reentrant extrasystolic grouping

For the above-described reentrant beats to occur, it is necessary that the heart rate be within a critical range.[9] At rates faster than this critical rate, the conduction pattern through the depressed area of tissue demonstrates a Wenckebach-like characteristic; that is, the velocity of conduction through this area becomes slower and slower as the heart rate increases until it fails altogether. When conduction is slow enough to outlast the effective refractory period of the normal myocardium, a reentrant beat results.

At rates slower than the critical rate there is less conduction delay within the depressed tissue, and 1:1 conduction results with no reentrant beats. As the heart rate increases, so do the Wenckebach-like conduction characteristics of the ischemic zone.

In the experiments conducted by El-Sherif and others[9,10] it was found that trigeminal and quadrigeminal groupings resulted from 3:2 and 4:3 Wenckebach-like periods, which would convert to 2:1 conduction at faster rates, resulting in a bigeminal rhythm. A higher degree of block in the reentrant pathway offers no chance for reentry, or reentry may be concealed.[10,11] For example, when there were 3:2 Wenckebach-like periods, the first beat of the series would experience depressed but adequate conduction through the ischemic area. The next two beats would suffer progressively deteriorating conduction through the ischemic tissue until conduction was blocked altogether by the third beat, after which the sequence would begin again. During this sequence of three beats the second beat in the series would produce the premature beat as illustrated in Fig. 7-5, A.

After beat 1, the normal impulse is able to enter all paths into the ischemic area and cancel any slowly propagating abnormal currents. After beat 2, conduction through the ischemic tissue has so deteriorated that the normal impulse cannot gain entry into every path at the perimeter of the ischemic tissue because of one-way conduction. However, the impulse may exit from the ischemic area. This exit is possible provided the impulse is sustained within the ischemic zone long enough for the surrounding normal tissue to repolarize. Then the wave front, trapped within the ischemic zone because of slow conduction and protected from extinction by one-way block, may find nonrefractory tissue and be propagated to produce a premature beat. After beat 3 (the premature beat), conduction through the ischemic area fails altogether, at which time the Wenckebach-like sequence begins again, resulting in a pattern in which every third beat is ectopic. Fig. 7-5, B and C, illustrates 2:1 and 4:3 Wenckebach-like conduction.

Trigeminal and quadrigeminal groupings were the result of 3:2 and 4:3 Wenckebach-like periods, which would convert to 2:1 conduction patterns at faster rates, resulting in a bigeminal rhythm. A higher degree of block in the reentrant pathway offers no chance for reentry, or reentry may be concealed.[10]

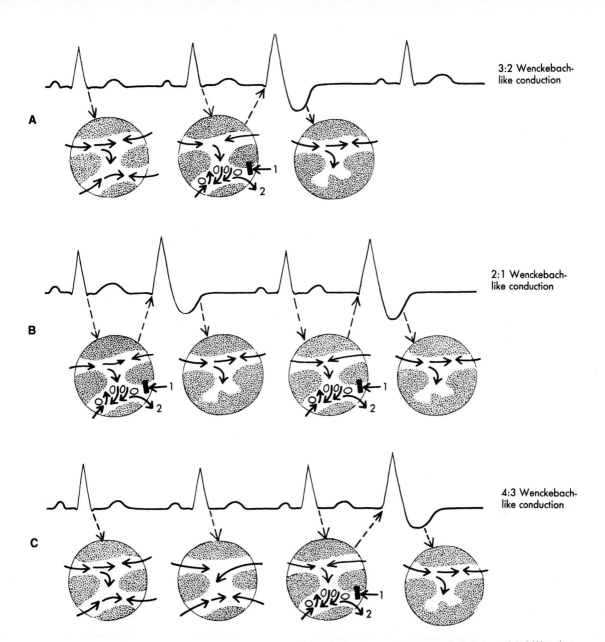

Fig. 7-5. Schematic representation of conduction disorders in infarction zone, leading to 3:2, 2:1, and 4:3 Wenckebach-like periods. **A,** 3:2 Wenckebach-like conduction, producing a ventricular ectopic beat every third beat. After beat 1, normal impulse enters all pathways into ischemic area to cancel the slowly propagating impulses within. After beat 2, ischemic tissue has deteriorated, and normal impulse is prevented from entering all pathways *(1)*, leaving avenues of exit available for the slowly propagating impulse, which exits *(2)* to produce a ventricular ectopic beat. After beat 3 (the ectopic beat), conduction through ischemic area fails completely. **B,** 2:1 Wenckebach-like conduction, producing a ventricular ectopic beat every other beat. After every normal beat, depressed conduction within the ischemic area produces slow conduction, and the impulse is prevented from entering all pathways *(1)*. This permits the reentry *(2)* of the slowly propagating impulse. After the ventricular ectopic beat, the impulse successfully invades all perimeters of ischemic tissue to cancel the slowly propagating impulse. **C,** 4:3 Wenckebach-like conduction, producing a ventricular ectopic beat every fourth beat. After the first two normal beats, currents enter all pathways into the ischemic tissue, although conduction within this tissue progressively deteriorates with each impulse. After the third normal beat, conduction deterioration permits reentry as described in **A.** After the premature beat, complete block through the ischemic area is present, and the sequence begins again.

Concealed reentry

Concealed reentry takes place when an impulse makes a circus movement through a loop of depressed fibers but does not reenter and reexcite the heart.[2] The reentrant pathway is thus rendered refractory without the impulse returning to its site of origin and declaring itself on the ECG. Such an event would be noted only because of its effect on the next impulse to invade the same loop.

The term "concealed reentry" was first used in 1950[12] and again in 1955[13] by Langendorf and others, who suggested that impulse propagation could be blocked within the reentrant pathway.

Later Cranefield, Wit, and Hoffman[14] demonstrated concealed reentry in vitro using a depressed loop of canine Purkinje fiber. El-Sherif and co-workers[10] documented concealed reentry in dogs, demonstrating rate-related concealed reentry caused by one of two mechanisms:

1. The reentrant impulse may be entrapped in the normal myocardial tissue bordering the ischemic zone if it leaves the reentrant pathway at the same time that the wave front from the next supraventricular beat reaches the area. This entrapment may occur when the heart rate is such that the conduction time through the reentrant pathway is approximately the same as or exceeds the basic cardiac cycle.
2. The reentrant wave front may never leave the depressed zone if the heart rate exceeds conduction through the reentrant pathway and the normal tissue has already been activated by the time the reentrant wave front is ready to emerge.

Concealed bigeminy

In 1961 and 1963 Schamroth and Marriott[15,16] coined the term "concealed bigeminy" as an explanation for an apparently haphazard distribution of extrasystoles.

Fig. 7-6 is an example of a ventricular bigeminy that may be intermittently latent (concealed). Although the distribution of extrasystoles at first appears to be haphazard, the number of sinus beats intervening between consecutive ectopic beats is always an odd number—1, 3, 5, 7 etc.

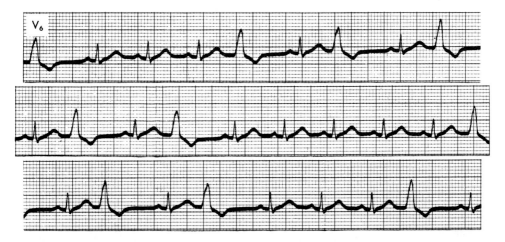

Fig. 7-6. Concealed ventricular bigeminy—a short sample from a much longer strip in which the number of sinus beats intervening between consecutive ectopics is always an odd number. The tendency to bigeminy is apparent in this sample, in which the intervening sinus beats consecutively number 3, 1, 1, 1, 1, 5, 1, 1, 3.

Reentry within the bundle branches and His bundle (macroreentry)

Macroreentry is applicable when the wave front enjoys a wider fascicular sweep (e.g., when both bundle branches and the His bundle are involved in the reentry circuit) or when, in the Wolff-Parkinson-White syndrome (Chapter 10), both the AV junction and the accessory pathway are traversed by the circulating wave.

As a rule, when ventricular tachycardia repeatedly recurs, macroreentry apparently is not the mechanism.[17] However, when it is, it is difficult to differentiate from a supraventricular tachycardia with aberrant ventricular conduction.[17] Even with a His bundle electrogram both tachycardias may have a His bundle spike preceding the QRS complex, and both mechanisms may demonstrate a 1:1 relationship between the atrial and the ventricular deflections.

Fig. 7-7 illustrates the possible pathways of reentry involving both bundle branches, the bundle of His, and the AV node.

In Fig. 7-7, *A*, the coupling interval between the basic and the premature beats is long. Thus conduction proceeds at a normal velocity retrogradely up the bundle branches, bundle of His, and AV node, leaving no opportunity for reentry.

In Fig. 7-7, *B* to *D*, the coupling intervals are shorter, and three possible mechanisms are illustrated for reentry.

In *B* retrograde conduction from the premature ventricular stimulus is initially blocked in the right bundle branch (RBB) but not in the left bundle branch (LBB). By the time the impulse travels slowly up the LBB, the RBB is able to conduct that impulse anterogradely to produce a reciprocal beat.

In *C* the premature ventricular stimulus is blocked in the LBB in both directions. The impulse still travels slowly up the bundle of His and into the node, where it turns around and propagates anterogradely down both bundle branches to produce a reciprocal beat. The resulting complex would, of course, be of normal configuration as long as there were no aberrancy.

In *D* the premature ventricular stimulus is blocked in the retrograde direction in the LBB. It therefore reaches the LBB through its retrograde pathway up the RBB and then descends the LBB to produce a reciprocal beat.

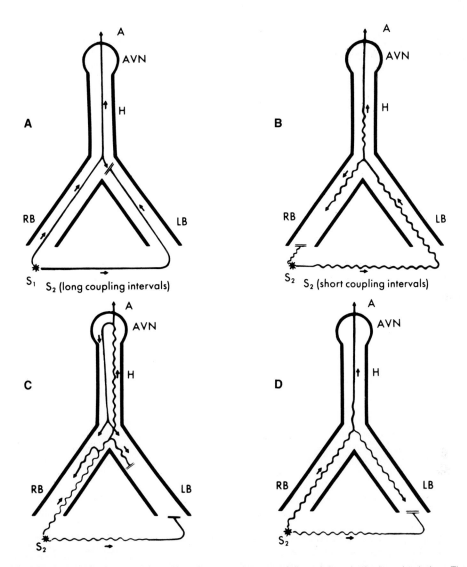

Fig. 7-7. Diagrammatic representation of events that may follow right ventricular stimulation. The possible sites of block and the circuits of reentry are depicted. *AVN*, AV node; *H*, bundle of His; *RB*, right bundle branch system; *LB*, left bundle branch system; *S₁*, basic ventricular drive stimulus; *S₂*, premature ventricular stimulus. (From Akhtar M and others: Circulation 50:1150, 1974.)

Summary

Reentry is undoubtedly one of the common mechanisms of ventricular ectopy. Ventricular tachycardia may be supported by a microreentry loop through Purkinje fibers or by a macroreentry loop involving the bundle branches, His bundle, and ventricular myocardium. Ventricular bigeminy, trigeminy, and quadrigeminy may result from reentry through ischemic myocardial tissue.

REFERENCES

1. Sasyniuk BS and Mendez C: A mechanism for re-entry in canine ventricular tissue, Circ Res 28:3, 1971.
2. Wit AL, Hoffman BJ, and Cranefield PF: Slow conduction and re-entry in the ventricular conducting system. I. Return extrasystole in canine Purkinje fibers, Circ Res 30:1, 1972.
3. Wit AL, Cranefield PF, and Hoffman BF: Slow conduction and re-entry in the ventricular conducting system. II. Single and sustained circus movement in networks of canine and bovine Purkinje fibers, Circ Res 30:11, 1971.
4. Mayer AG: Rhythmical pulsation in scyphomedusae, Carnegie Institution of Washington, Publ No 47, 1906.
5. Schmitt FO and Erlanger J: Directional differences in the conduction of the impulse through heart muscle and their possible relation to extrasystolic and fibrillary contractions, Am J Physiol 87:326, 1928-1929.
6. Mines GR: On dynamic equilibrium in the heart, J Physiol (Lond) 46:349, 1913.
7. Garrey W: Nature of fibrillary contraction of the heart. Its relation to tissue mass and form, Am J Physiol 33:397, 1914.
8. El-Sherif N and others: Re-entrant ventricular arrhythmias in the late myocardial infarction period. 1. Conduction characteristics in the infarction zone, Circulation 55:686, 1977.
9. El-Sherif N, Hope RR, and Scherlag BJ: Re-entrant ventricular arrhythmias in the late myocardial infarction period. 2. Patterns of initiation and termination of re-entry. Circulation 55:702, 1977.
10. El-Sherif N and others: Re-entrant ventricular arrhythmias in the late myocardial infarction period. 3. Manifest and concealed extrasystolic grouping, Circulation 56:225, 1977.
11. Cranefield PF: The conduction of the cardiac impulse, Mt Kisco, NY, 1975, Futura Publishing Co, Inc.
12. Mack I and Langendorf R: Factors influencing the time of appearance of premature systoles (including a demonstration of cases with ventricular premature systoles due to reentry but exhibiting variable coupling), Circulation 1:910, 1950.
13. Langendorf R, Pick A, and Winternitz FM: Mechanisms of intermittent ventricular bigeminy. 1. Appearance of ectopic beats dependent upon length of the ventricular cycle, the "rule of bigeminy," Circulation 11:422, 1955.
14. Cranefield PF, Wit AL, and Hoffman BF: Genesis of cardiac arrhythmias, Circulation 47:190, 1973.
15. Schamroth L and Marriott HJL: Intermittent ventricular parasystole with observations on its relationship to extrasystolic bigeminy, Am J Cardiol 7:799, 1961.
16. Schamroth L and Marriott HJL: Concealed ventricular extrasystoles, Circulation 27:1043, 1963.
17. Akhtar M and others: Reentry within the His-Purkinje system. Elucidation of reentrant circuit using right bundle branch and His bundle recordings, Circulation 58:295, 1978.

CHAPTER 8

SA reentry, block, and sick sinus syndrome

SA node

The SA node is located superficially under the epicardium at the junction between the superior vena cava and the right atrium (Fig. 8-1). It is a crescent-shaped structure of specialized cells with a central body and tapering ends, and it may extend from epicardium to endocardium.

The SA node is the dominant pacemaker of the heart because the maximal diastolic membrane potential is low (-60 mV) and phase 4 is steep. The means by which SA nodal cells depolarize and reach threshold (-30 to -40 mV) is discussed on p. 40.

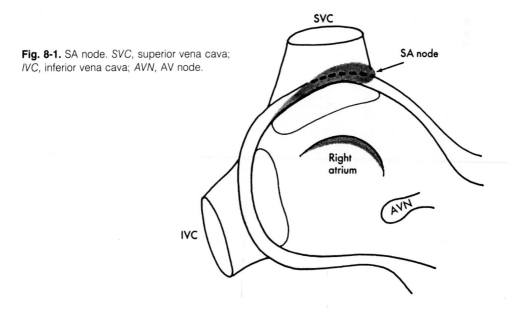

Fig. 8-1. SA node. *SVC*, superior vena cava; *IVC*, inferior vena cava; *AVN*, AV node.

The sinus nodal electrogram has enhanced understanding of sinus nodal automaticity and conduction. Gomes and Winters[1] have found that the sinus node has more than one pacing site within it and that this large reserve capacity for automaticity casts more suspicion on failure of SA conduction as the culprit in so-called "sinus arrest." Their study, involving 24 patients and the use of direct recordings of sinus nodal potentials, suggests that within the SA node itself are dominant and subsidiary pacing sites, which produce sinus P waves of different shapes and cycle lengths. The latent sinus pacemaker site has a longer cycle length than that of the dominant site.

Fig. 8-2 is a gross representation of pacemaker shifts in the human sinus node. Three shapes of sinus P waves result from shifts in pacing sites within the node. The primary site is in the upper portion of the sinus node; two distal sites are illustrated. A shift to the subsidiary sites for one to six beats was noted after atrial stimulation at close coupling intervals in 56% of patients and during carotid sinus massage in 75% of patients. In Gomes and Winters[1] study spontaneous sinus pacemaker shifts were infrequent, suggesting that the so-called "wandering atrial pacemaker," a change in P wave morphology after overdrive pacing, or an early atrial

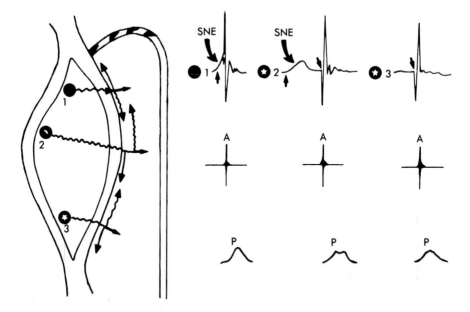

Fig. 8-2. Pacemaker shift to alternate sites within the sinus node results in different morphologies to the sinus node electrogram *(SNE)* and the sinus P wave. Dominant sinus pacemaker originates in the head end of the sinus node (position *1*). *A*, atrial potential; *P*, P wave. (From Gomes JA and Winters SL: J Am Coll Cardiol 9:150, 1987. Reprinted with permission from the American College of Cardiology.)

prematurebeat (APB) may represent a shift to another site within the sinus node rather than an atrial ectopic beat.

Another study,[2] using epicardial mapping on 14 patients at the time of surgery for Wolff-Parkinson-White (WPW) syndrome tachyarrhythmias, found multiple atrial pacemaker regions producing different patterns of global atrial activation and P waves of different shapes. A typical sinus beat originated posteriorly and medial to the sulcus terminalis at the junction between the superior vena cava and the right atria. Most of the patients in this study had more than one pacemaker site.

Perinodal fibers with electrophysiological characteristics distinct from those of atrial muscle and SA nodal cells have been found in the rabbit and are thought to be present in man.[3] Under pathological conditions these fibers may act as a conduction barrier. Conduction velocity in the sinus node and the perinodal zone becomes slower and slower in response to more and more premature atrial extrasystoles, exhibiting behavior comparable to AV nodal tissue.[4] Thus an atrial extrasystole may enter the perinodal zone and conduct slowly through it and the SA node, setting the scene for reentry. It may also rarely happen that the atrial extrasystole is early enough to arrive at the perinodal zone when the zone is in its absolute refractory period. In this case the rhythm of the SA node remains undisturbed and the next sinus beat appears on time, resulting in an interpolated APB.

BLOOD SUPPLY. The blood supply to the SA node is from a large central artery with a rich supply of collateral vessels that are dense toward the center and thinning toward the periphery of the node. The large central SA nodal artery originates from the right coronary artery in 55% of cases and from the circumflex artery in 45% of cases. The disproportionately large size of the SA nodal artery is considered physiologically important[5] in that its perfusion pressure may affect the sinus rate.[6,7] Distention of the artery slows the sinus rate, whereas collapse causes an increase in rate.[4]

Role of the autonomic nervous system in SA nodal function

Parasympathetic and sympathetic influences modify the rate of spontaneous depolarization in the SA node as well as SA conduction time.

Vagal stimulation prolongs SA conduction time[7] and causes sinus slowing,[8-11] an increase in intranodal conduction time, and lengthening of the effective and relative refractory periods of the SA node.[12]

Sympathetic stimulation shortens SA conduction time[4] and causes an increase in the sinus rate because of a steeper phase 4 depolarization.[11,13,14]

TEMPERATURE. Hypothermia inhibits the Na^+ pump, causing an accumulation of intracellular Na^+ and sinus slowing. Hyperthermia increases the sinus rate.

Paroxysmal sinus tachycardia caused by SA nodal reentry

The possibility of reentry through the SA node as a cause of paroxysmal sinus tachycardia was first suggested in 1943[15] and was conclusively documented by elaborate studies in the rabbit heart by Han, Malozzi, and Moe[16] in 1968. Experimental and clinical studies by others[17-27] have provided strong supportive evidence. Narula[21] in 1978 demonstrated SA nodal reentry as the underlying mechanism in 8% of patients with paroxysmal supraventricular tachycardia (PSVT). During programmed electrical stimulation of the heart the incidence ranged from 6% to 9.4% when a single atrial stimulus was introduced during the sinus rhythm.[23,24]

Gomes and others[25] found SA nodal reentry was the mechanism in 16.9% of 65 patients with symptomatic PSVT during a 4-year period. All 11 of these patients had a history of recurrent palpitation; nine had organic heart disease, four had syncope, and two had dizzy spells.

SA NODAL REENTRY MECHANISM. SA nodal reentry may develop without ectopic interference during a sinus rhythm or may be initiated by an APB that arrives at the SA node before it has completely recovered excitability (during its relative refractory period). The premature impulse is then conducted slowly through the node and reemerges to activate the atria in a normal manner. If the impulse then reactivates the incompletely recovered node, travels slowly through it, and again emerges, a reentry circuit is established (Fig. 8-3). Although reentry seems a likely mechanism, it is also possible that such a tachycardia could be caused by triggered activity from cells in the vicinity of the SA node; this is especially likely if there is also 2:1 AV block, ventriculophasic PP intervals, and digitalis is being taken.

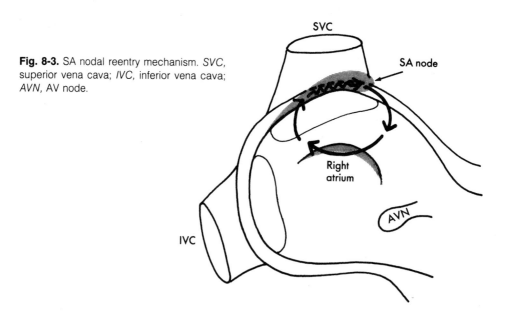

Fig. 8-3. SA nodal reentry mechanism. *SVC,* superior vena cava; *IVC,* inferior vena cava; *AVN,* AV node.

The paroxysmal tachycardia resulting from SA reentry usually has a rate between 100 and 150 beats/min, less than that of an AV reciprocating tachycardia.[22] It may go unnoticed by the patient, although in one study more than half the subjects complained of palpitations.

ECG FEATURES. This arrhythmia consists of what apparently is an inappropriate sinus tachycardia with sudden onset and ending. The P waves are usually similar to, but not always identical with, the sinus P waves and precede rather than follow the QRS complexes.[28] Most attacks do not last longer than 10 to 20 beats[29]; but they are repetitive and sensitive to changes in autonomic tone, including those changes associated with normal breathing,[26] making distinction from sinus arrhythmia sometimes impossible.

Fig. 8-4 is an example of repetitive paroxysmal sinus tachycardia. Most attacks go unnoticed or are only slightly bothersome. Others can cause angina, breathlessness, and syncope, especially when associated with heart disease and sick sinus syndrome.[29]

SA nodal reentry can masquerade as atrial tachycardia with block and sinus arrhythmia, and may even be mistaken for AV nodal reentry, although the P waves resemble sinus P waves. Gomes and others[25] found SA nodal reentry tachycardia to be responsive to intravenous ouabain, verapamil, or amiodarone.

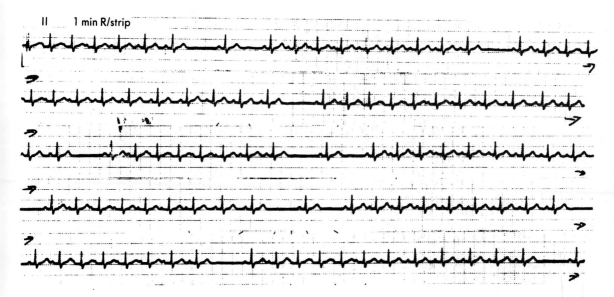

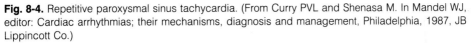

Fig. 8-4. Repetitive paroxysmal sinus tachycardia. (From Curry PVL and Shenasa M. In Mandel WJ, editor: Cardiac arrhythmias; their mechanisms, diagnosis and management, Philadelphia, 1987, JB Lippincott Co.)

SA block

SA block is exit block and occurs during the time between the actual discharge of the SA node and the arrival of the impulse in atrial tissue. The conduction barrier is assumed to be in the perinodal zone, and the block may be first, second, or third degree.

FIRST DEGREE SA BLOCK. First degree SA block is concealed since the actual firing of the SA node is not seen on the surface ECG and since all impulses are conducted at a fixed interval. Uncomplicated first degree SA block in the ECG is indistinguishable from normal sinus rhythm.

SECOND DEGREE SA BLOCK. Second degree SA block may be either type I or type II and is comparable to its second degree AV block counterpart.

Type I. In type I second degree SA block (sinus Wenckebach period) there is progressive lengthening of SA conduction time until finally a sinus beat is not conducted to the atria. Since the sinus discharge is a silent event, this arrhythmia can be inferred only because of a dropped P wave and the effect of the lengthening SA conduction times on the PP intervals. All the signs of AV Wenckebach, except the lengthening PR intervals, are present: (1) group beating, (2) shortening PP intervals, and (3) pauses that are less than twice the shortest cycle.

Fig. 8-5 is an example of SA Wenckebach with a 4:3 conduction ratio. Note the three above-mentioned clues to its diagnosis. The PR intervals are fixed, normal, and constant unless there is also a defect in AV conduction. The group beating is immediately apparent. The PP intervals shorten in classical Wenckebach fashion because the greatest increment in conduction time takes place between the first and the second beat. The pause of the dropped beat is less than two of the basic sinus cycles since conduction out of the SA node is better after the dropped beat than before it. Therefore the lengthened cycle is equal to two sinus cycles minus the conduction decrement out of the SA node. The cycle may be even further shortened if it ends with an escape beat (Fig. 8-6).

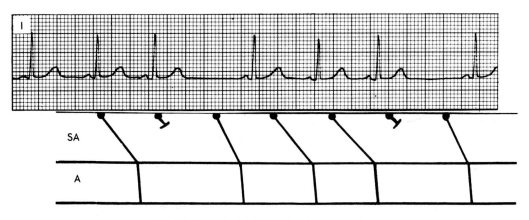

Fig. 8-5. Repeated 4:3 SA Wenckebach periods.

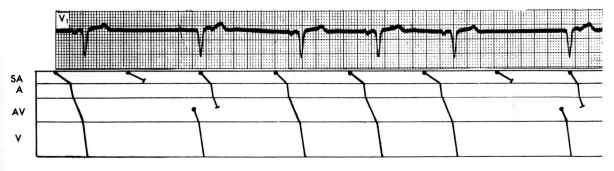

Fig. 8-6. Type I second degree SA block producing a 5:4 Wenckebach period. The two longer cycles of the dropped beats end with junctional escape beats (see laddergram.)

Type II. In type II SA block there are dropped P waves without previous progressive prolongation of conduction times and therefore without progressive shortening of PP intervals. The cycle of the dropped P wave is exactly equal to two of the basic sinus cycles, as illustrated in Fig. 8-7.

Sometimes two or more consecutive sinus impulses are blocked within the SA node, creating considerably longer pauses. In Fig. 8-8, *A*, the first pause equals four sinus cycles, and the second equals three. In Fig. 8-8, *B*, the long pause is interrupted by a junctional escape beat, probably without retrograde penetration of the SA node since the long PP interval equals exactly four sinus cycles, implying an uninterrupted constant SA nodal discharge rate with exit block.

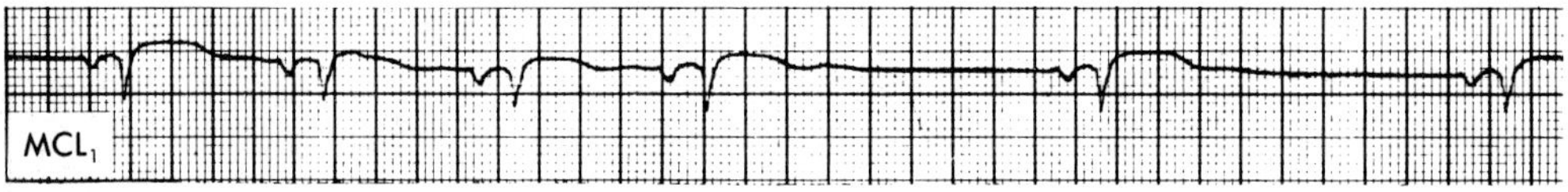

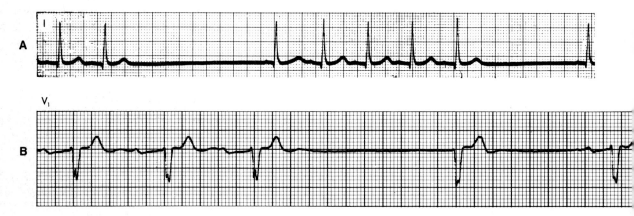

Fig. 8-7. Type II second degree SA block. The longer cycles equal exactly two of the basic sinus cycles.

Fig. 8-8. A, Type II second degree SA block. The first pause equals four sinus cycles (4:1 exit block), and the second pause equals three (3:1 exit block). **B,** Type II second degree SA block with 4:1 exit block. The long pause is interrupted by a junctional escape beat without retrograde conduction to the atria.

THIRD DEGREE SA BLOCK. Third degree SA block is usually compensated by an atrial escape rhythm. With complete block in SA conduction there are no sinus P waves, although the SA node continues to discharge at regular intervals. This cannot be differentiated clinically from sinus arrest, which is a total cessation of impulse formation within the SA node.

Sick sinus syndrome

HISTORY. As early as 1827 Adams,[30] and then Stokes[31] two decades later, described syncopal attacks in patients with permanent bradycardia. In 1954[32] Short presented the diverse clinical picture of SA nodal dysfunction in his classical paper on the syndrome of alternating bradycardia and tachycardia. The catchy alliterative title of *sick sinus syndrome* was coined by Lown[33] in 1967, was later popularized by Ferrer[34,35] and by Rubenstein and others,[36] and was first used to characterize the situation following cardioversion for atrial fibrillation when there was unstable SA activity in the form of sinoatrial arrest or exit block

Since that time many additional terms have been applied when SA nodal dysfunction is coupled with cerebral dysfunction, including "inadequate sinus mechanism," "sluggish sinus syndrome,"[37] "lazy sinus syndrome," and "sinoatrial syncope."[38]

ETIOLOGY. Sick sinus syndrome is usually encountered in the elderly, although it may be seen at any age, even in children and adolescents.[39-42] It is the result of a combination of abnormalities of the SA node itself (automaticity and SA conduction) and interdependence between these intrinsic properties and extrinsic factors such as the integrity of the autonomic nervous system, endocrine system, atrial muscle, and blood supply to the SA node.

Although sick sinus syndrome is most commonly idiopathic, it has been described as drug induced and in association with infiltrative disorders such as coronary atherosclerosis, atrial amyloidosis, diffuse fibrosis, collagen vascular disease, infectious processes, and pericardial disease.

During the acute stage of inferior and lateral wall myocardial infarction, sick sinus syndrome may be seen, especially in the form of profound sinus bradycardia or even sinus arrest.[43-45] It is not known whether it is secondary to ischemia or local edema or is the result of autonomic neural influences.

ECG FEATURES. Some of the ECG manifestations of sick sinus syndrome are as follows:

1. Sinus bradycardia that is persistent, severe, intermittent, or inappropriate
2. Sinus arrest with or without a new pacemaker arising
3. SA block
4. Failure of the sinus rhythm to follow termination of any supraventricular arrhythmia, whether the termination is spontaneous or electrically induced
5. Chronic atrial fibrillation with persistent slow ventricular rate in the absence of bradycrotic drugs
6. Alternating bradycardia and tachycardia (bradycardia-tachycardia syndrome)

Many patients with sick sinus syndrome may also have bundle branch block (BBB) and AV conduction abnormalities in the form of first degree or second degree AV block with prolonged AH interval.[46,47]

Fig. 8-9 illustrates SA nodal dysfunction in the form of the bradycardia-tachycardia syndrome. The first part of the tracing shows atrial fibrillation. When the paroxysm of atrial fibrillation ceases, a long pause ensues before the AV junction escapes.

Bradycardia-tachycardia is a frequent manifestation of the sick sinus syndrome; atrial tachycardia and atrial fibrillation are more frequently observed than atrial flutter. Other rhythms seen are accelerated junctional rhythm and AV nodal reentry tachycardia. These tachycardias terminate spontaneously. The response of the SA node and subsidiary pacemakers to this overdrive suppression is exaggerated, leaving the patient with a long period of asystole or bradycardia that may result in syncope.

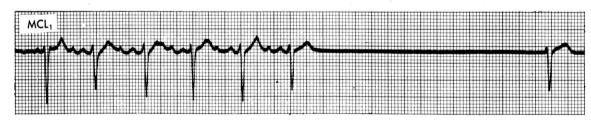

Fig. 8-9. Sick sinus syndrome in the form of bradycardia-tachycardia syndrome.

Fig. 8-10 shows an unusual form of sick sinus syndrome. The top strip portrays a relatively excitable node beating at a rate of approximately 125 beats/min. Yet, within a few seconds, the SA node becomes remarkably depressed and for several seconds perpetrates an irregular but marked bradycardia.

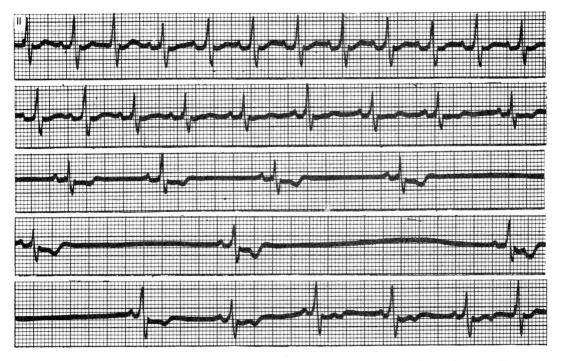

Fig. 8-10. Strips are continuous. Marked variation in rate manifested by a sick sinus node; soon after manifesting an excitable rate of approximately 125 beats/min, it rapidly slows to reach a maximal cycle length of 3 seconds (a rate of 20 beats/min).

Fig. 8-11 illustrates a sick sinus syndrome in the form of marked and inappropriate sinus arrhythmia. The top tracing shows a rather consistent sinus rate of 98 beats/min. Only a few seconds later there is a marked sinus arrhythmia with a cycle of almost 3 seconds in the bottom strip.

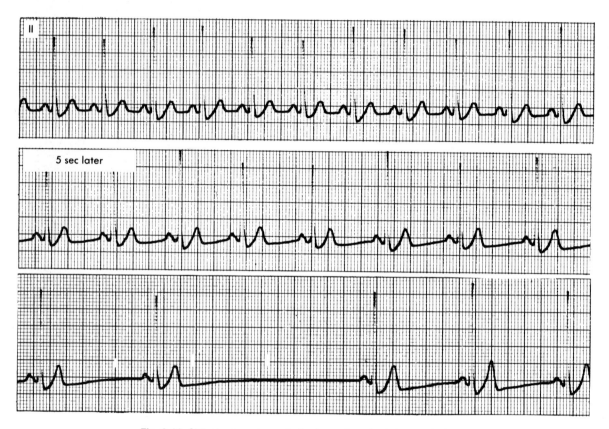

Fig. 8-11. Sick sinus syndrome in the form of marked sinus arrhythmia.

In Fig. 8-12 there is inappropriate overdrive suppression after an atrial premature beat. This patient also had SA Wenckebach and AV Wenckebach compounding the picture of sick sinus syndrome.

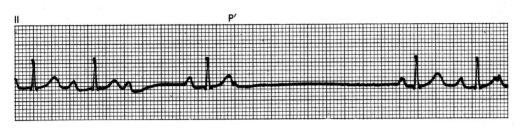

Fig. 8-12. Sick sinus syndrome with inappropriate overdrive suppression after an early atrial premature beat (in the T before the long pause). This patient also had AV and SA Wenckebach periods.

Summary

Arrhythmias originating in the SA node, other than the physiological ones (sinus tachycardia, bradycardia, and sinus arrhythmia), are SA nodal reentry, SA block, and the so-called sick sinus syndrome. SA nodal reentry is one of the mechanisms responsible for paroxysmal supraventricular tachycardia (PSVT), accounting for approximately 8% to 16% of symptomatic PSVT and often associated with organic heart disease. It is recognized because of its abrupt beginnings that are unrelated to respirations, and it is difficult to differentiate from triggered activity in the vicinity of the sinus node. SA block that can be noted on the surface ECG is second degree; in type I (SA Wenckebach) there are shortening PP intervals, pauses that are less than twice the shortest cycle, and group beating. In type II SA block there are dropped P waves without changes in PP intervals. Sick sinus syndrome, the term used with SA nodal dysfunction, is coupled with cerebral dysfunction. It usually involves not only the sinus node but a failure of adequate escape junctional beats as well.

REFERENCES

1. Gomes JA and Winters SL: The origins of the sinus node pacemaker complex in man: demonstration of dominant and subsidiary foci, J Am Coll Cardiol 9:45, 1987.
2. Boineau JP and others: Demonstration of a widely distributed atrial pacemaker complex in the human heart, Circulation 77:1221, 1988.
3. James TN and Nadeau RA: Sinus bradycardia during injections directly into the sinus node artery, Am J Physiol 204:9, 1963.
4. Jordan JL and Mandel WJ: Disorders of sinus function. In Mandel WJ, editor: Cardiac arrhythmias; their mechanisms, diagnosis, and management, Philadelphia, 1980, JB Lippincott Co.
5. James TN: Pulse and impulse formation in the sinus node, Henry Ford Hosp Med J 15:275, 1967.
6. Lang G and others: Effect of stretch on the isolated cat sinoatrial node, Am J Physiol 211:1192, 1966.
7. Brasil A: Autonomic sinoatrial block: a new disturbance of the heart mechanism, Arq Bras Cardiol 8:159, 1955.
8. West TC: Ultramicroelectrode recording from the cardiac pacemaker, J Pharmacol Exp Ther 115:283, 1955.
9. Harris EJ and Hutter OF: The action of acetylcholine on the movements of potassium ions in the sinus venosus of the heart, J Physiol 133:58, 1956.
10. Trautwein W, Kuffler SW, and Edward C: Changes in membrane characteristics of heart muscle during inhibition, J Gen Physiol 40:135, 1956.
11. Musso E and Vassalle M: Inhibitory action of acetylcholine on potassium uptake of the sinus node, Cardiovasc Res 9:490, 1975.
12. Hutter OF and Trautwein W: Vagal and sympathetic effects on the pacemaker fibers in the sinus venosus of the heart, J Gen Physiol 39:715, 1956.
13. Tsien RW: Effects of epinephrine on the pacemaker potassium current of cardiac Purkinje fibers, J Gen Physiol 64:293, 1974.
14. Kassebaum DG: Membrane effects of epinephrine in the heart. In Krays O and Kovarikova A, editors: Second International Pharmacologic meeting. vol 5. Pharmacology of cardiac function, Oxford, 1964, Pergamon Press.
15. Barker PS, Wilson FN, and Johnson FD: The mechanism of auricular paroxysmal tachycardia, Am Heart J 26:435, 1943.
16. Han J, Malozzi AN, and Moe GK: Sinoatrial reciprocation in the isolated rabbit heart, Circ Res 22:355, 1968.
17. Hoffman BF and Cranefield PF: Electrophysiology of the heart, New York, 1960, McGraw-Hill Book Co.
18. Paulay KL, Varghese PI, and Damato AN: Sinus node re-entry: an in vivo demonstration in the dog, Circ Res 32:455, 1973.
19. Coumel P, Attuel P, and Flammang D: The role of the conduction system in supraventricular tachycardias. In Wellens HJJ, Lie KI, and Janse MJ, editors: The conduction system of the heart, Philadelphia, 1976, Lea & Febiger.
20. Narula OS: Sinus node reentry: mechanism of supraventricular tachycardia (SVT) in man, Circ Res 32:455, 1973 (abstract).
21. Narula OS: Sinus node reentry: a mechanism for supraventricular tachycardia, Circulation 50:1114, 1974.
22. Paulay KL, Varghese PJ, and Damato AN: Atrial rhythms in response to an early atrial premature depolarization in man, Am Heart J 85:323, 1973.
23. Wellens HJJ: Role of sinus node re-entry in the genesis of sustained cardiac arrhythmias. In Bonke FIM, editor: The sinus node: structure, function, and clinical relevance, The Hague, 1978, Martinus Nijoff, Publisher.
24. Curry PVL, Evans TR, and Krikler DM: Paroxysmal reciprocating tachycardia, Eur J Cardiol 6:199, 1977.
25. Gomes JA and others: Sustained symptomatic sinus node reentrant tachycardia: incidence, clinical significance, electrophysiologic observations and the effects of antiarrhythmic agents, J Am Coll Cardiol 5:45, 1985.
26. Allessie MA and Bonke FIM: Re-entry within the sino-atrial node as demonstrated by multiple micro-electrode recordings in the isolated rabbit heart. In Bonke FIM, editor: The sinus node: structure, function, and clinical relevance, The Hague, 1978, Martinus Nijoff, Publisher.
27. Narula OS: Paroxysmal supraventricular tachycardia due to sinus node and intra-atrial reentry. In Narula OS, editor: Cardiac arrhythmias, Baltimore, 1979, The Williams & Wilkins Co.

28. Wu D and others: Clinical, electrocardiographic, and electrophysiologic observations in patients with paroxysmal supraventricular tachycardia, Am J Cardiol 41:1045, 1978.

29. Curry PVL and Shenasa M: Atrial arrhythmias: clinical concepts. In Mandel WJ, editor: Cardiac arrhythmias, their mechanisms, diagnosis, and management, Philadelphia, 1980, JB Lippincott Co.

30. Adams R: Cases of disease of the heart, Dublin Hosp Rep 4:353, 1827.

31. Stokes W: Observations on some cases of permanent slow pulse, Dublin J Med Sci 2:73, 1846.

32. Short DS: The syndrome of alternating bradycardia and tachycardia, Br Heart J 16:208, 1954.

33. Lown B: Electrical reversion of cardiac arrhythmias, Br Heart J 29:469, 1967.

34. Ferrer MI: Electrocardiographic notebook, ed 4, Mt Kisco, NY, 1974, Futura Publishing Co, Inc.

35. Ferrer MI: The sick sinus syndrome, Circulation 47:635, 1973.

36. Rubenstein JJ and others: Clinical spectrum of the sick sinus syndrome, Circulation 46:5, 1972.

37. Tabatznik B and others: Syncope in the "sluggish sinus node syndrome" Circulation 40 (suppl. III):200, 1969 (abstract).

38. Easley RM and Goldstein S: Sino-atrial syncope, Am J Cardiol 50:166, 1971.

39. Bharati S and others: The anatomic substrate for the sick sinus syndrome in adolescence, Am J Cardiol 46:163, 1980.

40. Radford DJ and Izukawa T: Sick sinus syndrome: symptomatic cases in children, Arch Dis Child 50:879, 1975.

41. Radford DJ and Izukawa T: Sick sinus syndrome in children, Arch Dis Child 51:100, 1976.

42. Yabeck SM, Swensson RE, and Jarmakani JM: Electrocardiographic recognition of sinus node dysfunction in children and young adults, Circulation 56:235, 1977.

43. Haden RF and others: The significance of sinus bradycardia in acute myocardial infarction, Dis Chest 44:168, 1963.

44. Adgey AJJ and others: Incidence, significance, and management of early bradyarrhythmia complicating acute myocardial infarction, Lancet 2:1097, 1968.

45. Rokseth R and Hattle L: Sinus arrest in acute myocardial infarction, Br Heart J 33:639, 1971.

46. Narula OS, Samet P, and Javier RP: Significance of the sinus node recovery time, Circulation 45:140, 1972.

47. Gupta PK and others: Appraisal of sinus nodal recovery time in patients with sick sinus syndrome, Am J Cardiol 34:265, 1974.

CHAPTER 9

AV nodal reentry

AV nodal reentry (AVNR) is the longitudinal dissociation of the fast and slow pathways within the AV node; when it repeatedly occurs, a reentry circuit develops. This appears to be the most common mechanism of paroxysmal supraventricular tachycardia (reciprocating tachycardia).[1-9] Knowledge of the structure of the AV node and bundle of His facilitates an understanding of the reciprocating mechanism, which in turn offers an approach to management.

Fig. 9-1 is a diagrammatic representation of the AV node and bundle of His. AV nodal tissue, with its special anatomical and electrophysiological characteristics, lends itself to nonuniform conduction.

Dual AV nodal pathways

The circus movement that supports the majority of paroxysmal supraventricular tachycardias is the result of functional longitudinal dissociation—meaning that current flow in parallel pathways within the AV node takes opposite directions.[3-5] Since 1956 two separate pathways through the AV node have been suggested[10-16] and later demonstrated[4,17] as the basis for this dissociation, although it is not known whether these are discrete anatomical pathways or whether the dissociation is purely functional.[18]

The two pathways, diagrammatically illustrated in Fig. 9-2, have different conduction times and different refractory periods. The pathway with slow conduction has a shorter refractory period, whereas the pathway with fast conduction has a longer refractory period.[3,10,12,17] The group of cells in the slow pathway have been called "alpha" cells,[12] and those cells in the fast pathway, "beta" cells.

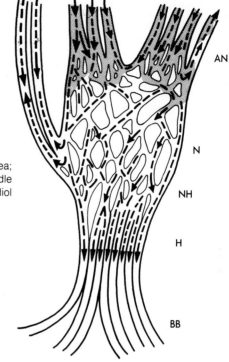

Fig. 9-1. AV junction. *AN,* atrionodal; *N,* nodal area; *NH,* nodal-His; *H,* bundle of His; *BB,* bundle branches. (From Sherf L and James TN: Am J Cardiol 29:529, 1972.)

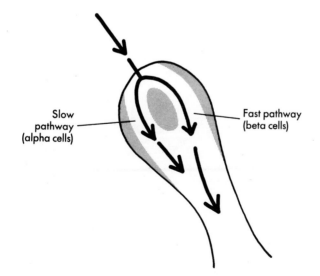

Slow pathway (alpha cells)

Fast pathway (beta cells)

Fig. 9-2. Diagrammatic representation of normal conduction down the slow and the fast pathways within the AV node. The cells of the slow pathway have been designated alpha cells, and those of the fast pathway, beta cells.

Mechanism of AV nodal reentry

Normally both the fast and the slow pathways within the AV node are invaded by the supraventricular impulse,[3-5] which reaches the His bundle first through the fast pathway (see Fig. 9-2). This is the usual sequence following a sinus beat or a relatively late atrial premature beat (APB). However, in the case of an early APB, anterograde conduction may be blocked in the pathway with the longer refractory period (the fast pathway) and be conducted to the ventricles through the pathway with the shorter refractory period (the slow pathway). The PR interval will thus be prolonged because of lengthening of the AH interval, and paroxysmal supraventricular tachycardia (PSVT) may be initiated if anterograde conduction down the slow pathway outlasts the refractory period of the fast pathway[2,3,5,19]; if this situation prevails, the impulse may return to the atria through the previously blocked fast pathway to produce an atrial echo (Fig. 9-3). The round trip may terminate with the atrial echo, failing anterograde transmission down the slow pathway again. However, a continuing circus movement may be established if the impulse returns again down the slow pathway and back up the fast pathway. The circus movement thus produced will result in PSVT (Fig. 9-4), and each time the distal AV node is activated, the impulse proceeds to the ventricles.

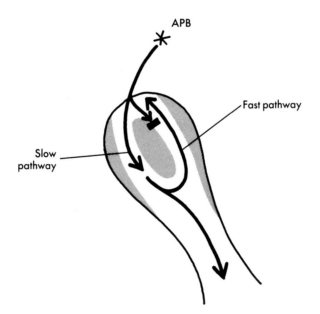

Fig. 9-3. Atrial premature beat *(APB)* may result in anterograde conduction down the slow pathway and retrograde conduction up the fast pathway to produce an atrial echo beat. Retrograde activation of the atria and anterograde activation of the ventricles are usually simultaneous.

Note in Fig. 9-4 that anterograde conduction to the ventricles and retrograde conduction to the atria are simultaneous during AVNR. This simultaneous action is almost always the case and permits differentiation of this usually benign supraventricular arrhythmia from the more threatening one seen in Wolff-Parkinson-White (WPW) syndrome. Because of simultaneous atrial and ventricular activation during AVNR, the P′ wave is buried within the QRS and not seen at all, or it peeks out at the end of the QRS, distorting it. If it shows itself at all, it looks like part of the QRS (an r′ in V_1 or an S in inferior leads; see Fig. 9-6).

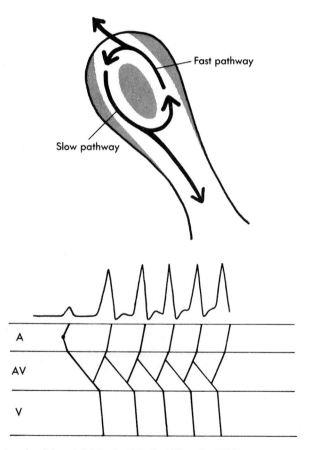

Fig. 9-4. If a reentry circuit is established within the AV node, PSVT results. Laddergram illustrates almost simultaneous activation of upper and lower chambers. Note that the P′ wave is partially hidden within the QRS and resembles an S wave as it peeks out at the end of the QRS.

Studies have shown that the atria may or may not be involved in the reentry circuit.[20] Fig. 9-5 diagrammatically illustrates an AVNR circuit without atrial *or* ventricular activation (concealed conduction). Note that such a circuit, once initiated, is not dependent on the atria or the ventricles for its perpetuation and could conceivably remain concealed to produce what apparently is complete AV block (pseudo-AV block[21]) as long as anterograde activation from the atria or retrograde activation from the ventricles does not interrupt the circuit.

AVNR may be initiated not only by an atrial premature beat but also by a junctional or even a ventricular premature beat (VPB), although when a VPB initiates PSVT, the mechanism usually involves an accessory pathway.[22]

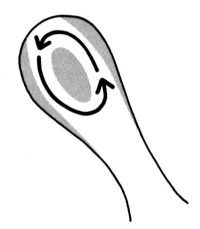

Fig. 9-5. AV nodal reentry without atrial or ventricular involvement.

ECG signs of common type of AVNR tachycardia

The paroxysm of narrow QRS tachycardia in Fig. 9-6 is an example of AVNR. Note the distortion at the end of the QRS during the tachycardia as compared to the sinus rhythm and the long P'R interval that initiates the tachycardia. The following summarizes the ECG of AVNR.[8,23-26]

1. The QRS is narrow.
2. Aberrancy is uncommon (in the AV reentry using an accessory pathway, aberrancy is common).
3. The initiating P'R interval is critically long (see Fig. 9-6), a requirement for the slow arm of the reentry circuit. This length is caused by conduction down the normally slow AV nodal pathway rather than by slow conduction through abnormal tissue.
4. The P' wave during the tachycardia is usually buried within the QRS and not seen at all, or it may be peeking out at the end of the QRS. The surest sign of a peeking P' is an r' wave (actually the P') in V_1 or a terminal s wave in leads II, III, or aVF. The diagnostic ECG features of AVNR are illustrated in Fig. 9-6. Notice that the initiating P'R interval is quite long (0.30 sec), reflecting conduction down the slow internodal pathway, and is necessary to permit the fast pathway time to repolarize so that retrograde conduction is possible; thus the reentry circuit is set up. Note also that the P' wave distorts the QRS during the tachycardia, looking like an s wave in lead II and an r' in lead V_1. When retrograde conduction to the atria fails (the last beat of the tachycardia), these "distortions" disappear.
5. The polarity of the P' wave (when it can be seen) is that of a retrograde P— negative in leads II, III, and aVF and isoelectric in lead I.

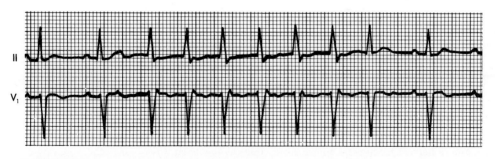

II

V_1

Fig. 9-6. PSVT caused by AV nodal reentry. Compare the ventricular complexes during the tachycardia with those of the sinus rhythm; note how the P' distorts the QRS of the tachycardia. The initiating P'R interval is at least 0.30 sec. (From Conover MB: Understanding electrocardiography, ed 5, St. Louis, 1988, The CV Mosby Co.)

Conduction ratio in AVNR. The conduction ratio is usually 1:1; that is, every time the ventricles are activated so are the atria. However, AVNR with 2:1 AV conduction is a possibility. The block in this case would be below the AV node—in the bundle of His so that with the microreentry circuit intact within the AV node, only every other beat gets through anterogradely at the bundle of His. Fig. 9-7 illustrates just such a case. Note that at the beginning of the tracing when the conduction ratio is 2:1, the P' wave is exactly midway between the two R waves, causing recollection of the Bix rule, which states that when this is the case, suspect a P wave hidden in the QRS. In this tracing, when the conduction ratio converts to 1:1, the first three beats are conducted with left bundle branch block (LBBB) aberration. During 1:1 conduction all P waves are hidden within the QRS.

Uncommon form of AVNR

There are two clinically distinct types of AVNR. The more common form has already been discussed, in which anterograde conduction is down the slow AV nodal pathway and retrograde conduction uses the fast AV nodal pathway, causing the P' waves to be hidden or to peek out just beyond the QRS. In the uncommon form of AVNR, anterograde conduction occurs through the fast AV nodal pathway and retrograde conduction through the slow pathway, not only causing separation of the P' wave from the QRS, but distancing from it as well (RP > PR). This PSVT would be identical in form to the so-called persistent, incessant, or junctional circus movement tachycardia. The differential diagnosis is made because the uncommon AVNR tachycardia would not dominate the patient's life as would incessant circus movement tachycardia, which is discussed in Chapter 10.

Maintenance and interruption of a reentry circuit

In 1908 Mayer[27] accurately described the conditions for reentry in the following words:

This wave will maintain itself indefinitely, provided the circuit be long enough to permit each and every point of the wave to remain at rest for a certain period of time before the return of the wave through the circuit. This single wave going constantly in one direction around the circuit may maintain itself for days traveling at a uniform rate. The circuit must, however, be long enough to allow each point to rest for an appreciable interval of time before the return of the wave. The wave is actually "trapped" in the circuit and must constantly drive onward through the tissue. The point . . . from which the . . . wave first arises is of no more importance in maintaining the rhythmical movement than is any other point on the ring.

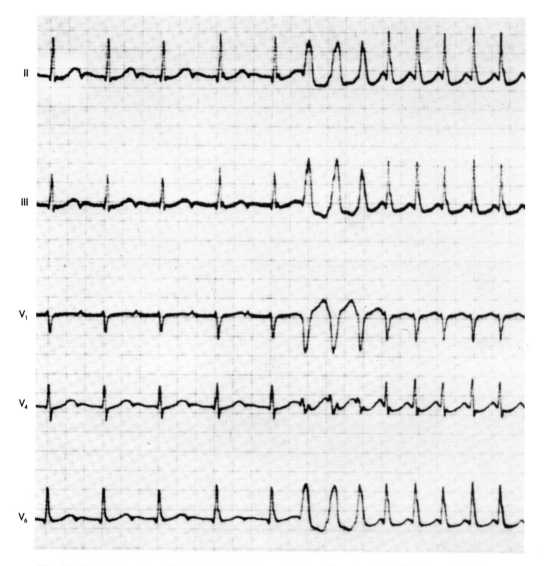

Fig. 9-7. AV nodal reentry with 2:1 and then 1:1 conduction. (Courtesy Hein JJ Wellens, MD, Maastricht, The Netherlands.)

A circus movement is interrupted if a well-timed impulse, natural or artificial, finds the gap between the head and the tail of the circulating wave and produces refractoriness. Fig. 9-8 illustrates how a circulating wave may thus be halted. A temporary pacemaker delivering rapid atrial stimulation is a tailor-made method of terminating any circus movement supraventricular tachycardia.

A vagal maneuver lengthens the refractory period of the AV nodal tissue and may upset the delicate balance between anterograde and retrograde conduction, thus terminating an AVNR mechanism. Pharmacological interventions are aimed at depressing AV nodal conduction and thus interrupting the circuit. Drugs that may depress the anterograde slow pathway include digitalis, propranolol, and verapamil.[19,28-30] However, digitalis is avoided if there is any possibility that the tachycardia owes its existence to an accessory pathway. Digitalis shortens the refractory period of an accessory pathway[31,32] and, if atrial fibrillation should develop, a shortened refractory period in the accessory pathway could lead to a fatally rapid ventricular response. Drugs that may depress the retrograde fast AV nodal pathway include procainamide and quinidine.[33]

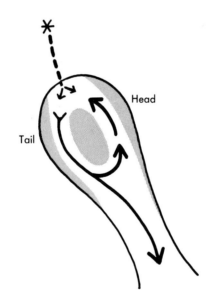

Fig. 9-8. AV nodal reentry circuit may be interrupted by inserting an impulse and producing refractoriness between the head and the tail of the wave front.

Differentiating the reciprocating supraventricular tachycardias

Electrophysiologists have adduced the following clues to help in differentiating the various types of supraventricular tachycardia (SVT):

1. The more common type of AVNR, using the slow pathway anterogradely and the fast pathway retrogradely, results in a P′ wave that usually coincides with the QRS and is therefore not seen at all or distorts the terminal QRS (Fig. 9-9, *A*).

2. An uncommon form of AVNR uses the fast pathway anterogradely and the slow pathway retrogradely, resulting in a P′ wave that is closer to the QRS that follows than it is to the preceding QRS (RP′ > P′R) (see Fig. 9-9, *A*).

3. In circus movement tachycardia using an accessory pathway (Chapter 10) the atria and ventricles are activated in sequence because of the relatively wide physical separation of the anterograde and retrograde pathways. Anterograde conduction is usually through the AV node and bundle of His, which takes longer than retrograde conduction through the rapidly conducting accessory pathway, resulting in P waves that immediately follow the QRS (RP′ < P′R) (Fig. 9-9, *B*).

4. In SA nodal reentry tachycardia P waves tend to precede rather than follow QRS complexes (Fig. 9-9, *C*). Also, conduction to the ventricles is not a necessary link in the maintenance of this reentry circuit as it is with the tachycardia using an accessory pathway.

5. In the so-called incessant, permanent, or persistent form of circus movement tachycardia, in which case there is slow retrograde conduction over an accessory pathway, the RP′ is greater than the P′R. Another feature of this condition is the persistent nature of the PSVT, which does not respond to antiarrhythmic drugs or vagal manuevers.

Reciprocal (echo) beats

AVNR may be an isolated occurrence, producing a single reciprocal or echo beat; a single impulse, having activated either the atria or the ventricles, returns to activate them for a second time. They were called "return extrasystoles" by Scherf and Shookhoff[34] in 1926. The term "reciprocal" was introduced in 1913 by Mines.[35]

Fig. 9-10 diagrammatically illustrates the three main forms of reciprocal beats, depending on their site of origin: the AV junction, the ventricles, or the atria.

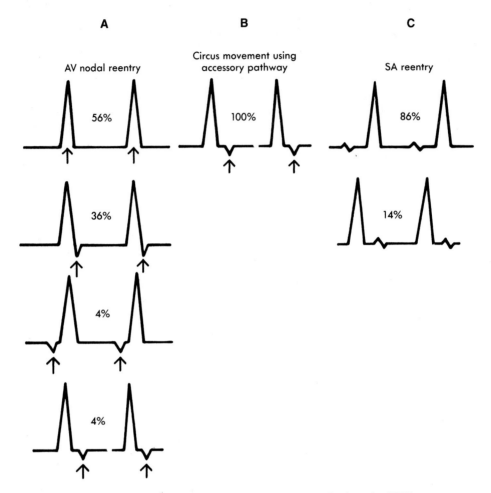

Fig. 9-9. Location of the P wave in the common mechanisms for PSVT.

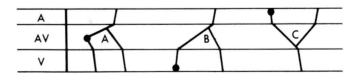

Fig. 9-10. Three forms of reciprocal beating: *A,* junctional rhythm with reciprocal beat; *B,* ventricular ectopic beat with reciprocal beat; *C,* reversed reciprocal beat.

AV JUNCTION (V-A-V SEQUENCE). Usually a reciprocal beat occurs when retrograde conduction to the atria from an ectopic junctional beat is long enough to permit reactivation of the ventricles. Fig. 9-11 is just such a case. The regular ectopic junctional rhythm, not preceded by a sinus P wave, is easy to spot (A, B, and C). Then what catches one's eye is a premature supraventricular beat that resets the junctional rhythm. The retrograde conduction following the junctional beats (A, B, and C) progressively lengthens (retrograde Wenckebach) until finally conduction is slow enough to permit reactivation of the ventricles.

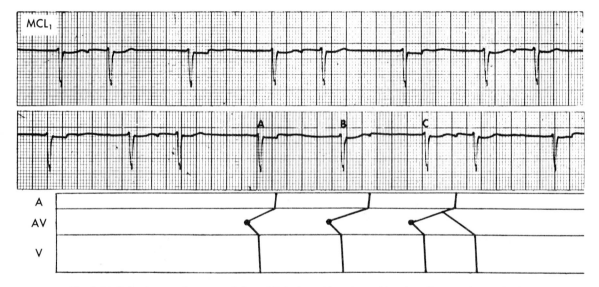

Fig. 9-11. Strips are continuous and show AV rhythm with reciprocal beating. Retrograde conduction is progressively delayed until, when the delay is sufficient, the impulse finds a responsive downward pathway and returns to reactivate the ventricles (see laddergram).

Reciprocal beating is one of the mechanisms that produce allorhythmia (i.e., a repeated arrhythmic sequence). Fig. 9-12 is an example of reciprocal beats producing an allorhythmia of three beats, each trio consisting of two junctional beats followed by a reciprocal beat.

VENTRICLES (V-A-V SEQUENCE). It is possible for a ventricular premature beat to initiate a PSVT. In Fig. 9-13 a ventricular premature beat with slow retrograde conduction to the atria produces a single ventricular echo or reciprocal beat.

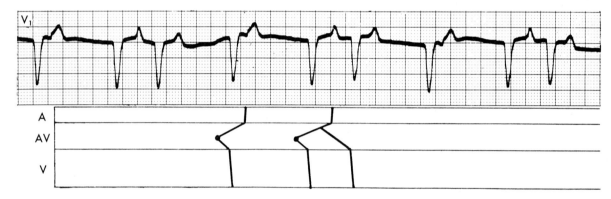

Fig. 9-12. AV rhythm with left bundle branch block and reciprocal beating. The allorhythmia consists of two junctional beats with lengthening retrograde conduction, the second of which is followed by a reciprocal beat. The three-beat sequence then repeats itself.

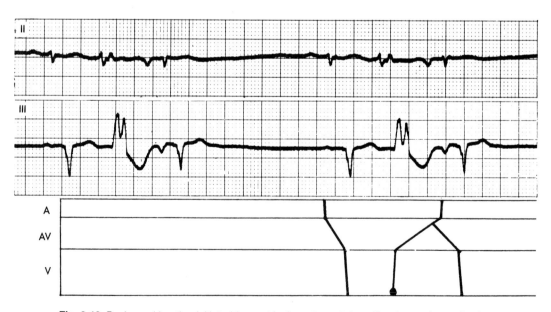

Fig. 9-13. Reciprocal beating initiated by ventricular extrasystoles with retrograde conduction.

Figs. 9-14 and 9-15 are examples of ventricular ectopic rhythms with retrograde Wenckebach conduction and ventricular echoes. In Fig. 9-14 the tracing begins with a run of ventricular tachycardia. Retrograde conduction from the first two beats lengthens until the third finally blocks (3:2 retrograde Wenckebach period). There are two sinus beats before the beginning of the next run of ventricular rhythm, which is interrupted after only two beats by a ventricular echo.

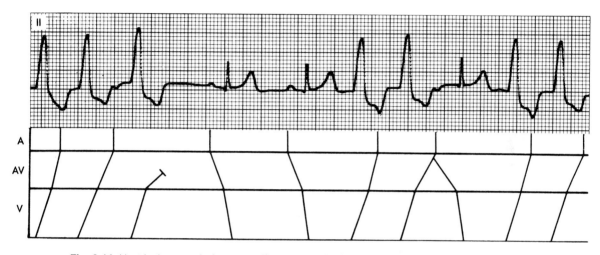

Fig. 9-14. Ventricular ectopic beats manifest retrograde Wenckebach conduction to the atria. The first group of ventricular ectopic beats have lengthening RP′ intervals until, after the third complex, retrograde conduction is blocked. The next group of ventricular ectopic beats also have retrograde Wenckebach conduction, but after the second complex, the impulse returns to the ventricles to produce a ventricular echo. (From Conover MH: Cardiac arrhythmias, ed 2, St. Louis, 1978, The CV Mosby Co.)

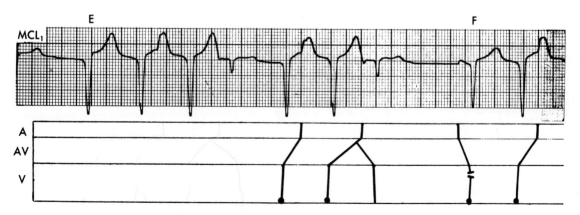

Fig. 9-15. Accelerated idioventricular rhythm with reciprocal beating. Two idioventricular beats are followed by increasingly delayed retroconduction to the atria (see laddergram). The delay following the second beat is sufficient to permit reentry and a reciprocal beat (ventricular echo). The first beats in the first and third groups (*E* and *F*) do not show retroconduction. Beat E does not probably because the sinus P wave is buried within it. Beat F is a fusion beat, with the sinus impulse therefore precluding retrograde conduction.

Fig. 9-15 is an example of accelerated idioventricular rhythm with progressively prolonging retrograde conduction culminating in a ventricular echo. If the retrograde P′ waves are elusive, follow the lines in the A tier of the laddergram—they point at the P waves.

These reciprocal beats do not change the management of these ventricular arrhythmias. They merely alert one to the possibility that a PSVT may develop.

In Figs. 9-16 to 9-18 more complex mechanisms are illustrated. In each tracing there is a ventricular tachycardia with retrograde conduction to the atria. In the first two tracings there is retrograde Wenckebach conduction, and when the RP′ interval is long enough, the impulse returns to the ventricles to produce a ventricular echo that fuses with the next expected ventricular ectopic beat.

In Fig. 9-16 (top tracing) there is ventricular tachycardia with 4:3 retrograde Wenckebach period. Note that the RP′ intervals get longer and longer until the impulse fails to reach the atria. In the bottom strip a laddergram is provided to illustrate a reciprocal beat with fusion. The second retrograde impulse spawns an anterograde impulse to the ventricles that fuses with the next beat of the ventricular tachycardia.

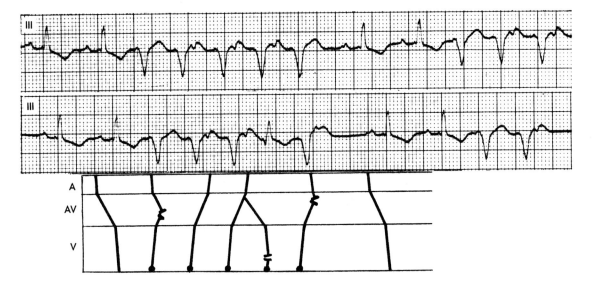

Fig. 9-16. Ventricular tachycardia (rate, 145 beats/min), with retrograde Wenckebach period in the top strip and a reciprocal beat in the lower strip.

In Fig. 9-17 there is a similar sequence. Since the lead is aVR, the retrograde P′ waves are upright. Here the third retrograde impulse turns down to reactivate the ventricles and fuse with the next ectopic impulse of the tachycardia.

In Fig. 9-18 every other beat is a fusion beat. The first ventricular ectopic beat on the tracing has retrograde conduction to the atria; meanwhile the impulse turns around in the AV node to reenter the ventricles just in time to fuse with the next ventricular ectopic beat and prevent its retrograde conduction. The sequence is then repeated again and again, masquerading as electrical alternans.

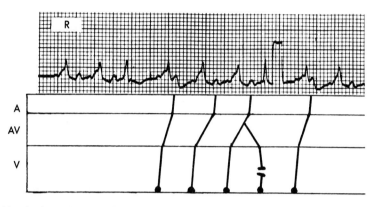

Fig. 9-17. Ventricular tachycardia (rate, 165 beats/min), with retroconduction and reciprocal beating. Five of the ectopic beats are diagrammed, of which the fourth represents fusion between the ectopic impulse and reentry from the third.

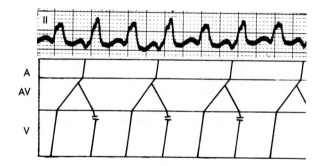

Fig. 9-18. Ventricular tachycardia at a rate of 105 beats/min. Every other beat is a fusion beat between the ectopic ventricular beat and a returning impulse from the preceding ectopic beat (see laddergram).

RP′ INTERVAL IN V-A-V SEQUENCES. In the last eight tracings illustrating V-A-V sequences the retrograde P′ that was followed by the ventricular reciprocal beat ended a long RP′ interval. This interval is usually 0.24 second or longer and may be as long as 0.60 second or more. Occasionally the RP′ is shorter than 0.24 second, and even with an RP′ interval of only 0.12 second, reciprocal beating may be possible. The shorter RPs are more often seen with junctional than with ectopic ventricular rhythms.

At first, it seems surprising that reentry can occur after a short RP interval since delayed conduction is an essential requirement for reentry and the short RP appears to indicate relatively rapid retrograde conduction. One must remember, however, that in AV junctional rhythms the RP interval is not a measure of retrograde conduction alone but represents, rather, the difference between anterograde and retrograde conduction times; thus very slow retrograde conduction, conducive to reentry, can be masked by correspondingly slow anterograde conduction, as illustrated diagrammatically in Fig. 9-19. Impulse b has considerable slowing of retrograde conduction, yet the masking effect of correspondingly slow anterograde conduction produces the same RP′ interval as that of the faster-conducted impulse, a. This masquerade is possible because the junctional discharge is a silent event, not seen on the surface ECG.

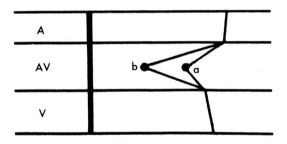

Fig. 9-19. RP interval of junctional beats remains unchanged, provided the difference between retrograde and anterograde conduction remains the same.

ATRIA (A-V-A SEQUENCE). When an atrial impulse is conducted with some delay (prolonged PR) through the AV junction (e.g., at the end of a Wenckebach cycle), it may return to the atria through another pathway to produce an atrial echo.[36,37]

In the top strip of Fig. 9-20 the sinus beats are conducted with PR intervals of 0.22 second, and the QRS complexes are followed closely by retrograde P' waves. In the bottom strip the same mechanism swings into a reciprocating tachycardia. Note the subtle differences between the sinus and the retrograde P waves. They are both diphasic, but as usual in V_1, the sinus diphasicity is $+-$ in contrast to the retrograde $-+$ pattern.

At times it is impossible to differentiate the atrial echo from a nonconducted atrial premature beat. Sometimes the fact that such a beat appears only after lengthening of the PR interval affords the necessary differential clue; for there is no reason why an atrial extrasystole should be dependent on lengthening AV conduction, whereas a measure of conduction delay is clearly a promoter of reentry.[2]

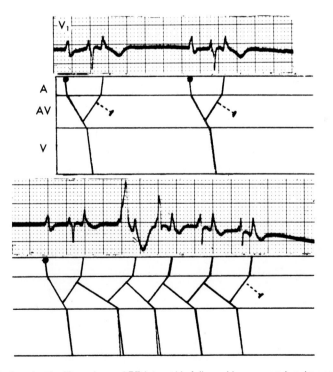

Fig. 9-20. Each sinus beat with prolonged PR interval is followed by reversed reciprocation-retroconduction to the atria, producing an atrial echo. Note that both sinus and retrograde P waves are diphasic. As is usual in V_1, the normal diphasic sinus P is $+-$, and the retrograde P' is $-+$. In the bottom strip, instead of a single atrial echo, a run of reciprocating tachycardia is initiated. (Courtesy Dr. Leo Schamroth, Johannesburg).

Fig. 9-21 illustrates the clue referred to above. In the top strip none of the beats with the shorter PR intervals are followed by an inverted P wave, but the one beat with a lengthened PR interval is. This establishes it as an echo rather than a non-conducted extrasystole. In each of the lower strips the third and last P wave of a 3:2 Wenckebach period is followed by a retrograde P wave without an intervening QRS complex. This undoubtedly represents an atrial echo as diagrammed below the bottom strip. Just as the anterogradely reciprocal beat (ventricular echo) can complete its circuit without activating the atria,[38,39] so the reversed reciprocal beat (atrial echo) can complete its return journey without involving the ventricles.[37,38]

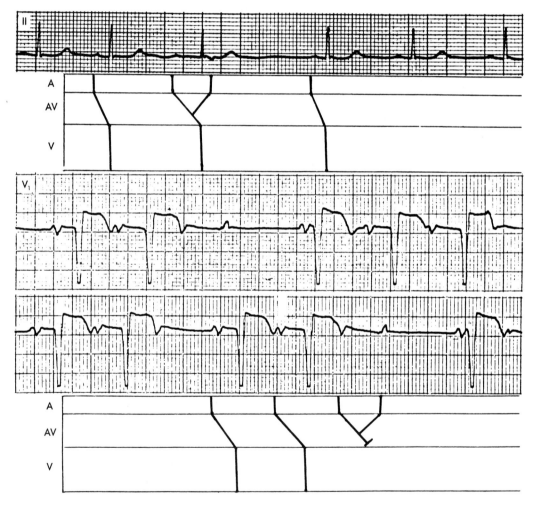

Fig. 9-21. Atrial echoes. Lead II illustrates an atrial echo resulting from lengthening of the preceding PR interval. The strips of V_1 are not continuous: each shows a 3:2 AV Wenckebach period in which the third and last sinus impulse, which fails to reach the ventricles, returns to the atria to produce an echo.

Summary

Because of normally slow conduction through the AV node, it is possible for this structure to support a reentry circuit without AV nodal pathology being present. This is especially true because of the dual pathways within the AV node, one with faster conduction velocity than the other. Because the faster conducting of the two pathways has the longest refractory period, an early APB may be conducted only down the slow pathway, resulting in a long P'R interval and giving the fast pathway time to complete its refractory period. The impulse, while passing anterogradely down the His-Purkinje system, also passes retrogradely up the fast pathway to activate the atria concurrently with ventricular activation. Because of these events, the AVNR circuit is reflected on the surface ECG by a PSVT that begins suddenly with a critically long P'R interval, after which the P' waves are buried within or are peeking out at the end of the QRS.

REFERENCES

1. Bigger JT and Goldreyer BN: The mechanism of supraventricular tachycardia, Circulation 42:673, 1970.
2. Goldreyer BN and Damato AN: The essential role of atrioventricular conduction delay in the initiation of paroxysmal supraventricular tachycardia, Circulation 43:679, 1971.
3. Denes P and others: Demonstration of dual AV nodal pathways in patients with paroxysmal supraventricular tachycardia, Circulation 48:549, 1973.
4. Rosen KM, Mehta A, and Miller RA: Demonstration of dual atrioventricular nodal pathways in man, Am J Cardiol 33:291, 1974.
5. Denes and others: Dual atrioventricular nodal pathways; a common electrophysiological response, Br Heart J 37:1069, 1975.
6. Wu D and others: Determinants of fast- and slow-pathway conduction in patients with dual atrioventricular nodal pathways, Circ Res 36:782, 1975.
7. Touboul P and others: Reciprocal rhythm in patients with normal electrocardiogram: evidence for dual conduction pathways, Am Heart J 91:3, 1976.
8. Sung RJ and others: Initiation of two distinct forms of atrioventricular nodal reentrant tachycardia during programmed ventricular stimulation in man, Am J Cardiol 42:404, 1978.
9. Akhtar M: Paroxysmal atrioventricular nodal reentrant tachycardia. In Narula OS, editor: Cardiac arrhythmias; electrophysiology, diagnosis, and management, Baltimore, 1979, The Williams & Wilkins, Co.
10. Moe GK, Preston JB, and Burlington H: Physiologic evidence for a dual A-V transmission system, Circ Res 4:357, 1956.
11. Mendez C and others: Some characteristics of ventricular echoes, Circ Res 16:562, 1965.
12. Mendez C and Moe GK: Demonstration of a dual A-V nodal conduction system in the isolated rabbit heart, Circ Res 19:378, 1966.
13. Rosenbluth A and Rubio R: Ventricular echoes, Am J Physiol 195:53, 1958.
14. Kistin AD: Multiple pathways of conduction and reciprocal rhythm with interpolated ventricular premature systoles, Am Heart J 65:162, 1963.
15. Watanabe Y and Dreifus LS: Inhomogeneous conduction in the A-V node. A model for reentry, Am Heart J 70:505, 1965.
16. Schuilenburg RM and Durrer D: Ventricular echo beats in the human heart elicited by induced ventricular premature beats, Circulation 40:337, 1969.
17. Wu D and others: Demonstration of dual atrioventricular nodal pathways utilizing a ventricular extrastimulus in patients with atrioventricular nodal re-entrant paroxysmal tachycardia, Circulation 52:789, 1975.
18. Bharati S and others: Congenital abnormalities of the conduction system in two patients with recurrent tachyarrhythmias, Circulation 59:593, 1979.

19. Wu D and others: The effects of propranolol in induction of A-V nodal reentrant paroxysmal tachycardia, Circulation 50:665, 1974.

20. Josephson ME and Kastor JA: Paroxysmal supraventricular tachycardia, Circulation 54:430, 1976.

21. Langendorf R and Pick A: Manifestations of concealed reentry in the atrioventricular junction, Eur J Cardiol 1:11, 1973.

22. Wellens HJJ: How to diagnose difficult arrhythmias, Miami, 1986, Medtronic.

23. Farré J and Wellens HJJ: The value of the electrocardiogram in diagnosing site of origin and mechanism of supraventricular tachycardia. In Wellens HJJ and Kulbertus HE: What's new in electrocardiography, The Hague, 1981, Martinus Nijhoff, Publishers.

24. Sung RJ and Castellanos A: Supraventricular tachycardia: mechanisms and treatment, Cardiovasc Clin 11:27, 1980.

25. Wu D and others: Clinical electrocardiographic and electrophysiologic observations in patients with paroxysmal supraventricular tachycardia, Am J Cardiol 41:1045, 1978.

26. Wellens HJJ: Value and limitations of programmed electrical stimulation of the heart in the study and treatment of tachycardias, Circulation 57:845, 1978.

27. Mayer AG: Rhythmical pulsation in scyphomedusae. II. In Papers from the Tortugas Laboratory of the Carnegie Institution of Washington, Pub no. 102, Part 7, 1908.

28. Wu D and others: The effects of ouabain on induction of atrioventricular nodal reentrant paroxysmal tachycardia, Circulation 52:201, 1975.

29. Wellens HJJ and others: Effect of digitalis in patients with paroxysmal atrioventricular nodal tachycardia, Circulation 52:779, 1975.

30. Wellens HJJ and others: Effect of verapamil studied by programmed electrical stimulation of the heart in patients with paroxysmal reentrant supraventricular tachycardia, Br Heart J 39:1058, 1977.

31. Wellens HJJ, Farré J, and Bar RWH: The WPW syndrome. In Mandel W, editor: Management of difficult arrhythmias, Philadelphia, 1980, JB Lippincott Co.

32. Wellens HJJ and Durrer D: Effect of digitalis on atrioventricular conduction and circus movement tachycardias in patients with Wolff-Parkinson-White syndrome, Circulation 47:1229, 1973.

33. Wu D and others: Effects of procainamide on atrioventricular nodal re-entrant paroxysmal tachycardia, Circulation 57:1171, 1978.

34. Scherf D and Shookhoff C: Experimentelle Untersuchungen über die "Umkehr-Extrasystole," Wien Arch Inn Med 12:501, 1926.

35. Mines GR: On dynamic equilibrium in the heart, J Physiol (Lond) 46:349, 1913.

36. Kistin AD: Atrial reciprocal rhythm, Circulation 32:687, 1965.

37. Pick A: Mechanisms of cardiac arrhythmias: from hypothesis to physiologic fact, Am Heart J 86:249, 1973.

38. Pick A and Langendorf R: Interpretation of complex arrhythmias, Philadelphia, 1979, Lea & Febiger.

39. Bix HH and Marriott HJL: Reciprocal beats masquerading as ventricular captures, Am J Cardiol 4:128, 1959.

CHAPTER 10

Preexcitation and its arrhythmias

Normally, supraventricular impulses gain access to the ventricles through the AV node and bundle of His, with the AV node providing the delay necessary to allow the atrial contribution to the ventricular end diastolic pressure. Some delay in AV conduction is also afforded because the impulse must traverse the entire His-Purkinje system before the ventricles can be activated because the His bundle and bundle branches are isolated from the septal myocardium.[1] A short circuit of this normal delay in AV conduction causes preexcitation.

Wolff-Parkinson-White (WPW) syndrome is the most common type of preexcitation. Since the accessory pathway can be surgically divided and because its arrhythmias can result in ventricular fibrillation, it is important to know how to make the diagnosis both when the condition is overt and when it is not. Many times, a patient who has been suffering for years with "palpitations" gets the first opportunity for a diagnosis when an informed, responsible physician or nurse obtains tracings in multiple leads during the tachycardia.

Terminology

Preexcitation. Activation of the ventricular myocardium earlier than would be expected if the activating impulse had traveled only normally through the AV junction.

Accessory AV connection. A muscular pathway between atrium and ventricle that excludes the conductive system.

Tract. A muscular pathway between atrium and ventricle with one end inserted into conductive tissue.

Delta wave. The slurred onset of the QRS, resulting from preexcitation and causing the QRS to be broad and the PR short.

Wolff-Parkinson-White (WPW) syndrome (overt). Short PR, broad QRS (caused by a delta wave), and a tendency to develop paroxysmal supraventricular tachycardia (PSVT); exists because of an accessory AV connection.

Wolff-Parkinson-White (WPW) syndrome (concealed). Normal PR and QRS, with a tendency to develop PSVT because of an accessory pathway that conducts only in the retrograde direction.

Wolff-Parkinson-White (WPW) syndrome (nonevident). Normal PR and QRS, with a tendency to develop both PSVT and atrial fibrillation with life-threatening ventricular rates caused by an accessory pathway that conducts in both directions.

Lown-Ganong-Levine syndrome. Short PR, normal QRS, and a tendency to develop PSVT[2]; exists because of an accessory atriofascicular connection originally described by Brechenmacher[3] or because of an intranodal bypass tract.

Kent bundle. Histologically specialized tissue anteriorly adjacent to the fibrous ring of the tricuspid valve; term often misassigned to the other AV connections responsible for WPW syndrome.[1]

Wolff-Parkinson-White syndrome

HISTORICAL BACKGROUND. The first examples of preexcitation were published in 1915 by Frank Wilson,[4] followed by Wedd[5] in 1921, Bach[6] in 1929, and Hamburger[7] in 1929, although their examples were not recognized as such. These investigators all thought that the broad QRS complex was atypical bundle branch block, as did Wolff, Parkinson, and White,[8] whose 1930 publication was entitled "Bundle branch block with short PR interval in healthy young people prone to paroxysmal tachycardia." They presented 11 cases without reference to AV bypass connections, although these muscular connections were actually described as early as 1876 by Paladino[9] and in 1893 by Kent,[10] who thought that they were the normal AV conduction pathways.

In 1914, Mines,[11] 30 years ahead of his time, suggested that the "bundles of Kent" provided a reentrant pathway for tachycardias. In 1929 de Boer[12] hypothesized that a circus movement could result from the presence of an anomalous pathway connecting the atria to the ventricles. It was, however, not until 1932[13] and 1933[14] that the concept of AV bypass connections capable of transmitting impulses from atria to ventricles in less than the normal AV conduction time was suggested.

By 1943 and 1944, Wood, Wolferth, and Geckeler[15] and Ohnell[16] had linked the ECG findings of short PR and broad QRS with postmortem histological confirmation of anomalous AV connections on both sides of the heart; theirs were the first demonstrations of the anatomical substrate of the WPW syndrome. The description in this study still applies to almost all left-sided accessory pathways.[1] At approximately the same time the experimental work of Butterworth and Poindexter[17] and the clinical observations of Wolff,[18] Harnischfeger,[19] and Langendorf, Lev, and Pick[20] suggested to clinical investigators that reentry could be the mechanism of the tachycardia of WPW syndrome.

In 1967, Durrer and others[21] used intracardiac electrical stimulation on four patients and applied all of the already known rules for a reentry mechanism to deduce that a circus movement using an accessory AV pathway was the cause of the PSVT common to patients with WPW syndrome.

CLINICAL SIGNIFICANCE. Clearly the clinical significance of WPW syndrome lies in its associated arrhythmias (i.e., the development of regular PSVT and/or atrial fibrillation, which may result in sudden death); atrial flutter is also a possibility, but it occurs less commonly than atrial fibrillation.

The incidence of WPW syndrome is not known, although it has been reported to appear in 0.1 to 3 per 1000 electrocardiograms.[22] The condition is undoubtedly underdiagnosed because it can be intermittent, latent, or concealed or because the examiner fails to recognize (1) the ECG signs of overt WPW syndrome during sinus rhythm, (2) the ECG signs of circus movement tachycardia using an accessory pathway, or (3) atrial fibrillation with conduction over an accessory pathway.

In one study, the incidence of arrhythmias (PSVT and atrial fibrillation) in a series of 265 patients with WPW syndrome was 89%.[22] WPW syndrome is the most important cause of PSVT with a regular rhythm, accounting for 57% of all patients with symptomatic PSVT. In patients in whom the PSVT first occurred before 21 years of age, the incidence of WPW syndrome as the underlying cause was as high as 73%![23]

ANATOMY. In the early stages of development the myocardium of the atria and ventricles is continuous. At the primitive AV junction there is a ring of histologically discrete tissue, which evolves into fibrous tissue and later interrupts the continuity of atrial and ventricular muscle fibers. When the continuity of one or more fibers fails to be divided by the evolving fibrous AV junction, a pathway exists, in addition to the AV node and His bundle, through which an impulse can pass from atria to ventricles. Since these accessory pathways are usually extensions of working myocardium,[1] they conduct faster than the AV node and are often responsible for ventricular preexcitation, although accessory pathways may be present without any preexcitation at all (e.g., latent WPW or concealed accessory pathway) and still provide an arrhythmogenic link. The arrhythmias experienced by patients with accessory pathways may be incapacitating or even life-threatening. Through the years intracardiac studies[21,24-26] and the development and improvement of standard surgical approaches to the severing of accessory AV connections[27] have greatly improved the prognosis for these patients, as has the epicardial approach and cryosurgery.[28] Once diagnosed, these patients have every chance at a normal life, especially if other cardiac abnormalities are absent. The problems arise because the diagnosis is often missed, even in the face of a long history of palpitations and an overt WPW syndrome pattern in sinus rhythm.

It is possible for one or more accessory AV connections to exist anywhere atrial and ventricular myocardial tissues are adjacent to each other. Left lateral pathways account for the most common locations (70%). Three other main locations are right lateral pathways (9%); right and left posteroseptal pathways (20%); and right and left anteroseptal pathways (1%). Fig. 10-1 shows the location of 28 bypass tracts in patients undergoing attempted surgical division.[29]

Fig. 10-2 is a photomicrograph *(A)* and a drawing *(B)* of a left-sided accessory pathway. The location of the majority of such pathways is outside of, but close to, the annulus fibrosus. Thus surgical interruption of a left lateral pathway involves dissection of the epicardial aspect of the AV groove. The location of right-sided ac-

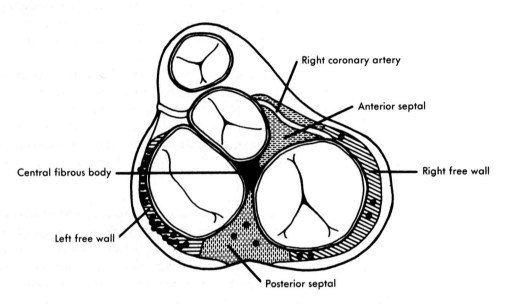

Fig. 10-1. Diagrammatic representation of location of 28 bypass tracts identified preoperatively or intraoperatively. Each black dot represents a bypass tract. (From Kirklin JK and others: Am Heart J 115:445, 1988.)

cessory pathways is not always as straightforward because, owing to the absence of a well-formed tricuspid fibrous ring, it passes directly through the fat that divides the atrial and ventricular muscle. Also, right-sided accessory pathways are frequently associated with Ebstein's malformation and as such may traverse the subendocardial tissues. The most difficult pathways to divide surgically are septal, which bridge the AV ring from the tricuspid to the mitral side and are behind the great vessels.[1]

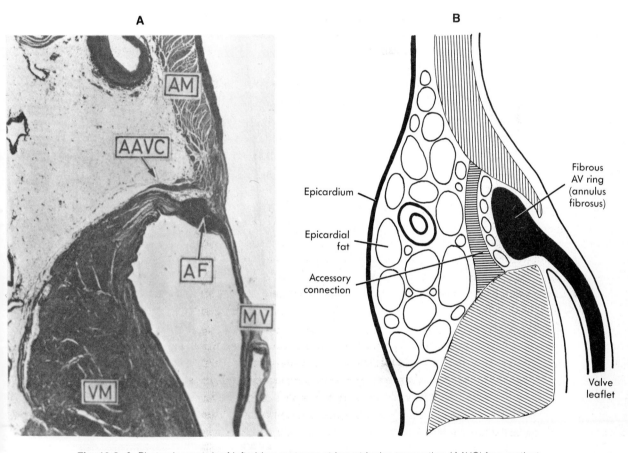

Fig. 10-2. A, Photomicrograph of left-side accessory atrioventricular connection *(AAVC)* from patient with preexcitation, showing its epicardial course relative to the annulus fibrosus *(AF)* of the mitral valve *(MV)*. *AM,* atrial myocardium; *VM,* ventricular myocardium. **B,** Left-sided accessory AV connection. (**A** from Anderson RH, Yen Ho S, and Becker AE: Gross anatomy and microscopy of the conducting system. In Mandel WJ: Cardiac arrhythmias, their mechanisms, diagnosis, and management, ed 2, Philadelphia, 1987, JB Lippincott Co.; **B** from Becker AE and others: Circulation 57:870, 1978. By permission of the American Heart Association, Inc.)

DEGREES OF PREEXCITATION. The degree of preexcitation refers to the amount of ventricular myocardium activated through the accessory pathway. This amount determines the duration of the PR interval and the width of the QRS complex and is itself determined by the following[22]:

1. *Location of the accessory pathway.* The distance between the site of impulse formation in the atria and the atrial insertion of the accessory pathway plays an important role in the degree of preexcitation. The closer the atrial insertion of the accessory pathway is to the sinus node, the sooner the sinus impulse will reach it, and the greater will be the degree of preexcitation. For example, a right-sided accessory pathway provides a greater degree of preexcitation than does a left-sided one if all else is equal; and a patient may have no preexcitation at all during sinus rhythm but may have a considerable degree with a premature atrial stimulus arising close to the accessory pathway.

2. *Intra-atrial conduction times.* The time it takes for the impulse to travel from the sinus node to both the accessory pathway and the AV node influences the degree of preexcitation, especially in the case of left laterally placed accessory pathways in which the distance from the sinus node to the accessory pathway is maximal. This time can be lengthened by atrial pathology and by drugs.

3. *Accessory pathway conduction time.* The length of time necessary for the impulse to transverse the accessory pathway is determined both by the length of the pathway, which may vary from 1 to 10 mm,[30] and by the velocity of conduction.

4. *AV nodal conduction time.* If the intranodal conduction time is short (AH intervals of <60 msec have been reported[22]), normal ventricular activation will occur before the impulse can traverse the accessory pathway, especially in left laterally located ones. The degrees of preexcitation from maximal to zero are illustrated in Fig. 10-3.

Maximal preexcitation. Fig. 10-3, *A*, illustrates the mechanism of maximal preexcitation through a right-sided accessory pathway. The sinus impulse rapidly reaches the nearby accessory pathway, traverses it, and activates the ventricles before the impulse arrives through the normal AV nodal route. In such a case the PR segment is nonexistent (P and delta waves overlap), and the QRS is totally the result of the delta force.

Preexcitation with fusion. Fig. 10-3, *B* and *C*, illustrates the mechanism of fusion beats resulting from right-sided *(B)* and left-sided *(C)* accessory pathways. In such a case the sinus impulse arrives in the ventricles through both the accessory and normal pathways, with the accessory pathway delivering first to produce the short PR, broad QRS, and delta wave.

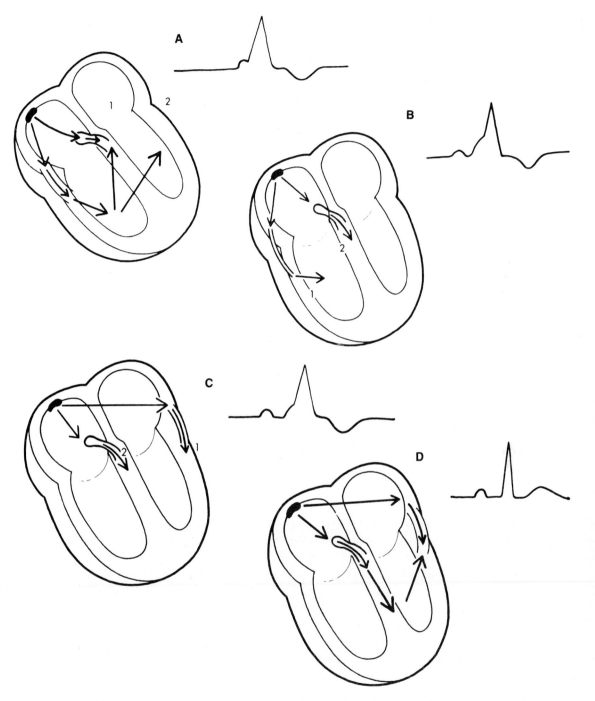

Fig. 10-3. Degrees of preexcitation from maximal to zero. **A,** Maximal preexcitation; ventricles are activated totally by delta force. **B** and **C,** Fusion beats. **D,** Zero preexcitation; impulse does not conduct rapidly enough over accessory pathway and is cancelled by the normally conducted impulse. The sequence of activation is indicated *(1, 2).*

WPW syndrome with zero preexcitation. Fig. 10-3, *D,* illustrates the mechanism of normal PR and normal QRS in the presence of an accessory pathway capable of conducting anterogradely. If a long conduction time from the sinus node to the top of, or across, the accessory pathway equals or exceeds that of the normal nodal-His route, the ECG in sinus rhythm would be perfectly normal (nonevident WPW syndrome). A short AV nodal conduction time would also contribute to nonevident or latent WPW syndrome.

ECG IN OVERT WPW SYNDROME. The classical ECG features of the syndrome originally described by Wolff, Parkinson, and White are seen only in the overt form—short PR, broad QRS, and delta wave. These signs may be intermittent and may require Holter monitoring to be documented.

PR interval. The PR interval is short because the sinus impulse partially avoids its normal delay in the AV node by travelling rapidly down the accessory pathway.

QRS complex. The sequence of intraventricular activation depends on how early the impulse arrives in the ventricles through the accessory pathway. Many factors influence the duration of its journey such as intra-atrial conduction time from the sinus node to the accessory pathway plus conduction time down the accessory pathway as compared with the conduction time from the sinus node to the ventricles through orthodox conduction pathways. Thus the QRS may be generated completely from the currents crossing the accessory pathway with no contribution through the AV node and bundle of His (maximal preexcitation), or the QRS may be the result of forces entering the ventricles through both the accessory pathway and the AV node–bundle of His axis (fusion beats).

Delta wave. Delta wave is the name given to the initial slurring of the QRS complex that results when the impulse first reaches the ventricles through the accessory pathway. The impulse arrives in the ventricles outside the conductive system and is therefore conducted more slowly. It is the delta wave that is responsible for the widening of the QRS (at the expense of the PR interval).

Secondary T wave changes. Because ventricular depolarization is abnormal, repolarization will also be abnormal, causing ST-T changes secondary to the degree and area of preexcitation.

Abnormal Q waves. Q waves are considered abnormal when they have an amplitude 25% of the succeeding R wave and/or a duration of 0.04 second or greater. These Q waves are often seen in the presence of an accessory AV pathway and may be misdiagnosed as myocardial infarction. They are actually negative delta waves, reflecting preexcitation and not myocardial necrosis. In some cases, the delta waves are very subtle. For example, there may be small q waves in the three inferior leads in a young patient with no history of myocardial infarction, but who is suffering from frequent "palpitations" (PSVT).

Fig. 10-4 is an example of overt WPW syndrome. The PR is only approximately 0.08 second when measured in the leads in which the delta wave is earliest. Note that in lead II the PR interval is normal because initial (delta) forces are isoelectric, illustrating the importance of evaluating all leads in the 12-lead ECG. In this patient the initial ventricular forces through the accessory pathway produce negative delta waves in the inferior leads; such a case may be mistaken by the uninformed observer as inferior wall myocardial infarction. Note also the negative delta wave in lead V_1.

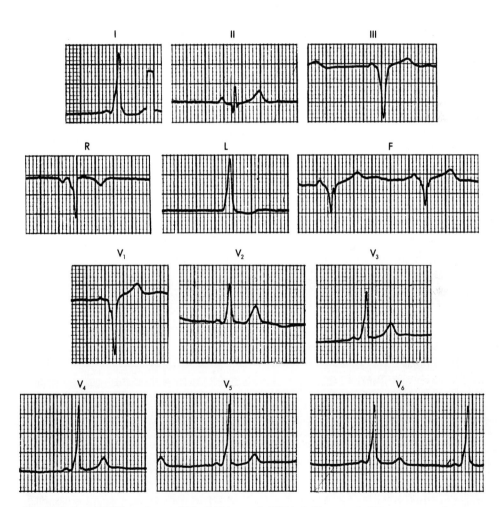

Fig. 10-4. Overt WPW syndrome. PR is 0.08 second; QRS is 0.12 second; delta waves can be seen well in most leads. In inferior leads delta waves are negative, mimicking inferior wall myocardial infarction.

Maximal preexcitation as seen in the ECG is illustrated in Figs. 10-5 and 10-6. In both cases the PR interval is only 0.09 second, and the QRS complex is very broad, with no well-defined ending to the delta wave. Except for the short PR and the broad R waves (>0.03 second) in the right precordial leads, these ECGs resemble left bundle branch block (LBBB).

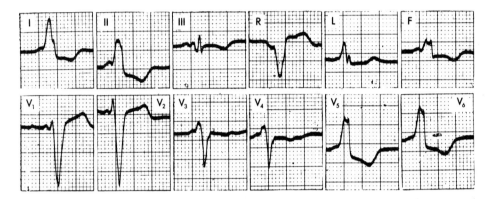

Fig. 10-5. Maximal preexcitation. P and delta waves overlap because of extremely rapid entry of sinus impulse into ventricles. This pattern could well be mistaken for left bundle branch block save for the short PR interval.

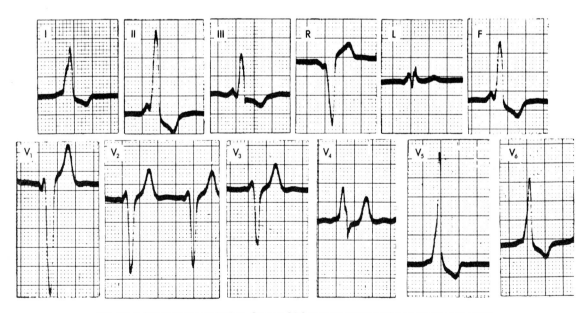

Fig. 10-6. Maximal preexcitation. Overall QRS pattern mimics left bundle branch block.

In Figs. 10-7 and 10-8 the PR intervals are 0.10 second, and the delta waves can be clearly seen in most leads. The QRS in these cases is a fusion complex—a lesser degree of preexcitation than that seen in Figs. 10-5 and 10-6. In Fig. 10-7 the delta wave is not seen in lead aVF because the delta force is perpendicular to the axis of that lead and the delta wave is therefore isoelectric—again illustrating the need to evaluate all 12 leads.

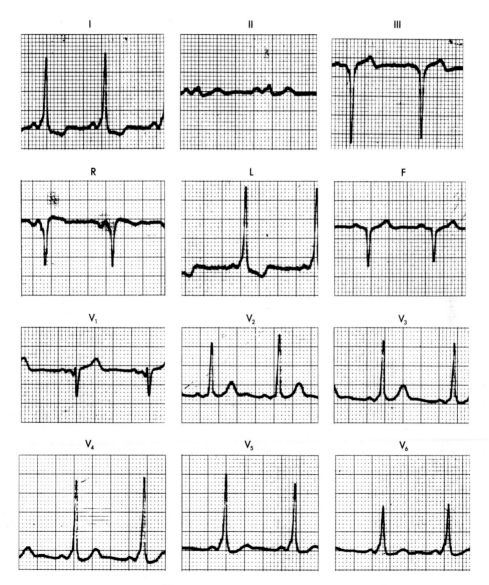

Fig. 10-7. Preexcitation with fusion.

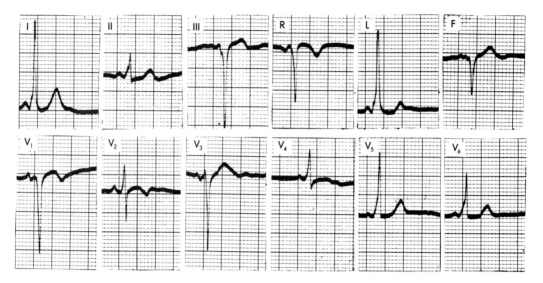

Fig. 10-8. Preexcitation with fusion.

CONCEALED ACCESSORY PATHWAY. The diagnosis of a concealed accessory pathway is made when the 12-lead ECG shows no evidence of preexcitation but electrophysiological studies demonstrate an accessory pathway capable of only retrograde conduction. Preexcitation is absent because only retrograde conduction is possible over the accessory pathway. Such a patient would be protected from the usual life-threatening heart rates experienced in overt or nonevident WPW syndrome should atrial fibrillation develop. However, there may be a history of regular paroxysmal supraventricular tachycardia (PSVT) caused by AV reentry in the form of orthodromic circus movement (anterograde conduction over the AV node and retrograde conduction through the accessory pathway). This condition should not be confused with nonevident WPW syndrome.

NONEVIDENT WPW SYNDROME. The term "nonevident (or latent) WPW syndrome" is actually a misnomer since there is zero preexcitation in control 12-lead ECG tracings; the preexcitation is demonstrated during electrophysiological studies, vagal maneuvers, or administration of calcium channel blockers. AV nodal block may reveal the preexcitation, demonstrating that both anterograde and retrograde conduction are possible through the accessory pathway. Because of one or of the factors listed in the section "Degrees of Preexcitation," the impulse arrives the ventricles through the normal AV nodal–His Purkinje axis before it can read the ventricles through the accessory pathway. This does not necessarily mean tha. such a patient would be protected from life-threatening arrhythmias; all of the arrhythmias associated with overt WPW syndrome are possible. During atrial fibrillation the effective refractory period in the accessory pathway, not the size of the delta wave, determines the ventricular rate. Distinction between nonevident WPW syndrome and a concealed accessory pathway is important because one (concealed WPW) is protected from excessively rapid ventricular rates during atrial fibrillation and the other (nonevident WPW) is not.

Fig. 10-9 is an example of nonevident WPW syndrome. The PR is 0.12 second with the sinus beats but only 0.09 second with an APB because the conduction time from the sinus node to the top of the accessory pathway is longer than from the site of the atrial ectopic focus. Thus the APBs in this case have unmasked a potentially lethal condition.

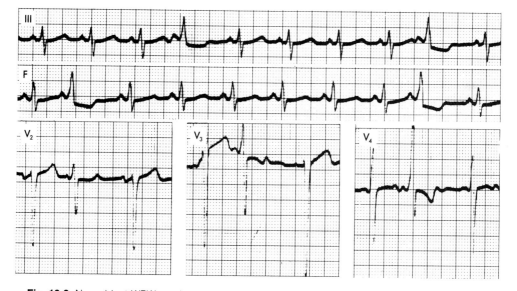

Fig. 10-9. Nonevident WPW syndrome. PR is normal until there is an atrial premature beat, at which time preexcitation is revealed.

CLASSIFICATION. The classification of preexcitation syndromes into either type A or type B has been abandoned for a more updated terminology. In 1945 Rosenbaum and others[31] had based their subdivisions of type A and type B on the QRS morphology in leads V_1, V_2, and V_E (positive electrode placed over the ensiform cartilage). In type A WPW syndrome there is a predominant R wave in these leads; in type B the predominant deflection is an S wave. Updated terminology based on extensive studies from Duke University refers not to type A or B, but to more precise locations—ECG determinations that can be made confidently only with maximal or nearly maximal preexcitation.[32]

LOCATING THE ACCESSORY PATHWAY

By means of the delta wave. In cases of maximal or nearly maximal preexcitation, the ventricular insertion of the accessory pathway can be determined fairly accurately by the polarity of the delta wave; the atrial insertion can be determined by the polarity of the P′ wave during orthodromic circus movement tachycardia (CMT). Fig. 10-10 illustrates some of the possible locations of the accessory pathway as determined by the polarity of the delta wave during sinus rhythm. Fig. 10-11 is an example of maximal preexcitation. Note that the delta wave actually interrupts the P′ wave. Consulting the table in Fig. 10-10, it can be said that there is a left posteroseptal accessory pathway because of the positive delta waves in all of the superior leads and the negative delta waves in all of the inferior leads. In Fig. 10-12 there is a right anteroseptal accessory pathway. Note the positive delta wave in I, aVL, and V_2-V_6.

Difficulties may arise in localizing the accessory pathway because of complicating conditions such as (1) multiple accessory pathways; (2) the presence of heart disease; (3) the distortion of the delta wave with the P wave; and (4) the influence exerted on ventricular activation by the location (endocardial versus epicardial) of the accessory pathway.[26]

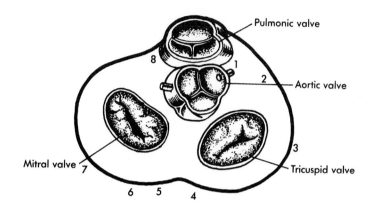

Delta wave polarity

	I	II	III	R	L	F	V₁	V₂	V₃	V₄	V₅	V₆
1	+	+	+	−		+		+	+	+	+	+
2	+	+	−	−	+	−		+	+	+	+	+
3	+		−	−	+			+	+	+	+	+
4	+	−	−	−	+	−		+	+	+	+	+
5	+	−	−	−	+		+	+	+	+	+	+
6	+	+		−		+	+	+	+	+	+	+
7	−		+	−	+	+	+	+	+	+	−	−
8	−	+	+	−	−	+	+	+	+	+	+	+

Fig. 10-10. Locating the accessory pathway from delta wave polarity. (Courtesy HJJ Wellens, MD.)

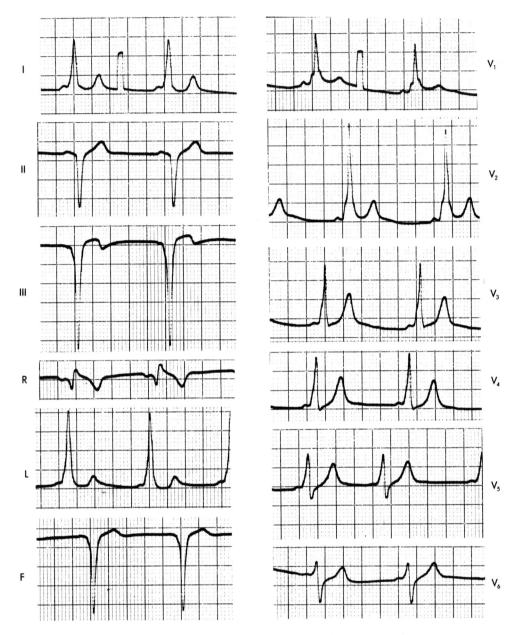

Fig. 10-11. WPW syndrome with a left posteroseptal accessory pathway.

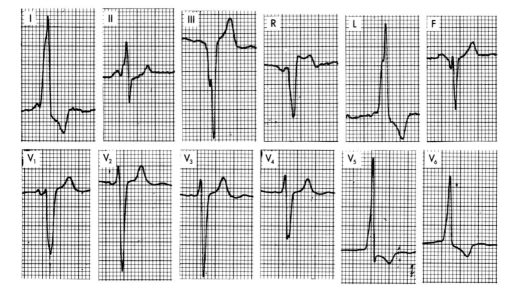

Fig. 10-12. WPW syndrome with a right anteroseptal accessory pathway.

By means of P′ polarity in CMT. In CMT, although retrograde, the P′ waves are not always inverted in the inferior leads. For example, a P′ wave resulting from retrograde conduction through a left ventricular accessory pathway is often negative in lead I. Its polarity in leads II and III depends on whether the left ventricular location is septal, posterior (negative P′), or left lateral (equiphasic or positive P′). CMT using a right ventricular free wall accessory pathway produces a positive or diphasic P′ wave in lead I and negative or diphasic P′ waves in V_1; the P′s may be positive in lead III and positive or equiphasic in lead II. A posteroseptal accessory pathway will produce a P′ wave that is bigger in aVR than in aVL during CMT.[33]

MASKING AND MIMICKING BY WPW SYNDROME. WPW syndrome can both mask or mimic ECG patterns of myocardial infarction, intraventricular block, or ventricular hypertrophy. Delta waves can be negative and resemble abnormal Q waves and myocardial infarction; the broad QRS can suggest bundle branch block (BBB); and the abnormal axis can cause the QRS to be excessively tall, prompting a diagnosis of ventricular hypertrophy.

ARRHYTHMIAS OF WPW SYNDROME. The arrhythmias associated with WPW syndrome are orthodromic CMT, atrial fibrillation, atrial flutter, and antidromic CMT.

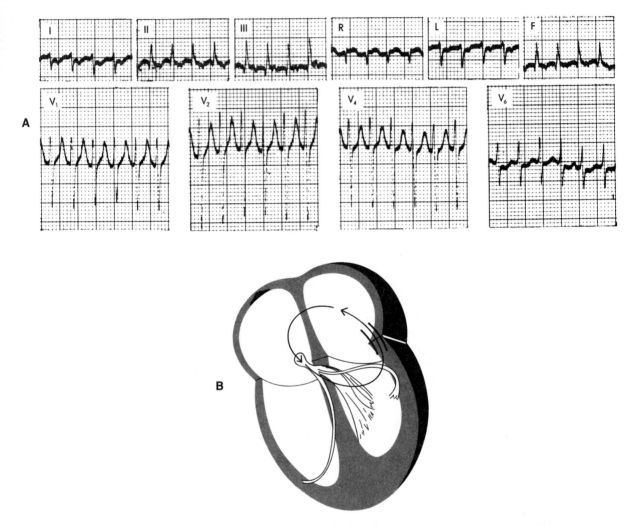

Fig. 10-13. A, Circus movement tachycardia using left-sided accessory pathway (note negative P′ in lead I); patient was 3-weeks-old. **B,** Mechanism of the tachycardia. Conduction is down AV node and up left-sided accessory pathway.

ORTHODROMIC CIRCUS MOVEMENT TACHYCARDIA. Orthodromic CMT is a regular PSVT caused by an AV reentry mechanism using the AV node in the anterograde direction (narrow QRS) and the accessory pathway in the retrograde direction. Fig. 10-13 demonstrates the mechanism of the most common arrhythmia experienced by patients with WPW syndrome—PSVT resulting from AV conduction through the AV node and VA conduction through the accessory pathway. This arrhythmia can be initiated by either an atrial premature beat (APB) or a ventricular premature beat (VPB). An APB that is blocked in the accessory pathway can travel (1) down the AV node and His-Purkinje system to activate the ventricles, (2) up the accessory pathway to activate the atria, and then (3) down the AV node again. A VPB that travels retrogradely up the accessory pathway to the atria can then go down the AV node to the ventricles, and so the circuit begins and is sustained. This circuit is repeated to produce a regular PSVT with a narrow QRS complex. Fig. 10-13 is an ECG from a 3-week-old baby; the sinus rhythm is shown in Fig. 10-14. During the tachycardia note that the P′ waves can easily be seen separate from the QRS. Note the negative P′ wave in the ST segment of leads I and aVL.

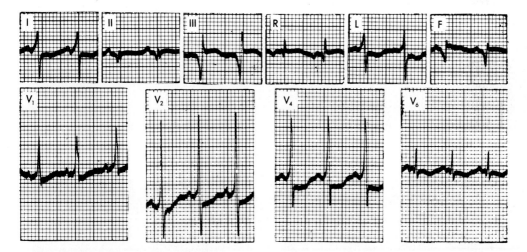

Fig. 10-14. Sinus rhythm from patient in Fig. 10-13. Note the marked delta waves (positive in leads I, aVL, and precordial leads; negative in the inferior leads).

DIFFERENTIAL DIAGNOSIS IN PSVT. The distinction between PSVT caused by orthodromic circus movement using an accessory pathway and that caused by AV nodal reentry can be made from the surface ECG mainly by observing the position of the P′ waves relative to the QRS and by looking for the presence of QRS alternans. These and other clues are listed below.

Position of the P′ waves. When an accessory pathway forms the retrograde arm of the tachycardia circuit, the P′ wave is always separate from the QRS, whereas in AV nodal reentry the P′ wave is usually buried within or peeking out at the end of the QRS complex (see Chapter 9). Fig. 10-15 illustrates two cases of PSVT. In Fig. 10-15, *A*, AV nodal reentry, note that the P′ wave is peeking out at the end of the QRS during the tachycardia, looking like an r′ wave in V₁ and an s wave in lead II. This distortion is more easily noted when the QRS of the tachycardia is compared with that of the sinus rhythm. In Fig. 10-15, *B*, CMT, the P′ waves are clearly sep-

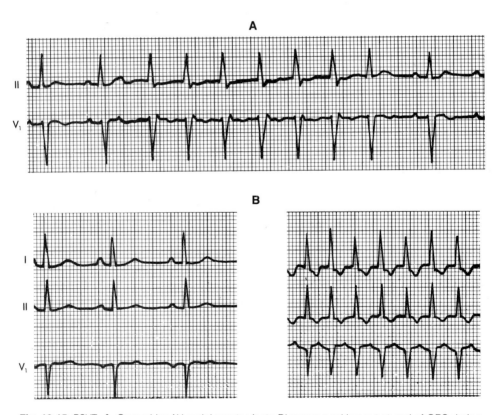

Fig. 10-15. PSVT. **A,** Caused by AV nodal reentry (note P′ waves peeking out at end of QRS during the tachycardia). **B,** Caused by AV reentry using accessory pathway (note P′ waves separate from QRS during the tachycardia). (From Conover M: Understanding electrocardiography, ed 5, St. Louis, 1988, The CV Mosby Co.)

arate from the QRS. They can be seen distorting the ST segment, especially when compared to the ST of the sinus rhythm.

QRS alternans. QRS alternans during narrow QRS tachycardia has a high degree of specificity (96%) for orthodromic CMT and is therefore helpful in differentiating this type of tachycardia from other types.[34,35] QRS alternans occurs in approximately 30% of CMTs and is rare in AV nodal reentry; look for it after the first 10 seconds of the tachycardia because it can occur before then in both mechanisms (CMT and AVNR).

The initiating P′R interval. The P′R interval of the APB that initiates the CMT is not as prolonged as it is in AV nodal reentry. In Fig. 10-15, *A*, note that the initiating P′R interval (P′ is in the second T wave) is long; a critical length is needed to initiate the AV nodal reentry mechanism, whereas in CMT, since the initiating impulse uses both AV nodal pathways (fast and slow), it is only the timing during the cycle that is critical. To initiate CMT the impulse must be blocked in one pathway (usually the accessory pathway) and not the other (AV node).

Aberrant ventricular conduction. Ventricular aberration is more common in CMT than it is in AV nodal reentry. Also, if the aberration is on the same side as the accessory pathway, the rate is often slower during aberrant ventricular conduction when compared to the tachycardia without aberration. This finding is not only diagnostic of CMT, but it also often identifies the accessory pathway as right-sided or left-sided. For example, slowing of the rate during CMT because of a right bundle branch block (RBBB) aberration indicates a right-sided accessory pathway; slowing because of a LBBB aberration indicates a left-sided accessory pathway. If the aberration is on one side and the accessory pathway on the other, there will be no slowing during aberration. This mechanism is illustrated in Fig. 10-16.

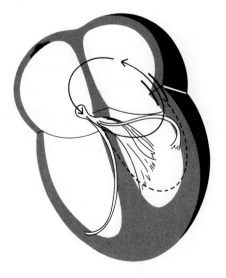

Fig. 10-16. When aberrant ventricular conduction occurs during CMT, if accessory pathway is on the same side as BBB, the longer circuit required to negotiate the functional BBB *(dotted line)* causes rate of the tachycardia to be slightly slower than it is without the aberration *(solid line)*. (From Conover MB: Understanding electrocardiography, ed 5, St. Louis, 1988, The CV Mosby Co.)

Rate of the tachycardia. A narrow QRS tachycardia with a rate in excess of 200 beats/min is suggestive of CMT.

AV block. AV block rules out CMT. When AV block is present, the atrial rate helps to make the differential diagnosis; rates of more than 250 beats/min suggest atrial flutter, and rates of less than that suggest atrial tachycardia. AV nodal reentry with 2:1 block below the AV node is rare, but it is a possibility.

P' wave axis. A frontal plane P' wave axis that is superior to inferior rules out both AV nodal reentry and CMT and indicates atrial tachycardia (often caused by digitalis toxicity). A frontal plane P' wave axis that is inferior to superior could be the result of either AV nodal reentry or CMT. On the horizontal plane, a right-to-left P' wave axis rules out AV nodal reentry, but it could be either atrial tachycardia or CMT; a left-to-right axis could be anything (CMT, AV nodal reentry, or left atrial tachycardia).

PERSISTENT CIRCUS MOVEMENT TACHYCARDIA. In the more common form of orthodromic CMT, conduction up the accessory pathway is fast, causing the RP' interval to be shorter than the P'R interval (RP' < P'R). In a very rare form of orthodromic CMT, the opposite is true (RP > P'R) because conduction up the accessary pathway is slow. This type of orthodromic CMT is commonly of a persistent (often called "incessant" or "permanent") nature and is illustrated in Fig. 10-17; it can be completely cured by surgery. If a diagnosis is not made and surgery is not performed, these patients suffer most of their lives, being in tachycardia more than in sinus rhythm; atrial damage and congestive heart failure are results.

Such an accessory pathway is usually posteroseptally located. It is thought to be AV nodal–like tissue, thus atropine, isuprel, and exercise all cause faster conduction.

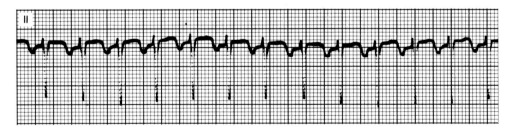

Fig. 10-17. Persistent CMT. Note that RP' is greater than P'R.

ANTIDROMIC CIRCUS MOVEMENT TACHYCARDIA. Antidromic CMT is a regular PSVT caused by an AV reentry mechanism using the AV node in a retrograde direction and the accessory pathway in an anterograde direction (broad QRS). This tachycardia is a much less common mechanism than orthodromic CMT and is impossible to distinguish from ventricular tachycardia on the surface ECG (Fig. 10-18). A similar pattern may be produced when there are two accessory pathways with anterograde conduction through one pathway and retrograde conduction through the other.[32,36,37]

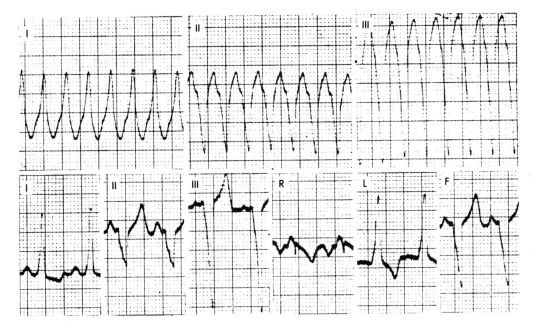

Fig. 10-18. Antidromic CMT. Conduction is down accessory pathway and up AV node, causing ventricular complexes to look identical to those of ventricular tachycardia.

Fig. 10-19 illustrates common potential for reentrant tachycardia caused by retrograde conduction into the accessory pathway after ventricular extrasystoles (in this case, interpolated). Most of the sinus beats have short PR intervals, prolonged QRS durations, and delta waves. However, the ventricular complexes after the extrasystoles are narrow and normally conducted, presumably because of concealed retrograde conduction from the extrasystole into the accessory pathway.

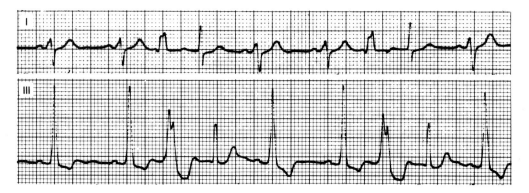

Fig. 10-19. Except for those beats that follow interpolated ventricular extrasystoles, sinus beats all have short PR intervals with delta waves. Those beats that follow extrasystoles are narrow and normally conducted, presumably because of concealed retrograde conduction from extrasystole into accessory pathway.

ATRIAL FIBRILLATION IN WPW SYNDROME. Atrial fibrillation is a fairly common arrhythmia in patients with WPW syndrome, being found in 18% of a series of 265 patients.[22] If conduction during atrial fibrillation occurs exclusively through an accessory pathway with a short refractory period, the ventricular rates can be very high (160 to 300 beats/min), and the rhythm can degenerate into ventricular fibrillation.[38,39] It is claimed that when RR intervals during atrial fibrillation are equal to or less than 205 msec, the atrial fibrillation is likely to degenerate into ventricular fibrillation.[39]

Figs. 10-20 and 10-21 illustrate the tachycardia that develops as a result of atrial fibrillation and an accessory pathway. The shortest RR intervals are 0.16 and 0.18 second, prime candidates for the development of ventricular fibrillation.

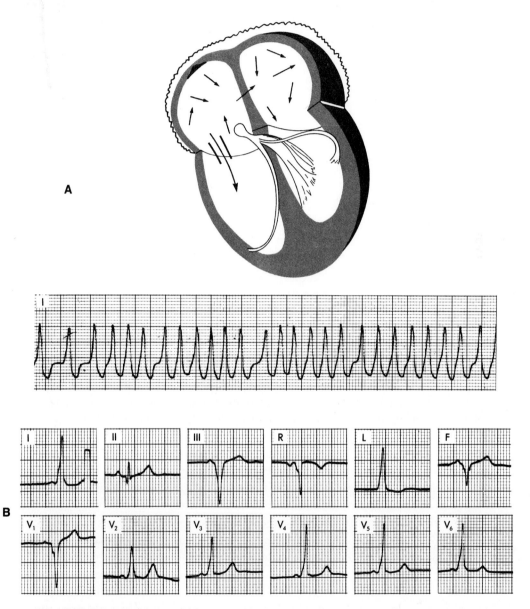

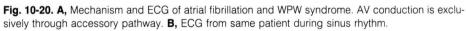

Fig. 10-20. A, Mechanism and ECG of atrial fibrillation and WPW syndrome. AV conduction is exclusively through accessory pathway. **B,** ECG from same patient during sinus rhythm.

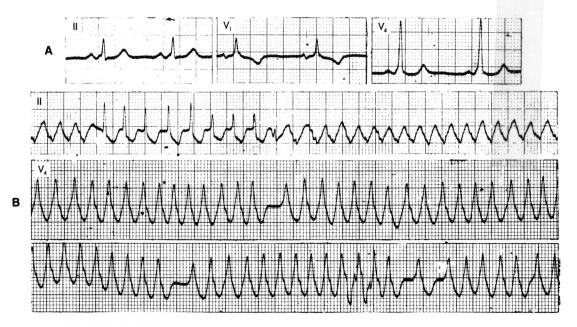

Fig. 10-21. A, WPW syndrome. **B,** Same patient during atrial fibrillation, with conduction exclusively through accessory pathway.

Fig. 10-21, *A,* shows a typical preexcitation pattern during sinus rhythm. In Fig. 10-21, *B,* the patient is in atrial fibrillation, with a ventricular response of 280 beats/min. Several beats in the first half of lead II are evidently conducted through normal pathways at a somewhat slower rate. Note the maximal preexcitation in the remaining complexes and the irregularity of the rhythm caused by the atrial fibrillation. This irregularity is often in a pattern of rapid rates alternating with slower rates. This pattern is thought to be caused by the rapid rates' shortening the refractory period in the accessory pathway and in the ventricular muscle.[26]

Fig. 10-22, *A,* is a sinus rhythm from an 18-year-old man. The signs of preexcitation are very subtle and difficult to identify with certainty; there are abnormal Q waves in the inferior leads and very small delta waves in leads I, V_3, and V_4. In spite of the essentially normal 12-lead ECG, this young man had an accessory pathway with a short effective refractory period, permitting rapid rates during atrial fibrillation. His admission tracing is seen in Fig. 10-22, *B.* As is often the case, the diagnosis was made during his arrhythmia, not during the sinus rhythm.

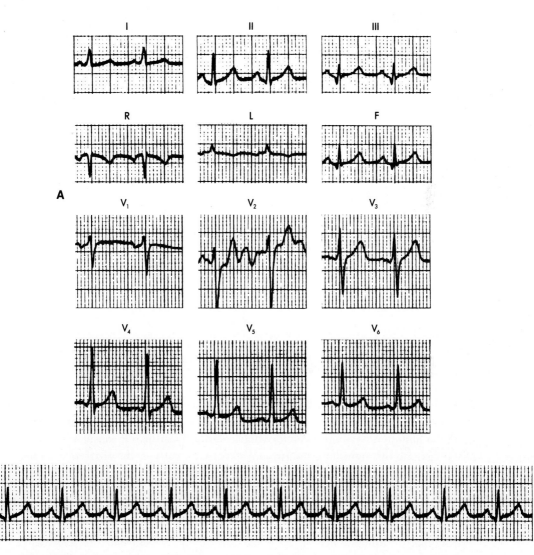

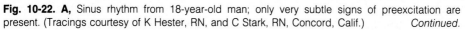

Fig. 10-22. A, Sinus rhythm from 18-year-old man; only very subtle signs of preexcitation are present. (Tracings courtesy of K Hester, RN, and C Stark, RN, Concord, Calif.)   *Continued.*

B

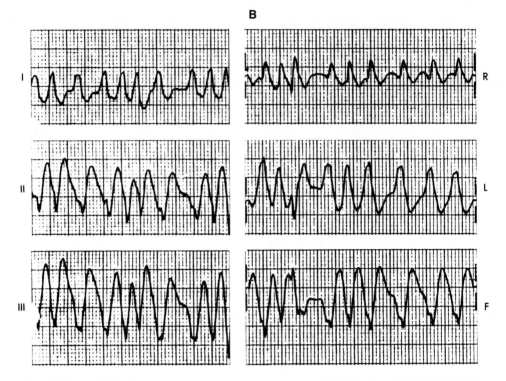

Fig. 10-22, cont'd. B, Admission tracings clearly show signs of atrial fibrillation and WPW syndrome.

DIFFERENTIAL DIAGNOSIS IN IRREGULAR WIDE QRS TACHYCARDIA. Because of maximal preexcitation during atrial fibrillation with an accessory pathway, this arrhythmia has often been mistaken for ventricular tachycardia. Of considerable diagnostic value in distinguishing the two are the clinical setting, the rhythm and rate, and the QRS morphology.

Clinical setting. If the victim is a septuagenarian in a coronary care unit, the arrhythmia is probably ventricular tachycardia; on the other hand, if he is a 22-year-old man in the emergency room, it is more likely preexcitation.

Rhythm. In the large majority of cases, the rhythm of ventricular tachycardia is perfectly regular,[40] whereas in atrial fibrillation and WPW syndrome, the rhythm is irregular; runs of very short cycles often alternate with runs of longer cycles. The longest cycle length is often more than twice the length of the shortest cycle; that is, variation is greater than 100%.

Rate. It is possible for ventricular tachycardia to achieve rates of more than 300 beats/min. However, in the presence of any rate much greater than 200 beats/min, a broad QRS, and an irregular rhythm, an accessory pathway must be suspected and ruled out.

QRS morphology. QRS morphology is identical to that of ventricular tachycardia (see Chapter 12) because the entry of the supraventricular impulse into the ventricles is through the accessory pathway, i.e., outside of the conduction system.

Lown-Ganong-Levine syndrome

In 1952 Lown, Ganong, and Levine[2] reported the syndrome of "short PR interval, normal QRS complex, and paroxysmal rapid heart action," which later became known as the Lown-Ganong-Levine (LGL) syndrome. Many favor the abandonment of this term for the more descriptive "short-PR–normal-QRS syndrome."[41,42] Fig. 10-23 illustrates this syndrome.

The anatomical substrate can be an intranodal bypass tract or an atriofascicular connection,[1] that is, fibers that insert directly through the fibrous AV ring into the penetrating bundle of His.[4] Of interest is the fact that the incidence of short PR intervals and of long PR intervals is exactly the same (1.3%) in a healthy young population, suggesting that neither is necessarily abnormal, but this incidence may represent the extremities of the bell curve of normal PR intervals.[43]

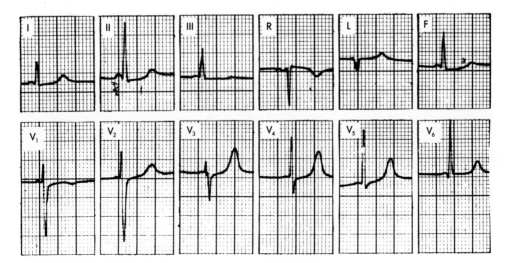

Fig. 10-23. Lown-Ganong-Levine sydrome.

Mahaim fibers

Mahaim and colleagues[44-46] first described anomalous conduction pathways connecting the AV node or His-Purkinje system to the ventricle. Mahaim fibers can connect a fascicle with the ventricle or the atria with a fascicle. These fibers, along with nodoventricular fibers, are illustrated in Fig. 10-24. The existence of nodoventricular fibers has recently come into question.[47] Electrophysiological studies[47] and observations during surgical resection[48-50] indicate that many of these pathways may actually represent atriofascicular or atrioventricular connections with decremental conduction. A nodofascicular Mahaim fiber is also thought a possibility.[51]

The ECG during sinus rhythm depends on the location and length of the fiber. The expected pattern has a small delta wave, which increases the QRS width less than in WPW syndrome; for the same reason the PR is not so short. Preexcitation due to Mahaim fibers is, however, indistinguishable from minimal preexcitation through an accessory AV pathway. Mahaim fibers potentially provide one arm of an AV reentry circuit, and their presence can result in PSVT.[52,53]

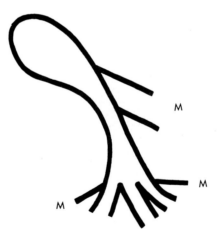

Fig. 10-24. Mahaim fibers *(M)*.

Summary

The most common form of preexcitation is the WPW syndrome. In this condition there is an accessory pathway connecting the atria with the ventricles. In its overt form the PR is short and the QRS broad. However, in its nonevident or concealed form, the ECG may be perfectly normal. The clinical significance of WPW syndrome lies in its arrhythmias, which may cause ventricular fibrillation and death. Patients with WPW are prone to develop PSVT because of a reentry circuit that uses the AV node and the accessory pathway. They can also develop atrial fibrillation with exceedingly rapid ventricular rates. Often the diagnosis is first made as a result of the ECG during the arrhythmias. An ECG diagnostic of PSVT using an accessory pathway depends on finding the P' wave separate from the QRS complex; QRS alternans may also be present and can be used as a diagnostic clue after the first 10 seconds of the tachycardia. The ECG diagnosis of atrial fibrillation with WPW syndrome is made because of a rapid, broad QRS tachycardia that is irregular.

REFERENCES

1. Anderson RH, Yen Ho S, and Becker AE: Gross anatomy and microscopy of the conducting system. In Mandel WJ: Cardiac arrhythmias, their mechanisms, diagnosis, and management, ed 2, Philadelphia, 1987, JB Lippincott Co.
2. Lown B, Ganong WF, and Levine SA: The syndrome of short P-R interval, normal QRS complex and paroxysmal rapid heart action, Circulation 5:696, 1952.
3. Brechenmacher C: Atrio-His bundle tracts, Br Heart J 37:853, 1975.
4. Wilson FN: A case in which the vagus influenced the form of ventricular complex of the electrocardiogram, Arch Intern Med 16:1008, 1915.
5. Wedd AM: Paroxysmal tachycardia. With reference to nomotopic tachycardia and the role of the extrinsic cardial nerves, Arch Intern Med 27:571, 1921.
6. Bach R: Paroxysmal tachycardia of 48 years duration and right bundle branch block, Proc Royal Soc Med 22:412, 1929.
7. Hamburger WW: Bundle branch block. Four cases of intraventricular blocks showing some interesting and unusual clinical features, Med Clin North Am 13:343, 1929.
8. Wolff L, Parkinson J, and White PD: Bundle branch block with short P-R interval in healthy young people prone to paroxysmal tachycardia, Am Heart J 5:685, 1930.
9. Paladino G: Contribuzione a l'anatomia, istologia e fisiologia del cuore, Moiv Med Chir (Napoli) 8:428, 1876.
10. Kent AFS: Researches on structure and function of mammalian heart, J Physiol 14:233, 1893.
11. Mines GR: On circulating excitation in heart muscles and their possible relation to tachycardia and fibrillation, Trans R Soc Can Ser 8(3):43, 1914.
12. de Boer S: Herzwuhlen, Flimmern, Flattern, gehaufte extrasystolie, parozysmale tachyKardie, Pflugers Arch 187:193, 1921.
13. Holzman M and Scherf D: Uber Elektrokardiogramme mit vorkurzten vorhol Kammer-Distanz und positiven P-Zacken, Z Klin Med 121:404, 1932.
14. Wolferth CC and Wood FC: The mechanism of production of short P-R intervals and prolonged QRS complexes in patients with presumably undamaged hearts. Hypothesis of an accessory pathway of auriculoventricular conduction (bundle of Kent), Am Heart J 8:297, 1933.
15. Wood FC, Wolferth CC, and Geckeler GD: Histological demonstration of accessory muscular connections between auricle and ventricle in a case of short P-R interval and prolonged QRS complex, Am Heart J 252:454, 1943.
16. Ohnell RF: Preexcitation, a cardiac abnormality, Acta Med Scand 152(supp):74, 1944.

17. Butterworth JS and Poindexter CA: Short P-R interval associated with a prolonged QRS complex; clinical and experimental study, Arch Intern Med 69:437, 1942.
18. Wolff L: Anomalous ventricular excitation (Wolff-Parkinson-White syndrome), Circulation 19:14, 1959.
19. Harnischfeger WW: Hereditary occurrence of the preexcitation (Wolff-Parkinson-White) syndrome with re-entry mechanism and concealed conduction, Circulation 19:28, 1959.
20. Langendorf R, Lev M, and Pick A: Auricular fibrillation with anomalous A-V excitation (WPW syndrome) imitating ventricular paroxysmal tachycardia, Acta Cardiol (Brux) 7:241, 1952.
21. Durrer D and others: The role of premature beats in the initiation and termination of supraventricular tachycardia in the Wolff-Parkinson-White syndrome, Circulation 36:644, 1967.
22. Wellens HJJ, Farré J, and Bar FWHM: The Wolff-Parkinson-White syndrome. In Mandel WJ: Cardiac arrhythmias, their mechanisms, diagnosis, and management, ed 2, Philadelphia, 1987, JB Lippincott Co.
23. Wellens HJJ: Paroxysmal supraventricular tachycardia. Recognition by the general practitioner, Rev Lat Cardiol 1:51, 1980.
24. Wellens HJJ: Contribution of cardiac pacing to our understanding of the Wolff-Parkinson-White syndrome, Br Heart J 37:231, 1975.
25. Durrer D and Roos JP: Epicardial excitation of the ventricles in a patient with Wolff-Parkinson-White syndrome (type B), Circulation 35:15, 1967.
26. Castellanos Jr A and others: His-bundle electrograms in two cases of WPW (pre-excitation) syndrome, Circulation 41:399, 1970.
27. Sealy WC and others: An improved operation for the definitive treatment of the Wolff-Parkinson-White syndrome, Ann Thorac Surg 17:107, 1974.
28. Guiraudon GM and others: Surgical repair of Wolff-Parkinson-White syndrome: a new closed-heart technique, Ann Thorac Surg 37:67, 1984.
29. Kirklin JK and others: Intermediate-term results of the endocardial surgical approach for anomalous atrioventricular bypass tracts, Am Heart J 115:444, 1988.
30. Becker AE and others: The anatomical substrates of Wolff-Parkinson-White syndrome, Circulation, 57:870, 1978.
31. Rosenbaum FF and others: Potential variations of the thorax and the esophagus in anomalous atrioventricular excitation (Wolff-Parkinson-White syndrome), Am Heart J 29:281, 1945.
32. Gallagher JJ and others: The preexcitation syndromes, Prog Cardiovasc Dis 20:285, 1978.
33. Garcia-Civera R and others: Retrograde P wave polarity in reciprocating tachycardias utilizing lateral bypass tracts, Eur Heart J 1:137, 1980.
34. Green M and others: Value of QRS alternation in determining the site of origin of narrow QRS supraventricular tachycardia, Circulation 68:368, 1983.
35. Bar FW and others: Differential diagnosis of tachycardia with narrow QRS complex (shorter than 0.12 second), Am J Cardiol 54:555, 1984.
36. Gallagher JJ and others: Multiple accessory pathways in patients with the preexcitation syndrome, Circulation 54:571, 1976.
37. Wellens HJJ, Farré J, and Bar RW: Stimulation studies in the Wolff-Parkinson-White syndrome. In Narula O, editor: Clinical electrophysiology, Philadelphia, 1979, FA Davis Co.
38. Dreifus LS and others: Ventricular fibrillation, a possible mechanism of sudden death in patients with the Wolff-Parkinson-White syndrome, Circulation 43:520, 1971.
39. Bashore TM and others: Ventricular fibrillation in the Wolff-Parkinson-White syndrome, Circulation 53:II187, 1976.
40. Wellens HJJ, Bar FWHM, and Lie KI: The value of the electrocardiogram in the differential diagnosis of a tachycardia with a widened QRS complex, Am J Med 64:27, 1978.
41. Sherf L and Neufeld HN: The pre-excitation syndrome: facts and theories, New York, 1978, Yorke Medical Books.
42. Wellens HJJ, Lubbers WJ, and Losekoot TG: Preexcitation. In Roberts NK and Gelband H, editors: Cardiac arrhythmias in the neonate infant and child, New York, 1977, Appleton-Century-Crofts.
43. Marriott HJL: Preexcitation "syndromes." In Contemporary electrocardiography, vol 2, no 7, Baltimore, 1980, The Williams & Wilkins Co.
44. Mahaim I and Benatt A: Nouvelles recherches sur les connexions superieures de la branche gauche du faisciau de His-Tarawa avec cloison interventriculaire, Cardiologia 1:61, 1938.

45. Mahaim I and Winston RM: Recherches d'anatomie comparee et de pathologie experimentale sur les connexions hautes du faisceau de His-Tawara, Cardiologia 5:189, 1941.
46. Mahaim I: Kent's fibers and the A-V paraspecific conduction through the upper connections of the bundle of His-Tarawa, Am Heart J 33:651, 1947.
47. Tchou P and others: Atriofascicular connection or a nodoventricular Mahaim fiber? Electrophysiologic elucidation of the pathway and associated reentrant circuit, Circulation 77: 837, 1988.
48. Gillette PC and others: Prolonged and decremental antegrade conduction properties in right anterior accessory connections: wide QRS antidromic tachycardia of left bundle block pattern without Wolff-Parkinson-White configuration in sinus rhythm, Am Heart J 103:66, 1982.
49. Gallagher JJ and others: Surgical interruption of nodoventricular Mahaim fibers with preservation of normal A-V conduction, J Am Coll Cardiol 7:133A, 1986 (abstract).
50. Klein G and others: The "nodoventricular" accessory pathway: evidence for a distinct accessory AV pathway with AV node-like properties, J Am Coll Cardiol 11:5, 1988.
51. Bardy GH and others: Surface electrocardiographic clues suggesting presence of a nodofascicular Mahaim fiber, J Am Coll Cardiol 3:1161, 1984.
52. Gallagher JJ and others: Role of Mahaim fibers in cardiac arrhythmias in man, Circulation 64:176, 1981.
53. Tonkin AM and others: Role of Mahaim fibers in cardiac arrhythmias in man, Circulation 64:176, 1981.

CHAPTER 11

Proarrhythmic actions of antiarrhythmic drugs

Antiarrhythmic drugs are generally thought to have actions that suppress arrhythmias, although it has been known for many years that digitalis and quinidine both have arrhythmogenic effects,[1,2] as do class I antiarrhythmic drugs, which may cause sinus node dysfunction.[3] In recent years, because of new information about antiarrhythmic drugs and their cell receptors, the clinical significance and the frequency of occurrence of the drug-induced arrhythmias have been appreciated, and data are being collected that will help treat arrhythmias more effectively.[4-13] This serious side effect, proarrhythmia, is common to all drugs in use or under investigation. With increasing numbers of patients being treated with antiarrhythmics, it is imperative that those patients susceptible to their proarrhythmic effects be identified. Indeed, it seems that the very patients at greatest risk for developing life-threatening arrhythmias, those with severe heart disease, are also most at risk for proarrhythmic effects of antiarrhythmics.[14-15]

Antiarrhythmic drugs act by binding to specific sites on the cell membrane. For example, fast sodium channels are blocked by local anesthetics, and slow calcium channels are blocked by verapamil; phase 3 repolarization is modified by drugs such as quinidine; the electrophysiological function of the heart is changed by beta adrenergic blockers; digitalis binds to the membrane in place of the potassium in the enzyme, sodium-potassium ATPase; and vagal input to the heart is enhanced either directly by digitalis, which increases acetylcholine release, or indirectly by edrophonium, which inhibits acetylcholinesterase and thus reduces the breakdown of acetylcholine.

Medical personnel have learned to anticipate arrhythmias caused by digitalis and by drugs that lengthen the QT interval, but the arrhythmias that are difficult to identify as drug related are those that result from a change in resting membrane potential and conduction velocity. Although antiarrhythmic drugs may further depress and disarm troublesome tissue, by the same mechanism they may also change slightly depressed cells into active foci for abnormal automaticity or reentry circuits and thus be proarrhythmic.

Membrane channel

The membrane channel illustrated in Fig. 11-1 was described in detail in Chapter 3 and is briefly reviewed here. The channel is a pore surrounded by protein and imbedded in the membrane's lipid bilayer. A selectivity filter is near the outside of the pore, and gates are toward the inside; the binding site for local anesthetic drugs is between these two structures. The selectivity filter permits ions to pass according to their size, shape, and charge; the fast sodium channel admits mainly sodium (Na^+) and some hydrogen (H^+). The local anesthetic drugs are too big to be admitted through this filter and gain access to the channel directly through the membrane's lipid bilayer and protein channel or through the lipid bilayer, the cytosol, and the channel gates, depending on the drug's lipid solubility. The gates open and close in response to voltage and time, admitting or blocking the entrance of Na^+. The cell's excitable (resting) phase is electrical diastole, during which time the "m" gate is closed and the "h" gate open. The m gate is the activation gate; it opens when electrical systole begins and voltage reaches threshold potential. The h gate is the inactivation gate; it closes when voltage becomes more positive. This transition from electrical diastole to electrical systole is illustrated in Fig. 11-1. During electrical systole the m gate is open, and Na^+ enters the cell before the h gate can close. Once the h gate closes, a certain voltage must be attained, a certain time must pass, and a condition of ionic disequilibrium must be achieved before the channel can

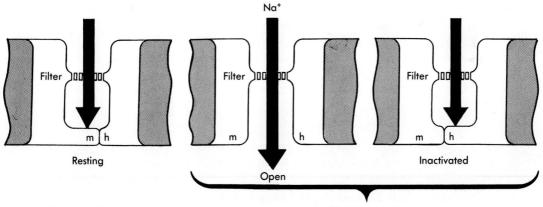

Fig. 11-1. States of the fast sodium channel during different phases of the action potential. The resting state is seen during phase 4 of the action potential and constitutes electrical diastole. Both the open state and the inactivated state occur during electrical systole; the open state is during phase 0, and the inactivated state is during phase 2 and part of phase 3. The selectivity filter determines the size and shape of molecule that will be admitted; the "m" and "h" gates open and close in response to voltage and time. (Modified from Rosen MR and Wit AL: Am J Cardiol 59[11]:10E, 1987.)

return to its resting state, ready to initiate another action potential. Although the channels generally respond together, there is a "randomness" to their opening and closing[9] so that some channels may be able to respond to a second stimulus before others can.[16]

Fast Na$^+$ channel blockade by local anesthetic antiarrhythmics

All local anesthetic drugs have a common function: they block the fast sodium channels. Their antiarrhythmic effect is attributed to this action. Clinically useful agents do not usually block resting channels but have a preference for their activated and/ or inactivated state. If this were not the case, the drug would be arrhythmogenic since it would cause conduction block in normal tissue. For example, quinidine blocks activated (open) channels, amiodarone blocks inactivated channels, and lidocaine blocks both.[17] This function in turn determines which tissue will be affected relative to action potential duration. A drug that mostly blocks open channels, although strongly voltage dependent, is not affected by action potential duration since its only entry into the channel is during phase 0. On the other hand, a drug that blocks inactivated channels exerts its effect for a longer time—during the plateau of the action potential—and thus would have more effect on Purkinje fibers, in which the action potential duration is longest, than on atrial tissue, in which the action potential duration is shortest.

In addition to these considerations, the effectiveness of channel blockade is dependent on (1) whether the plasma molecule of the drug is uncharged or ionized, (2) the membrane potential, (3) whether or not there is acidosis, and (4) the molecular weight and shape of the drug.[9]

Drugs exist in the extracellular space in both the nonionized and ionized forms, given a physiological pH. Fig. 11-2 illustrates how the local anesthetic drugs gain access to the channel. In the nonionized form (D) they have high lipid solubility and can traverse the lipid bilayer of the cell membrane and reach binding sites between the selectivity filter and the channel gates from both directions—straight through the lipid bilayer and channel protein and also through the lipid bilayer into the cytosol and through the gates when they are briefly open during phase 0 of the action potential (Fig. 11-2, B).

The ionized form (D$^+$), on the other hand, does not have the high lipid solubility of the nonionized molecule and must move slowly through the lipid bilayer toward the cytosol, in which it can move freely. Thus the ionized form of the drug reaches its binding site from an intracellular position during electrical systole when the gates are briefly open (Fig. 11-2, B); access is closed to the ionized molecule at all other times in the cardiac cycle (Fig. 11-2, A and C). Hence such a drug would be more effective at faster heart rates since there is more blocking during tachycardia than during bradycardia. The term "use dependence" expresses this fact.[9,16,18-21] That is, drug-induced reduction of channel availability is caused by use of the channels by the ionized molecules.[17] The term "tonic blocking" actions applies to the uncharged molecules that gain access to their channel binding sites directly through the lipid bilayer and channel protein, regardless of the position of the gates.[9,20] Thus tonic block can occur in open and inactivated channels alike.[17]

Some of the variables that influence channel blockade are (1) membrane potential, (2) pH, and (3) molecular weight and structure.

1. Block of transmembrane ionic channels is both time and voltage dependent. Lidocaine, for example, binds more readily to the channel when the membrane is depressed; this explains its greater effectiveness in depressing conduction in infarcted tissue and suppressing arrhythmias in diseased (depolarized) tissue, while having only minimal effects on conduction in normal cardiac tissue.[9,12,22]

2. Although most local anesthetic antiarrhythmics are weak bases that exist in both forms (cationic and neutral) at physiological pH, acidosis, as it occurs in ischemic tissue, increases the proportion of the ionized form of the drug molecule and causes it to disassociate more slowly from the channel receptor site. Thus the drug selectively depresses conduction in acidotic tissue at any given heart rate. If the pH changes, so do the actions of the drug. For example, if the plasma becomes alkaline, the neutral form of the drug dominates, and sodium-channel blockade is reduced.[17,23,24]

3. Drugs with higher molecular weight bind to the channel more persistently than do those with lower molecular weight.[9,25,26]

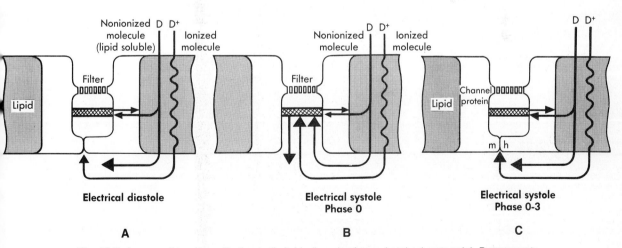

Fig. 11-2. Access of local anesthetics to their binding site *(cross-hatched rectangle).* D represents nonionized molecules, which easily gain access to the channel binding site from both directions and during all channel states (resting, open, and inactivated). D⁺ represents ionized molecules, which traverse the lipid bilayer poorly but, after gaining access to the aqueous cytosol, can readily enter the channel when it is open but not when it is closed. (Modified from Rosen MR and Wit AL: Am J Cardiol 59[11]:10E, 1987.)

Abnormal conduction caused by cardiac disease

An action potential from a normal fiber is compared to that from a depolarized fiber in Fig. 11-3. As the fiber is depolarized, the number of fast sodium channels decreases, phase 0 does not rise as rapidly or as steeply, and conduction velocity slows. Fig. 11-4 illustrates the depolarization of a fiber after coronary occlusion. As the membrane potential is reduced, conduction velocity slows, and reentry circuits may be established (Chapter 6). The membrane potential is reduced from its normal of approximately −90 mV to a depressed fast response within 5 minutes and to a slow response within 7 minutes. The slow response action potential is devoid of all fast sodium channels and not only conducts slowly, but may also be a focus for abnormal automaticity even though it never possessed the capability for automaticity in health.

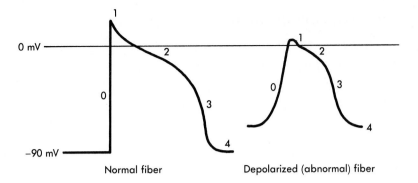

Fig. 11-3. Effect of cardiac disease on cardiac action potential. Normal Purkinje fiber has a resting membrane potential of −90 mV and a tall phase 0 with a large overshoot. Depolarized fiber has a resting membrane potential of −70 mV and very small overshoot; conduction velocity will be slow in this fiber.

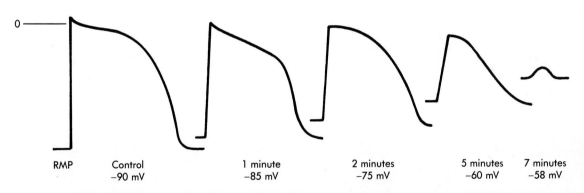

Fig. 11-4. Effect of ischemia on cardiac action potential. *RMP*, resting membrane potential.

Abnormal conduction caused by antiarrhythmic drugs

When antiarrhythmic drugs cause arrhythmias, they do so because of a process different from that of cardiac disease or ischemia, but the end result is the same—the modification of conduction. Whereas cardiac disease may cause failure of the sodium-potassium ATPase pump[10] and ischemia causes K^+ loss because of the effects of lactate and phosphate generated by the ischemic cell,[10,27] antiarrhythmic drugs depolarize the fiber by blocking the fast sodium channels. In both cases, conduction velocity slows. Therapeutically, the antiarrhythmic drug causes a two-way block in an area of one-way conduction and thus obliterates the reentry circuit. Fig. 11-5, A, illustrates the modification of conduction by lidocaine and lidocaine-like drugs. In the arrhythmogenic state there is a depressed fast response action potential in an area of ischemia, resulting in anterograde block through the area, slow one-way conduction in the retrograde direction, and a reentry circuit resulting in tachycardia. The lidocaine further depresses the area, terminating the tachycardia. In Fig. 11-5, B, there is another area of ischemia that is not as depressed as that of A. Conduction has been slowed, but anterograde conduction persists, and no arrhythmia results. The administration of the antiarrhythmic drug further blocks the fast Na^+ channels in the borderline tissue and depresses the fiber, modifying conduction so that reentry results and a new arrhythmia appears.

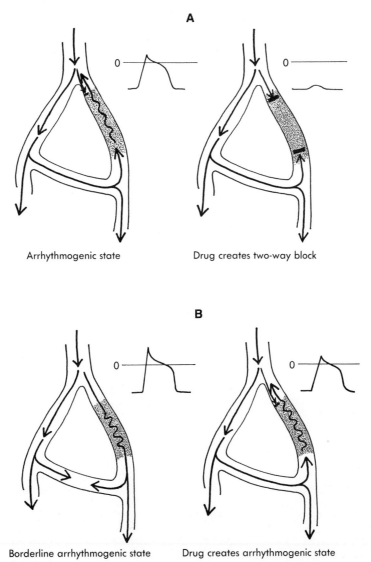

A

Arrhythmogenic state   Drug creates two-way block

B

Borderline arrhythmogenic state   Drug creates arrhythmogenic state

Fig. 11-5. Modification of conduction by an antiarrhythmic drug. **A,** In the arrhythmogenic state a reentry circuit and tachyarrhythmia are established through depressed fibers because of an area of slow, one-way conduction; the drug further depresses the fibers, producing two-way block and interrupting the reentry circuit. **B,** Fiber to the left is only slightly depressed; conduction is slow but adequate. The antiarrhythmic drug further depresses the fiber, creating the arrhythmogenic state seen in **A.** (Modified from Rosen MR and Wit AL: Am J Cardiol 59[11]:10E, 1987.)

Proarrhythmic effects of prolonging the refractory period

Besides the effect on borderline arrhythmogenic foci, there is another way through which drugs can alter conduction velocity—as a secondary effect of prolongation of the refractory period. Fig. 11-6, *A* and *B*, illustrates two possible effects of lengthening the refractory period (e.g., as would occur with use of quinidine and quinidine-like drugs). In Fig. 11-6, *A*, an ectopic beat occurs during phase 3 repolarization, causing conduction velocity to be slow through that area of the heart, and reentry circuits may result; when the refractory period is lengthened, the ectopic focus is suppressed. In Fig. 11-6, *B*, the ectopic beat occurs during diastole, and

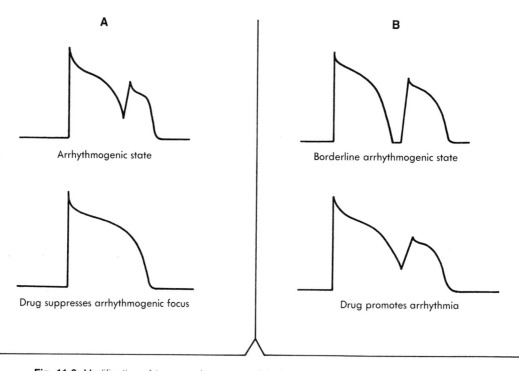

Fig. 11-6. Modification of transmembrane potential characteristics by prolonging repolarization. **A,** An arrhythmogenic state exists because an ectopic focus discharges during phase 3 when the membrane potential is depressed, contributing to slow conduction. When the refractory period is lengthened by an antiarrhythmic drug, the premature action potential is obliterated. **B,** A premature beat propagates normally; when an antiarrhythmic drug is given to lengthen the refractory period, the premature beat arrives during phase 3 and propagates abnormally. (Modified from Rosen MR and Wit AL: Am J Cardiol 59[11]:10E, 1987.)

although it is premature, it propagates normally. When the refractory period is lengthened by the antiarrhythmic drug, the ectopic firing occurs during phase 3 repolarization, creating the same arrhythmogenic situation that existed in A.

Drugs that lengthen the refractory period are capable not only of modifying conduction velocity, but also of causing early afterdepolarizations that can initiate triggered activity. In fact, even quinidine concentrations within the therapeutic range are capable of this effect.[10,28-30] Early afterdepolarizations and triggered activity have already been discussed in Chapters 4 and 5.

Drug-induced supraventricular arrhythmias

The term "proarrhythmia" indicates that an antiarrhythmic agent has aggravated existing arrhythmias by increasing their duration and/or frequency, has caused new arrhythmias to develop, or has caused cardiac arrest.[31]

Of the supraventricular disturbances induced by antiarrhythmic drugs, those caused by digitalis toxicity (Chapter 5) are most common and include atrial tachycardia with block, accelerated idiojunctional rhythm and junctional tachycardia, sinus bradycardia, SA block, and AV block.

Drug-induced ventricular tachyarrhythmias

Ventricular proarrhythmia has been described in one study of patients with mixed cardiac disease and chronic ventricular arrhythmias as having the following characteristics[32]:

1. Threefold increase in ventricular ectopics when baseline ventricular extrasystole frequency is more than 100/hour.
2. Tenfold increase in ventricular ectopics when that frequency is less than 100/hour.

Lown and co-workers have proposed other criteria[33]:

1. Fourfold increase in frequency of ventricular premature beats (VPB).
2. Tenfold increase in repetitive forms (couplets or runs of ventricular tachycardia [VT]).
3. Onset of sustained VT or ventricular fibrillation (VF) not present during the control period.

Although drug toxicity is the cause of many arrhythmias (e.g., digitalis dysrhythmias and torsade de pointes), proarrhythmia does not necessarily occur because of toxicity or because blood levels of the drug are too high but may simply be a result of the known "therapeutic" action of the drug on borderline arrhythmogenic foci.

UNIFORM SPONTANEOUS AND SUSTAINED VT OF NEW ONSET OR IN-CREASED FREQUENCY. The onset of spontaneous, sustained VT shortly after starting or increasing the dosage of an antiarrhythmic drug for the treatment of sporadic ventricular ectopy certainly attracts one's attention. The cause of this arrhythmia may be the drug itself, or it may be simply a coincidence. If the arrhythmia fails to occur for a reasonable period after the drug is discontinued and then recurs when the drug is restarted, there is a high degree of certainty that the drug is the culprit. When the onset of the VT occurs late in the course of drug therapy, it is more difficult to know the cause because the evolution of the disease process and inadequate or excessive drug plasma concentrations then come into question.[34]

With increased frequency of uniform spontaneous, sustained VT, it is difficult to know if the cause is the drug itself or failure of the drug to suppress the already existing VT. Since one cause would call for discontinuation of the drug and the other for an increase in the drug, it is necessary to ascertain the answer by alternately giving and withholding the drug until a clear-cut difference in frequency of attacks is demonstrated.[33]

NEW PERSISTENT VT WITH TOXIC CONCENTRATIONS OF CLASS IA OR IC ANTIARRHYTHMICS. Persistant VT (nonsustained VT interrupted by only a few sinus beats) occurs with toxic concentrations of class IA or IC antiarrhythmic drugs.[5,12,34-37] Even in patients with normal hearts, high concentrations of quinidine, procainamide, or tricyclic antidepressant drugs can cause persistent VT. The persistent VT that occurs soon after administering an increased dosage of, or starting, a class IC drug such as encainide, flecainide, propafenone, or moricizine is almost certainly an adverse drug effect.[34] This VT usually looks and acts differently from the VT seen before drug administration; it is wider, slower, and difficult to terminate with cardioversion, converting to sinus rhythm for only one or two beats. Use of drugs to treat this VT only compounds the situation. Factors predisposing to this type of persistant VT with class IC antiarrhythmic drugs are a history of spontaneous sustained VT and a left ventricular ejection fraction <30%. The patient is usually on high doses of antiarrhythmic drugs, the dosage of which has been rapidly increased.[14,37]

ACCELERATED IDIOVENTRICULAR RHYTHM. Accelerated idioventricular rhythm (AIVR) is digitalis arrhythmia that is often fascicular (rate 90 to 160) and that may develop into bidirectional VT. Typically there is an incomplete right bundle branch block (RBBB) pattern, right or left axis deviation, a QRS of <0.14 second, and a rate of 140 to 180 beats/min. Fig. 11-7 illustrates the accelerated fascicular rhythm caused by digitalis toxicity; it is further discussed and illustrated in Chapter 5.

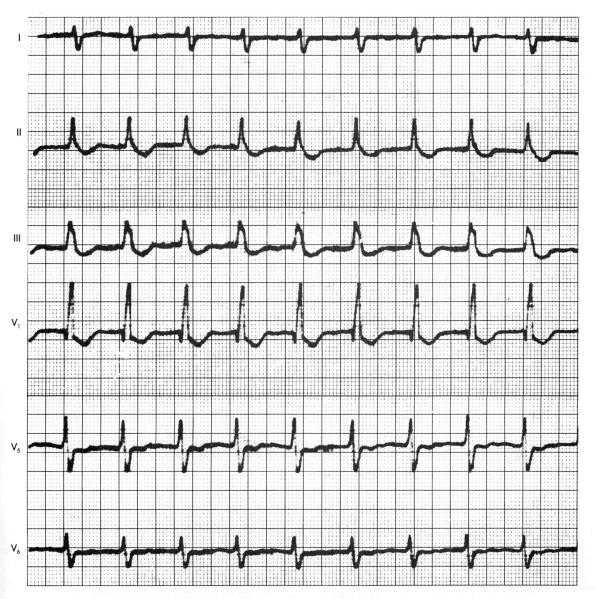

Fig. 11-7. Accelerated fascicular rhythm caused by digitalis toxicity. Note the typical incomplete right bundle branch block pattern and the right axis deviation indicating a superior fascicular focus. (From Josephson ME and Wellens HJJ: How to approach complex arrhythmias, Miami, 1987, Medtronic.)

TORSADES DE POINTES. Torsades de pointes (twisting of the points) is a type of paroxysmal VT (rate 200 to 250 beats/min) characterized by QRS complexes that appear to twist around the isoelectric line (Fig. 11-8) and show varying polarity and changing amplitudes; the paroxysm is initiated by a long-short cycle sequence. Torsades de pointes typically is accompanied by a long QT interval, although, according to Rosen,[38] its occurrence spans the range of QT intervals, and the degree of QT prolongation that predicts it is not known. In quinidine-induced torsades de pointes the QT intervals have exceeded 0.60 second.[31] This arrhythmia can be a precursor to ventricular fibrillation and sudden death.

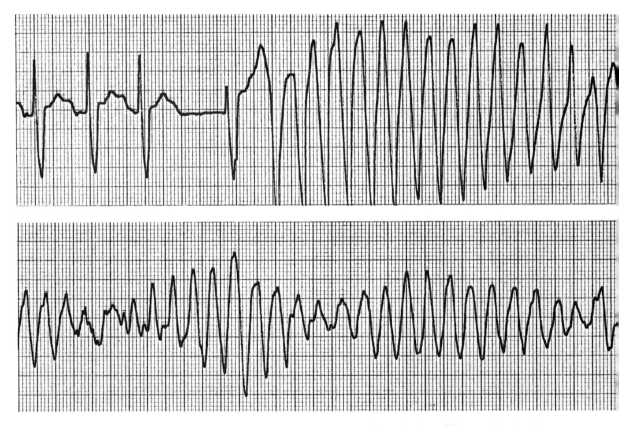

Fig. 11-8. Torsades de pointes caused by use of quinidine. Note the long QT interval during sinus rhythm. (Courtesy Dr. Alan Lindsay.)

Clinical characteristic. An important clinical characteristic of the class I antiarrhythmic drug-induced torsades de pointes is that it appears to occur early in the drug course, permitting in-hospital detection and treatment.[34] Certainly, progressive lengthening of the QT interval and the development of a prominent U wave are an important warning that the appearance of the arrhythmia itself requires only a change in cycle length and/or a change in the autonomic nervous system.[39]

Torsades de pointes is more common in women, who represent almost half of the cases even though they constitute the minority of patients receiving antiarrhythmic drugs for ventricular arrhythmias.[34,40] Torsades de pointes that is the result of electrolyte disturbances and drugs tends to recur with high frequency until the underlying cause is corrected, which usually takes from several hours to several days.

Causes. The most common cause of torsades de pointes is class I antiarrhythmic drug toxicity.[34] Among the drugs that prolong the action potential duration of Purkinje fibers are quinidine, procainamide, disopyramide, and amiodarone, which not only prolong the QT interval but also slow intraventricular conduction and increase QRS duration. Quinidine is especially effective in prolonging the action potential duration during bradycardia or hypokalemia, both of which themselves prolong repolarization. Sotalol is an investigational drug that lengthens the QT by inhibiting repolarizing potassium currents with essentially no effect on the duration of the QRS, but which may also cause torsades de pointes. In one study drug-induced torsades de pointes was almost always preceded by sinus bradycardia or a pause[41]; this finding was less consistent with torsades de pointes that was not drug related. Although it is true that quinidine-induced torsades de pointes often occurs against a background of long QT interval, it is also true that the arrhythmia may occur at low plasma drug concentrations that do not cause QRS prolongation.[10,42]

Other causes of torsades de pointes besides class I antiarrhythmic drugs, hypokalemia, and severe bradycardia are as follows:

Congenital long QT interval[43]
Hypomagnesemia
Low-protein diets[44-46]
Tricyclic antidepressants
Antihistamines
Phenothiazines[44]
Insecticide poisoning (organophosphorus, a replacement for DDT)[47]
Chui-Feng-Su-Ho-Wan[48] (a traditional Chinese herbal medicine for upper respiratory symptoms)
Hypothyroidism[49]
Myocardial ischemia[50]
Contrast injections into a coronary artery[31]

Torsades de pointes has also occurred in clinically stable patients without electrolyte disturbance or antiarrhythmic drugs and with normal or minimally prolonged QT intervals.[42]

Electrophysiology. When the refractory period is lengthened, early afterdepolarizations can occur and produce triggered activity (Fig. 11-9). Torsade de pointes may result from this mechanism,[10] or it may be the result of reentry.

Mechanism. The mechanism of the distinctive ECG pattern of torsades de pointes is not known, although reentry with changing epicardial breakthrough sites and triggered activity caused by early afterdepolarizations are two suspects. Dessertenne,[51] who originally described the arrhythmia, favored the theory that two competitive automatic ventricular pacemakers were alternately controlling the heart. Later studies have shown, with epicardial mapping, that there is a shift in the epicardial breakthrough site with each change in QRS morphology.[37,52,53] Electrophysiological studies from Josephson's laboratory[44] support the thesis that the typical ECG pattern of torsades de pointes results from changing exit sites or local conduction block from a rapid reentrant focus. The exit block would in turn be secondary to the rapid rate.

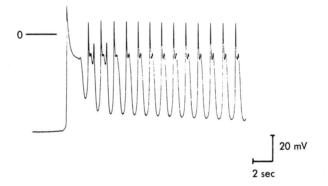

Fig. 11-9. Early afterdepolarizations causing triggered activity. Note that the onset of the rhythm is quite regular, requiring no period of warm-up. (Modified from Damiano BP and Rosen MR: Circulation 69:1013, 1984.)

PERSISTENT VT CAUSED BY CLASS IC DRUGS. When incessant VT develops after starting drugs such as encainide, flecainide, propafenone, or moricizine, the mechanism is almost certainly a proarrhythmic drug effect. Characteristics of persistent VT caused by class IC drugs are as follows[33]: a history of spontaneous sustained VT and a low left ventricular ejection fraction; sustained tachycardia that occurs spontaneously soon after starting the drug; sinusoidal morphology of the tachycardia that differs from previous spontaneous VT morphologies; and the VT either cannot be terminated by cardioversion or programmed ventricular stimulation or it resumes immediately after termination.

DRUG-INDUCED VENTRICULAR FIBRILLATION. Minardo and others[54] have reported 40 episodes of drug-induced ventricular fibrillation in 30 patients. The drugs involved were quinidine, procainamide, disopyramide, and a variety of other ones. The events were not necessarily associated with or predicted by QT prolongation.

RISK FACTORS. The clinical predictors of the development of arrhythmias caused by antiarrhythmic drugs are sustained VT, ventricular fibrillation, hypokalemia, left ventricular ejection fraction of <35%, and use of diuretics.[55,56]

Data from clinical studies with flecainide and encainide identified those patients with risk factors associated with proarrhythmias and death.[55] Patients with sustained ventricular tachycardia in association with serious structural heart disease and hypokalemia are at higher risk for developing arrhythmias after the use of antiarrhythmic drugs, particularly class IA drugs. Patients with a clinical history of sustained VT or ventricular fibrillation are 3.4 times more likely to have worsening arrhythmias after antiarrhythmic drug therapy. These patients already have the potential substrate to support a reentry circuit. Altering conduction velocity or refractoriness through the use of antiarrhythmic drugs may convert borderline tissue into areas of reentry.[56]

In a study performed by Slater and others[56], patients with a left ventricular ejection fraction of <35% had a risk of worsening arrhythmias that was twice that of those patients with an ejection fraction of >35%. Use of diuretics was also found to be a factor. Normokalemic patients who were taking diuretics were 2.2 times more likely to develop worsening arrhythmias than those not requiring diuretics.

Summary

Local anesthetic antiarrhythmic drugs act by blocking membrane channels; other antiarrhythmics prolong refractory periods and cause triggered activity. Many factors such as myocardial state and preexisting arrhythmias work together to contribute to the proarrhythmic actions or toxicity of antiarrhythmic drugs. Other factors such as pH, heart rate, and molecular size and shape of the drug influence the binding and release of the local anesthetic antiarrhythmic drugs at their receptor sites. The arrhythmias promoted by antiarrhythmic drugs are not unlike those induced by myocardial disease and ischemia, although the mechanisms differ. It is possible for an antiarrhythmic drug, through the very mechanism that causes it to suppress an arrhythmogenic focus, also to cause arrhythmias by converting adequately propagating ectopic foci into more depressed, slowly propagating tissue. Information about the proarrhythmic mechanisms presented in this chapter have been derived from the latest in cellular electrophysiology and clinical evidence; much work is still needed to prove the relationship between drug toxicity, long QT intervals, and triggered activity.

CHAPTER 12

Aberrant ventricular conduction

As early as 1910, Sir Thomas Lewis[1] described aberrant ventricular conduction of atrial premature beats and during atrial fibrillation and flutter. He stated: "I term the . . . beats aberrant because they are caused by impulses which have gone astray." Since that time "aberrancy," "aberrant ventricular conduction," and "ventricular aberration" have become interchangeable terms.

Lewis also illustrated bundle branch block (BBB) as a form of permanent ventricular aberration. Although the term aberration is now reserved for transient BBB, these early studies correctly identified the mechanism.

In 1947 Gouaux and Ashman[2] further defined the mechanism of ventricular aberration by relating it to the refractory period and the cycle length in atrial fibrillation. Although the cycle length of the bundle branches during atrial fibrillation cannot be known from the surface ECG because of the prevalence of concealed conduction into the bundle branches, the concept of the long-short phenomenon is still valid, although less so when applied to atrial fibrillation. Thus their statement was correct: "Aberration occurs (may occur) when a short cycle follows a long one because the refractory period varies with cycle length." Much to their credit, Gouaux and Ashman, through deductive reasoning, arrived at the conclusion that the right bundle branch has a longer refractory period than the left bundle branch so that right bundle branch block (RBBB) aberration is the more common form, a fact later verified by the experimental studies of Moe, Mendez, and Han.[3]

Further delineating the type of BBB involved in ventricular aberration, Wellens, Bar, and Lie[4] found that out of 70 episodes of aberration, 69% were RBBB. Sandler and Marriott[5] have reported the incidence of RBBB aberration is as high as 80% to 85%. In a relatively sick population (e.g., in a coronary care facility) left bundle branch block (LBBB) aberration assumes greater prominence and accounts for perhaps a third of the aberrant conduction encountered; Wellens' group[4] found 31% were LBBB aberration. In the study by Kulbertus and others[6] RBBB accounted for a smaller-than-expected proportion of the aberration produced exper-

Table 12-1. Relative frequency of experimental aberration

	Percent	
RBBB	24	i.e.:
RBBB + LAHB	18	RBBB = 52%
LAHB	15	LAHB = 33%
RBBB + LPHB	10	LPHB = 19%
LPHB	9	LBBB = 14%
LBBB	9	
ILBBB	5	
Trivial changes	6	
Marked anterior displacement	4	

From Kulbertus HE and others: Br Heart J 38:549, 1976.

imentally, whereas left posterior hemiblock occurred with surprising frequency. By inducing premature atrial beats in 44 patients, 116 aberrant configurations were produced. The results of this study are presented in Table 12-1.

Mechanism

Conduction velocity depends on, among other things, the rate of rise of phase 0 of the action potential (dV/dt) and the height to which it rises (V_{max}), which are in turn dependent on the membrane potential at the time of stimulation. The more negative the membrane potential is, the more fast sodium channels available and the more the influx of sodium (Na^+) into the cell during phase 0.

Fig. 12-1 illustrates that if a stimulus occurs either during phase 3 or during phase 4 of the action potential, the membrane potential at the time of stimulation is reduced, and conduction is compromised—hence the terms "phase 3" aberration and "phase 4" aberration.

In Fig. 12-1, *A*, the ECG shows an atrial premature beat (APB) conducted with aberration. The action potential of the right bundle branch (RBB) is shown above the ECG tracing and indicates that aberration occurs because the stimulus reaches the RBB during phase 3 when the membrane potential is −65 mV. At this time only approximately half of the fast sodium channels are available for activation. The resulting action potential is a slow channel response; thus conduction fails.

In Fig. 12-1, *B*, the ECG shows a long cycle ending with RBBB. The action potential of the RBB indicates enhanced automaticity so that by the time the impulse arrives in the RBB, the membrane potential has been reduced. The resulting action potential is a slow channel response; thus conduction fails.

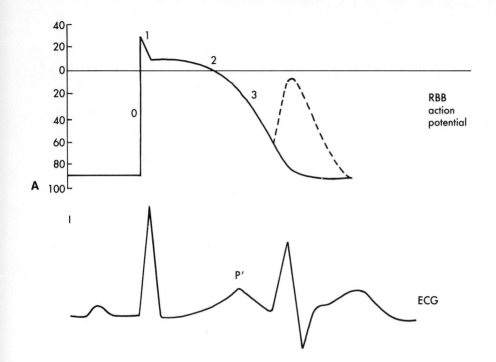

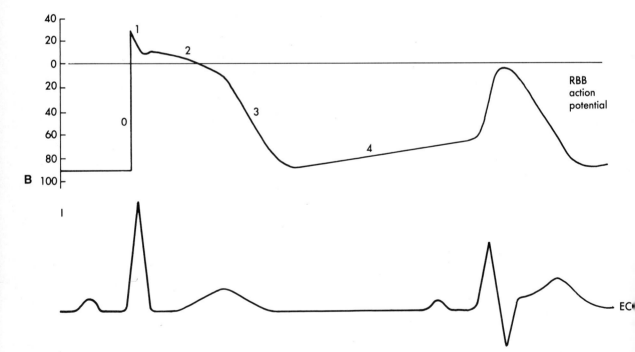

Fig. 12-1. Phase 3 and phase 4 block. **A,** An atrial premature beat is conducted with phase 3 right bundle branch block (RBBB) aberration. **B,** Phase 4 RBBB aberration. *RBB,* Right bundle branch.

Phase 3 aberration

Functional or physiological phase 3 aberration (BBB) can occur in normal fibers if the impulse is premature enough to reach the fiber during electrical systole of the preceding beat when the membrane potential is still reduced. This is the common form of aberration that often accompanies very early APBs.

Phase 3 aberration may also occur pathologically if electrical systole and/or the refractory period are abnormally prolonged and the involved fascicle is stimulated at a relatively rapid rate. Thus the terms "systolic block" or "tachycardia-dependent BBB" are sometimes used. In the case of abnormal prolongation of the refractory period, refractoriness extends beyond the action potential duration or the QT interval.

Although the supernormal period is a part of phase 3, very early premature beats can occur before the period of supernormal excitability, a property not exhibited by all fibers. Fig. 12-2 illustrates the abrupt onset of supernormal excitability

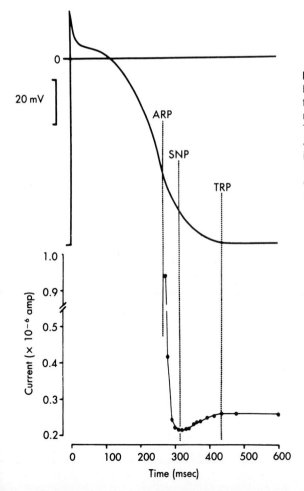

Fig. 12-2. Excitability determination in a canine Purkinje fiber. Excitability curve is displayed beneath the action potential and represents the minimal depolarizing current necessary to evoke a response at the time indicated. *TRP,* Total refractory period; *ARP,* absolute refractory period; *SNP,* minimal current requirements to excite the fiber during the supernormal period. (From Spear JF and Moore N: In Wellens HJJ, Lie KI, and Janse MJ, editors: The conduction system of the heart, Hingham, Mass, 1976, Martinus Nijhoff, Publisher.)

and the small portion of the action potential actually involved. Spear and Moore[7] found that intraventricular conduction times of very early premature beats could be decreased as well as increased.

Fig. 12-3 illustrates examples of phase 3 RBBB aberration after an APB. In these cases it is often difficult or impossible to make the distinction between physiological phase 3 BBB and a pathological one involving lengthening of the refractory period.

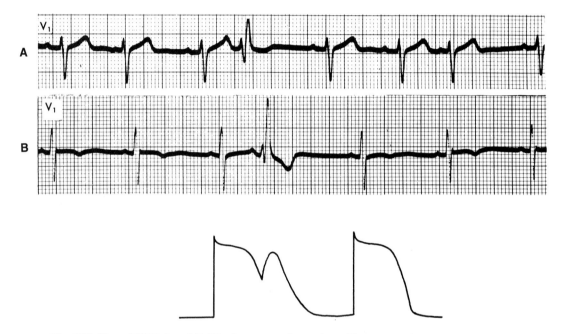

Fig. 12-3. Phase 3 BBB. **A** and **B,** After three normally conducted beats, an atrial extrasystole arises, and its impulse arrives at the RBB, which is still refractory; it is therefore conducted with RBBB aberration. In **A,** the second and seventh beats are also extrasystoles, but they are less premature and are therefore conducted normally. The action potentials illustrate the mechanism.

Fig. 12-4 gives two more examples of phase 3 aberration. In Fig. 12-4, *A*, there is RBBB, and in Fig. 12-4, *B*, LBBB. Both develop in response to a gradual shortening of the cycle length until it becomes shorter than the refractory period of one of the bundle branches, whereupon aberrant conduction develops and persists until the cycle lengthens enough for normal conduction to recur. The BBB seen in these two tracings is secondary to a pathological prolongation of the action potential and/ or refractory period in the respective bundle branches.

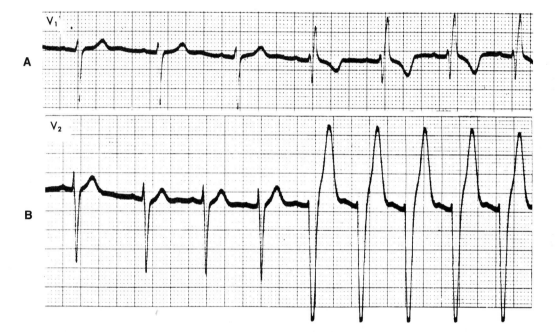

Fig. 12-4. Phase 3 BBB. **A,** From a 19-year-old student nurse. As her sinus rate accelerates and the cycle shortens in response to gentle exercise, progressively increasing degrees of RBBB develop ("critical-rate" or "rate-dependent" RBBB). **B,** From a 64-year-old man with severe coronary disease. As his sinus rate accelerates, the cycles shorten; LBBB develops at a critical rate of just over 100 beats/min.

Phase 4 aberration

Phase 4 aberration is one of the theories offered to explain the development of abnormal intraventricular conduction only at the end of a lengthened cycle. Since better conduction would be expected at the end of a longer diastole, this form of aberration is known as *paradoxical critical rate*. It is also sometimes referred to as *bradycardia-dependent BBB*, but this is unsatisfactory as an inclusive term because it is not always necessary to achieve a rate that merits the designation bradycardia.

Phase 4 block occurs late in diastole and is associated with the cyclical reduction in resting membrane potential typical of latent pacemaker cells. If these cells are activated when their membrane potential is thus reduced, conduction disturbances can result like those that develop when activation occurs during phase 3.[8-10]

This type of aberration would be expected in the setting of bradycardia or enhanced normal automaticity (enhanced automaticity of pacemaker cells). However, in spite of the fact that bradycardia is common and cells with phase 4 depolarization are abundant, phase 4 block is not frequently seen, and most reported cases are associated with organic heart disease. Singer and Cohen[10] offer this explanation: in normal fibers conduction is well maintained at membrane potentials greater than -70 to -75 mV. Significant conduction disturbances are first manifested when the membrane is below -70 mV at the time of stimulation, and local block appears at -65 to -60 mV. Since the threshold potential for normal His-Purkinje fibers is -70 mV, spontaneous firing would take place before the membrane could actually be reduced to the potential necessary for conduction impairment or block. Therefore phase 4 block is always pathological when it does occur and requires one or more of the following:

1. The presence of slow diastolic depolarization, which need not be enhanced.
2. A decrease in excitability (shift in threshold potential toward zero) so that, in the presence of significant bradycardia, enough time elapses before the arrival of the impulse for the bundle branch fibers to reach a potential at which conduction is impaired.
3. A deterioration in membrane responsiveness so that significant conduction impairment develops at -75 mV instead of -65 mV. This occurrence would also negate the necessity for such a long cycle before conduction falters.

Membrane responsiveness is determined by the relationship of the membrane potential at excitation to the maximal height of phase 0. Thus hypopolarization (the loss of maximal diastolic potential) is an important factor in phase 4 block since it itself causes both a decrease in excitability and enhanced automaticity.[11]

Two examples of phase 4 BBB can be seen in Fig. 12-5. In Fig. 12-5, *A,* the longer sinus cycles end with LBBB; in Fig. 12-5, *B,* the lengthened postextrasystolic cycles end with RBBB conduction.

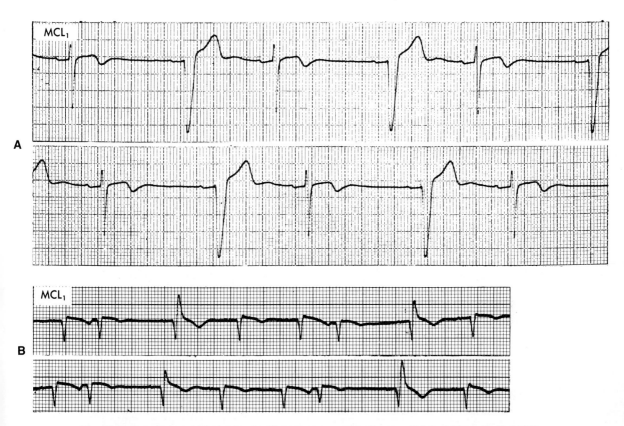

Fig. 12-5. Paradoxical critical rate. **A,** All the longer cycles (range, 138 to 142) end with LBBB, whereas the shorter cycles (range, 107 to 110) end with improved, virtually normal, intraventricular conduction. The alternately longer and shorter sinus cycles are presumably caused by a 3:2 sinus Wenckebach period. **B,** Sinus rhythm is repeatedly interrupted by atrial extrasystoles. Conducted beats ending the lengthened postextrasystolic cycles all show RBBB, whereas the shorter sinus cycles and the even shorter extrasystolic cycles show more normal intraventricular conduction.

Rate-dependent and critical rate BBB

Rate-dependent BBB is the term used when the block comes and goes with changes in heart rate. *Critical rate* is the term given to the rate at which the BBB develops during acceleration or disappears during slowing. It is of interest that rate-dependent BBB develops at a critical rate faster than the rate at which it disappears. Note in Fig. 12-6 that although rate-dependent BBB develops when the rate reaches 66 beats/min (cycle equals 91), normal conduction is not restored until the rate falls to 56 beats/min (cycle equals 108).

There are two reasons for this phenomenon. First, as the heart rate accelerates, the refractory period shortens; because of this response, normal conduction tends to be preserved. Conversely, as the heart rate slows, the refractory period lengthens. It is thus necessary for the heart rate to slow down more than would be expected to reestablish normal intraventricular conduction.

Second and more importantly is the fact that once BBB is established, the depressed bundle branch will be activated late transseptally through the still conducting bundle branch. The operative sequence is illustrated in Fig. 12-7. Once BBB is established, the actual cycle for the blocked branch does not begin until approximately halfway through the QRS complex. For example, in the case of the rate-dependent LBBB (see Fig. 12-6) it takes approximately 0.06 second for the impulse to negotiate the unaffected right bundle and the septum and reach the depressed left branch. Therefore the left branch actually begins its cycle 0.06 second after the right branch. It follows that for normal conduction to resume, the cycle during deceleration—as measured from the beginning of one QRS to the beginning of the next QRS—must be longer than the "critical" cycle during acceleration by at least 0.06 second.

Two more examples of phase 3 BBB can be seen in Fig. 12-8. This time the fact that the BBB is rate dependent is revealed only because of the pause following ventricular premature beats (VPBs) in Fig. 12-8, *A*, and a nonconducted APB in Fig. 12-8, *B*. In each case the complex ending the pause achieves better intraventricular conduction.

Phase 3 and phase 4 AV blocks

Phase 3 and phase 4 AV blocks can also cause intermittent AV block whenever the necessary conditions exist in the only available AV connection. For example, in a patient with complete LBBB and hypopolarization of the right bundle, complete heart block could conceivably be precipitated by a critical slow rate (phase 4 AV block). On the other hand, if this same patient had abnormal lengthening of the refractory period in the right bundle, complete heart block could result from a critical increase in heart rate (phase 3 AV block).

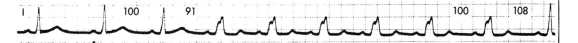

Fig. 12-6. Rate-dependent LBBB. As the sinus rhythm accelerates, LBBB develops when the rate exceeds 60 beats/min (cycle length <100); but for normal conduction to resume, the rate must fall below 60 beats/min (cycle length >100).

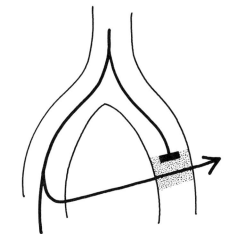

Fig. 12-7. Diagram to illustrate one of the two mechanisms responsible for the fact that the "critical rate" is different (faster) during acceleration from what it is during deceleration (see text).

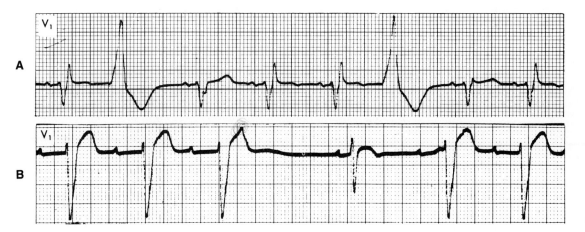

Fig. 12-8. Examples of postextrasystolic revelation of rate-dependent BBB. **A,** After each of the ventricular extrasystoles, the returning sinus beat manifests a lesser degree of RBBB than do the sinus beats ending the normal (shorter) sinus cycles. **B,** After three sinus beats conducted with first degree AV block and LBBB, a nonconducted atrial extrasystole results in a prolonged ventricular cycle, at the end of which the returning sinus beat is conducted with normal PR and normal intraventricular conduction, demonstrating that both the AV delay and the LBBB are rate dependent.

Morphology of aberration

Since aberrant ventricular conduction is either RBBB and/or hemiblock or LBBB, its recognition is determined by the ability to recognize the typical ECG patterns in these conditions. The morphology of RBBB and LBBB aberration are discussed below; the differential diagnosis in broad QRS tachycardia with application of all of the current and past rules is covered in Chapter 13.

RBBB ABERRATION. In 1965 and 1970 the RBBB pattern in V_1 (rSR′) was described as 10:1 in favor of aberration.[5,12] RBBB aberration is recognized because of the classical triphasic rSR′ pattern in V_1 and qRS pattern in V_6. Fig. 12-9 illustrates these two patterns. Note the narrow little q wave in V_6 that reflects normal septal activation. This q wave is a strong indicator of RBBB aberration but only if the pattern in V_1 is upright. In Table 12-2 Wellens and associates' study[4,13] shows the classical RBBB pattern in V_1 (rSR′; complex number 4) to be strongly in favor of aberration. This pattern was also demonstrated by Gulamhusein and others[14] who studied patients with atrial fibrillation, whereas the nonclassical RBBB pattern in V_1 (complex number 3) in Wellens and associates' study indicated aberration in 19 of 22 cases. In Table 12-3 note complex number 1; this classical triphasic RBBB pattern in V_6 (qRs) is strong evidence of aberration, but the rule can only be applied when the complex is upright in V_1.

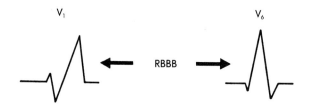

Fig. 12-9. Classical RBBB pattern in V_1 and V_6.

Table 12-2. Findings of Wellens and associates

Complex	V_1	Aberrant	Ventricular tachycardia
1		—	15
2		11	17
3		19	3
4		38	3
5		—	7
6		1	16
7		—	4
		$\overline{69}$	$\overline{65}$

From Wellens HJJ, Bar, and Lie: Am J Med 64:27, 1978, and Wellens HJJ and others: Am J Cardiol 49:187, 1982.

Table 12-3. Findings of Wellens and associates

Complex	V$_6$	Aberrant	Ventricular tachycardia
1		44	3
2		21	15
3		4	27
4		—	16
5		—	3
6		—	1
		69	65

From Wellens HJJ, Bar, and Lie: Am J Med 64:27, 1978, and Wellens HJJ and others: Am J Cardiol 49:187, 1982.

LBBB ABERRATION. Recent findings by Kindwall, Brown, and Josephson[15] indicate that the classical pattern of LBBB is a good clue to the presence of LBBB aberration. Thus signs seen in the initial part of the QRS in V_1 and V_2 are the key to the diagnosis of LBBB aberration. In such a case, the typical pattern of LBBB is also seen in lead V_6. If an r wave is present in either V_1 or V_2, in LBBB aberration it is narrow (<0.03 second), and the downstroke of the S wave is clean and swift (no slurs or notches). Because of the narrow r and/or the clean downstroke, the distance from the beginning of the QRS to the nadir of the S wave is 0.06 second or less. Fig. 12-10 illustrates the typical LBBB patterns that can be used to diagnose aberrant ventricular conduction. Hemiblock aberration is, of course, diagnosed by axis deviation with or without RBBB aberration.

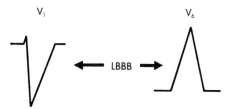

Fig. 12-10. Classical LBBB pattern in V_1 and V_6.

Additional helpful clues

In addition to the classical RBBB and LBBB patterns in V_1, V_2, and V_6, other signs of aberration are a normal axis, a QRS of less than 0.14 second in duration, preceding atrial activity, an anomalous second-in-the-row beat, and, in the RBBB pattern, the initial deflection in V_1 identical with that of conducted beats. AV dissociation, morphology of ectopic beats, history and physical examination, and other clues useful in the differential diagnosis of broad QRS tachycardia are discussed in Chapter 13.

QRS DURATION. A QRS of 0.14 second or less supports a diagnosis of aberration.[4,13] An exception to this rule is the fascicular VT of digitalis toxicity in which the QRS is usually narrower than 0.14 second.

NG ATRIAL ACTIVITY. Atrial ectopic beats before the broad complex in helpful in differentiating aberration from ectopy. However, an atrial beat can initiate VT, somewhat limiting the value of this clue.[16-23] In Figs. 1 and 12-12 APBs can be seen at the onset of the broad QRS tachycardia, suggesting a supraventricular mechanism.

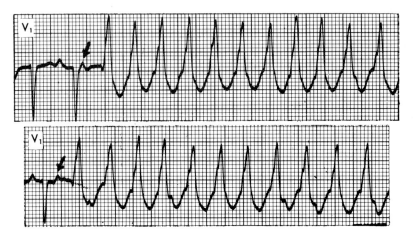

Fig. 12-11. Supraventricular tachycardia with RBBB aberration. P' waves are clearly visible at the onset of the tachycardia and clinch the diagnosis.

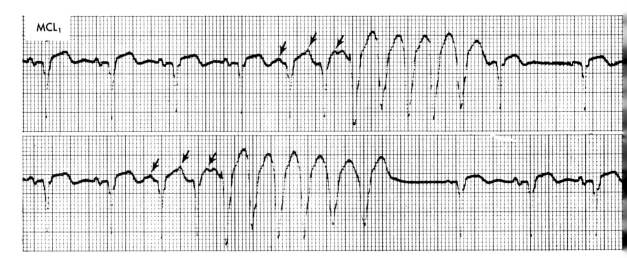

Fig. 12-12. Each strip contains a brief run of supraventricular tachycardia with LBBB aberration. Diagnosis is made because of antecedent P' waves, the width of the QRS (0.12 second), and the rate (200 beats/min). Note the momentary shift of pacemaker after each burst of tachycardia—the returning P' wave differs from the sinus P waves.

INITIAL DEFLECTION IDENTICAL WITH THAT OF CONDUCTED BEATS. This rule applies only to RBBB aberration because the initial forces in uncomplicated RBBB are normal (septal) and are best seen in V_1 and in the lateral leads I, aVL, and V_6. Fig. 12-13 contains both RBBB and LBBB aberrations. Note that the initial deflections of the RBBB aberration are almost the same as the sinus conducted beats, whereas those of the LBBB aberration are not. The presence of P′ waves in front of the anomalous complexes secures the diagnosis of aberration.

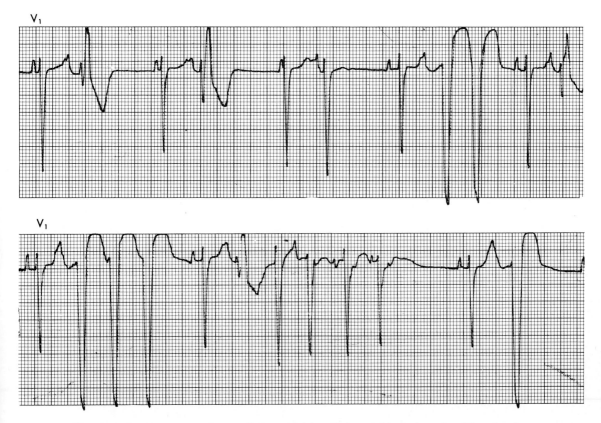

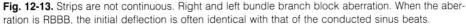

Fig. 12-13. Strips are not continuous. Right and left bundle branch block aberration. When the aberration is RBBB, the initial deflection is often identical with that of the conducted sinus beats.

SECOND-IN-THE-ROW ANOMALY. The reason the second in a row of rapid beats is most likely to be aberrant is that it is the only beat that ends a relatively short cycle preceded by a relatively long one. The duration of the action potential and hence the refractory period are directly related to the cardiac cycle. As the cycle lengthens or shortens, so does the refractory period (this is reflected in the QR interval, which shortens as the heart rate increases).

Fig. 12-14 illustrates short bursts of supraventricular tachycardia (SVT) in which only the first beat of the tachycardia (second in the row, counting the preceding sinus beat) is anomalous. The first premature beat shortens the cycle, causing itself to be conducted with RBBB aberration. Then the aberrant beat itself ends a relatively short cycle, creating a short refractory period for itself and giving the next beat a better chance for normal conduction. Unfortunately, according to the "rule of

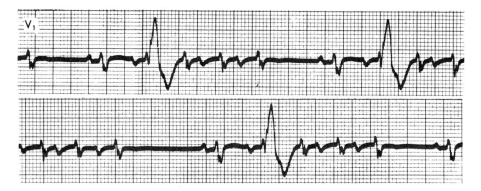

Fig. 12-14. Strips are continuous. Three short bursts of supraventricular tachycardia in which only the first beat (second in the row) develops ventricular aberration.

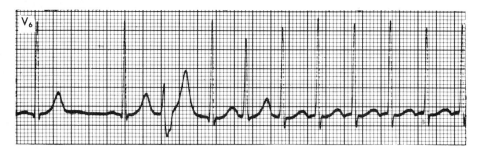

Fig. 12-15. Second in the row of rapid beats can be, and is diagrammed as, a ventricular extrasystole initiating a run of AV reciprocating tachycardia.

bigeminy,"[24] a lengthened cycle tends to precipitate a VPB; therefore the longer-shorter cycle sequence is inconclusive, and the morphology and presence of a P′ wave preceding the onset of tachycardia are clearly of more help in making the diagnosis of aberration (as illustrated in Fig. 12-14). In Fig. 12-15 the alternative mechanism is illustrated—a VPB initiates circus movement tachycardia. In this tracing the second in the row is also anomalous. However, the morphology of the anomalous beat (RS) and the absence of visible ectopic atrial activity strongly support a diagnosis of a VPB initiating circus movement tachycardia. The VPB is conducted up the accessory pathway to activate the atria and down the AV node to the ventricles.

Fig. 12-16 is another tracing in which the diagnosis of aberration of a single broad beat is mainly dependent on preceding atrial activity. In each of the three strips the second in a row of rapid beats is anomalous. The decision as to whether this broad beat is aberrant or ventricular ectopic is made on the basis of the P′ wave in front of all four of the broad beats. Carefully compare the T waves preceding the anomalous complexes with those of the other sinus beats—a superimposed P′ wave is clearly seen distorting the T wave before the broad beat. The mechanism of the paroxysmal supraventricular tachycardia (PSVT) that follows may be AV nodal reentry. In the first two tracings P′ waves are distorting out at the end of the QRS. In the bottom tracing the rhythm develops into atrial flutter (note the change of pattern and rate; the flutter waves look like elevated PR segments).

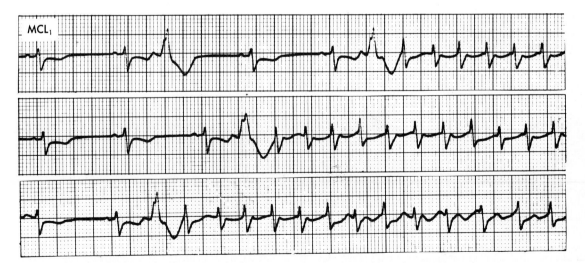

Fig. 12-16. Frequent atrial premature beats that initiate supraventricular tachycardia (SVT). The second in a row is aberrant. In the top two tracings the SVT is caused by AV nodal reentry. In the bottom tracing the mechanism is more likely atrial flutter.

Aberrancy in atrial fibrillation

Since there is always preceding atrial activity in atrial fibrillation, one relies heavily on morphology to distinguish between aberration and ectopy. This reliance is justified by the His bundle studies of Vera and co-workers[25] who used His bundle electrography to examine 1100 abnormal QRS complexes (750 ectopic, 350 aberrant) in patients with chronic atrial fibrillation. V_1 was the most helpful lead in differentiating aberration from ectopy, with the rSR' pattern affording 24:1 odds in favor of aberration. Gulamhusein and others[4] arrived at the same conclusion in 1985.

Ashman's phenomenon. The application of Ashman's phenomenon in atrial fibrillation is precarious since, because of concealed conduction, one never knows from the surface ECG exactly when a bundle branch is activated. It is known that the rampant electrical activity during atrial fibrillation incompletely penetrates the bundle of His and bundle branches (concealed conduction) and that the irregular ventricular rhythm during atrial fibrillation is one result. Thus there are often pauses longer than the actual refractory period of the AV conduction system. Therefore, if an aberrant beat does end a long-short cycle sequence during atrial fibrillation, it may be because of refractoriness of a bundle branch secondary to concealed conduction into it rather than because of changes in the length of the ventricular cycle. In more than 400 cases of chronic atrial fibrillation and 1100 anomalous beats, Vera and associates[25] did not find the Ashman's phenomenon helpful in differentiating aberration from ectopy. Gulamhusein and associates[14] examined 1068 wide QRS complexes in chronic atrial fibrillation and did not find Ashman's phenomenon specific for SVT.

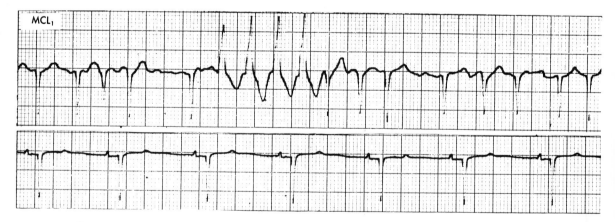

Fig. 12-17. Top strip shows atrial fibrillation with rapid ventricular response complicated by a four-beat run of aberrant conduction of RBBB type. Bottom strip was taken 30 minutes after 0.75 mg of digoxin was administered intravenously.

An equally important point establishing the invalidity of applying Ashman's phenomenon to atrial fibrillation is the "rule of bigeminy,"[24] which states that a long cycle tends to precipitate a VPB. Thus a long-short sequence ending with an anomalous beat is of no distinguishing value.

Fig. 12-17 shows an example of atrial fibrillation complicated by a rapid ventricular response (approximately 160 beats/min). Toward the middle of the top strip four beats are conducted with RBBB aberration. Although in the lead shown the morphology of these anomalous beats may be either aberrant or ectopic, a width of only 0.10 second in the QRS supports a diagnosis of aberration. Lead V_6 is often very helpful in such a case; a qRS pattern strongly indicates SVT.

The temptation is to misdiagnose and mistreat this short run of apparent ventricular tachycardia; but if one yields to this temptation, the result can be similar to the effect on the patient in Fig. 12-19. The proper treatment aims at restoring a normal ventricular rate—the golden rule of antiarrhythmic therapy—and it applies whether the anomalous beats are aberrant or, in fact, ectopic ventricular. In either situation the four available options are the use of digitalis, propranolol, verapamil, or cardioversion. In this case the bottom strip in Fig. 12-17 illustrates the prompt effect of 0.75 mg of digoxin administered intravenously.

In Fig. 12-18, A, there are a single anomalous beat, a classical triphasic RBBB pattern with the initial deflection the same as in the normally conducted complexes, and a QRS width of only 0.12 second—all signs in favor of aberration. In Fig. 12-18, B, there is a run of RBBB aberration and two isolated RBBB complexes.

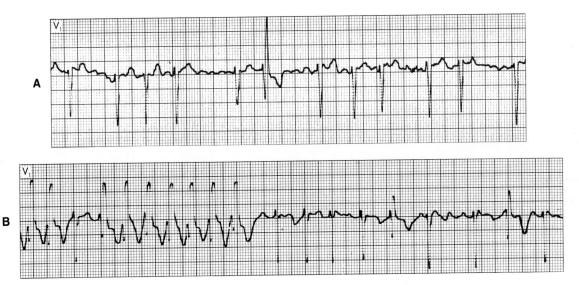

Fig. 12-18. RBBB aberration in atrial fibrillation.

rrancy in atrial tachycardia

Fig. 12-19 illustrates aberration that was misdiagnosed and thus led to gross mismanagement. The top strip shows the patient's rhythm on admission: atrial tachycardia with 2:1 AV conduction (note the nonconducted P waves partially hidden in the ventricular complexes). This patient was started on digitalis and by the next morning (second strip) frequently manifested 4:1 conduction ratios. Because of this satisfactory "impairment" of conduction, digitalis was discontinued, and quinidine was started. The bottom strip was taken the following morning and shows the situation that developed at approximately midnight and led to night-long erroneous therapy for ventricular tachycardia; the bottom strip, in fact, represents atrial tachycardia with 1:1 AV conduction and RBBB aberration. The quinidine—perhaps partly through its antivagal effect but certainly through its slowing effect on the atrial rate (from 210 to 192 beats/min)—enabled the AV junction to conduct all the ectopic atrial impulses. The resulting much-increased ventricular rate (from approximately 90 to 192 beats/min) produced a dangerous hypotension from which the patient was finally rescued by the administration of a combination of a pressor agent and countershock.

In 1958 Rosenblueth[26] documented the effect of atrial rate on normal AV conduction by pacing the atria of normal dogs. He found that at an average rate of 257 beats/min the animals developed Wenckebach periods and began to drop beats; and at an average rate of 285 beats/min they developed constant 2:1 conduction. Consider what this means in terms of ventricular rate. At an atrial rate of 286 beats/min

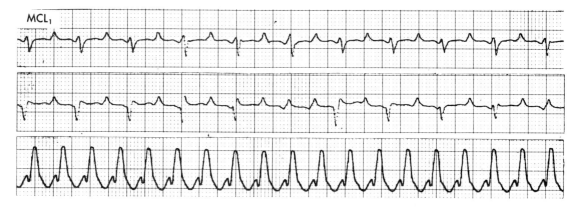

Fig. 12-19. Strips are not continuous. Top strip (on admission) shows atrial tachycardia with 2:1 AV conduction. Middle strip (next day) shows 2:1 and 4:1 conduction. Bottom strip (24 hours later) shows a slower atrial rate with 1:1 conduction and RBBB aberration—mistaken and treated for hours as ventricular tachycardia.

the ventricular rate is 143 beats/min. If the atrial rate slows by only 30 beats/min (to 256), conduction will be 1:1 with a ventricular rate of 256 beats/min. Thus, with slowing of the atrial rate by only 30 beats/min, the ventricular rate increases by 113 beats/min. This is why it can be so dangerous to give atrial slowing drugs such as lidocaine, quinidine, or even procainamide in the presence of atrial flutter or fibrillation when the ventricular response is already uncomfortably fast.[27] For example, if atrial flutter at a rate of 300 beats/min is associated with a 2:1 response, producing a ventricular rate of 150 beats/min, and a drug such as lidocaine is administered, the atrial rate may slow to 250 beats/min, and AV conduction may increase to 1:1, producing a dangerous ventricular rate of 250 beats/min.

Aberrancy in atrial flutter

From a therapeutic point of view an important form of aberration may complicate atrial flutter. Uncomplicated and untreated atrial flutter usually manifests a 2:1 AV conduction ratio. If digitalis or propranolol is then administered, the conduction pattern often changes to alternating 2:1 and 4:1, producing alternately longer and shorter cycles (Fig. 12-20). At this stage the beats that end the shorter cycles may develop aberrant conduction; and if the patient is receiving digitalis, ventricular bigeminy secondary to digitalis toxicity is likely to be diagnosed. The drug is then wrongfully discontinued when, in fact, the situation calls for more digitalis to reduce conduction still further to a constant 4:1 ratio and a *normal ventricular rate*— always the immediate goal of therapy.

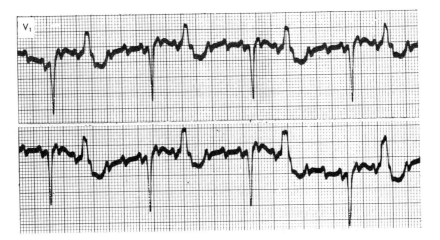

Fig. 12-20. Atrial flutter with alternating 2:1 and 4:1 conduction and RBBB aberration of the beats that end the shorter cycles—readily mistaken for ventricular bigeminy.

Alternating aberrancy

It is not uncommon to see both RBBB and LBBB aberration in the same patient. This is the case in Figs. 12-13 and 12-21. An interesting feature of each of these tracings is the abrupt switch from one BBB form of aberration to the other after a single intervening normally conducted beat. The mechanism of this phenomenon is unexplained but is sufficiently characteristic to assist in differentiating bilateral aberration from bifocal ectopy. It is of interest that the first published example of ventricular aberration (Lewis in 1910[1]) was alternating aberration complicating atrial bigeminy. This tracing is shown in Fig. 12-22. A contemporary example of a similar alternating aberration is in Fig. 12-23.

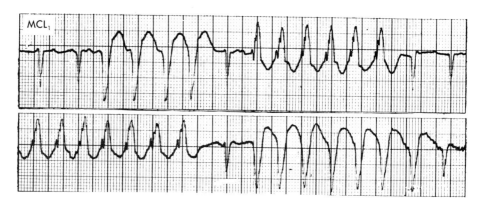

Fig. 12-21. Both strips illustrate the abrupt change from one BBB aberration to the other BBB, with a single intervening normally conducted beat.

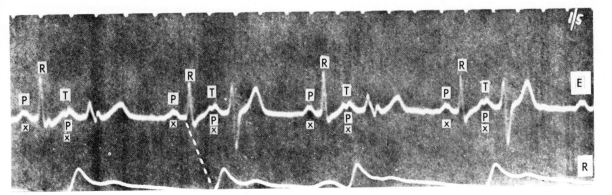

Fig. 12-22. First published example of ventricular aberration (Lewis in 1910[1]). Sinus rhythm with atrial bigeminy; each extrasystole is conducted aberrantly, but the form of aberration alternates. *E,* electrocardiogram; *R,* radial pulse.

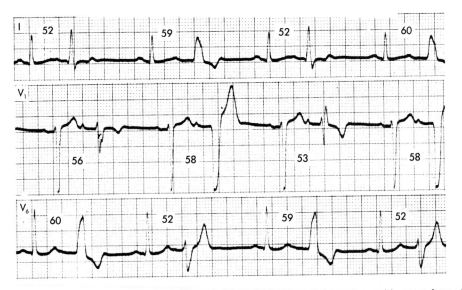

Fig. 12-23. Sinus rhythm with atrial bigeminy. The shorter extrasystolic cycles end in some form of RBBB aberration, whereas the longer ones end with LBBB aberration. Beats with RBBB, as evidenced by the slightly increased height of the R waves in lead I and the rS pattern in V$_6$, presumably manifest bifascicular aberration (RBBB plus left anterior hemiblock). In V$_1$ the first atrial extrasystole shows only the earliest sign of RBBB, namely notching of the terminal upstroke.

Clinical implications

RBBB aberration is often considered physiological by many (secondary to tachycardia or sudden shortening of the cycle). Phase 4 and/or LBBB aberration, on the other hand, are thought to indicate underlying cardiac disease. Whatever the cause, aberration is always secondary to another primary disturbance and of itself never requires treatment.

It is important to recognize ventricular aberration because it may be mistaken for ventricular ectopy, causing the administration of unnecessary drugs and delaying the treatment and the diagnosis of the mechanism of supraventricular tachycardia.

Summary

Aberrant ventricular conduction is a form of transient BBB and/or hemiblock, occurring most often as phase 3 aberration but also at times as phase 4 aberration. The morphological clues that identify ventricular aberration are the classical forms of RBBB and LBBB as seen in leads V_1, V_2, and V_6. When the complex is mainly upright in V_1, an rSR' in that lead or a qRs complex in V_6 indicates RBBB aberration. When the complex is mainly negative in V_1, a sharp, narrow r (if one is present) and a smooth, quick downstroke to the S indicate LBBB aberration.

Other indicators of aberrant ventricular conduction are a QRS width of 0.14 second or less, preceding atrial activity, initial deflection identical with that of conducted beats in the RBBB pattern, and second-in-the-row anomaly.

REFERENCES

1. Lewis R: Paroxysmal tachycardia, the result of ectopic impulse formation, Heart 1:262, 1910.
2. Gouaux JL and Ashman R: Auricular fibrillation with aberration simulating ventricular paroxysmal tachycardia, Am Heart J 34:366, 1947.
3. Moe GK, Mendez C, and Han J: Aberrant AV impulse propagation in the dog heart: a study of functional bundle branch block, Circ Res 16:261, 1965.
4. Wellens HJJ, Bar FWHM, and Lie KI: The value of the electrocardiogram in the differential diagnosis of a tachycardia with a widened QRS complex, Am J Med 64:27, 1978.
5. Sandler IA and Marriott HJL: The differential morphology of anomalous ventricular complexes of RBBB type in lead V_1: ventricular ectopy versus aberration, Circulation 31:551, 1965.
6. Kulbertus HE and others: Vectorcardiographic study of aberrant conduction, Br Heart J 38:549, 1976.
7. Spear JF and Moore EN: Supernormal excitability and conduction. In Wellens HJJ, Lie KI, and Janse MJ, editors: The conduction system of the heart; structure, function, and clinical implications, Philadelphia, 1976, Lea & Febiger.
8. Singer DH, Lazzara R, and Hoffman BF: Interrelationships between automaticity and conduction in Purkinje fibers, Circ Res 21:537, 1967.
9. Singer KH, Yeh BK, and Hoffman BF: Aberration of supraventricular escape beats, Fed Proc 23:158, 1967 (abstract).
10. Singer DH and Cohen HC: Aberrancy: electrophysiologic aspects and clinical correlations. In Mandel WJ, editor: Cardiac arrhythmias, Philadelphia, 1987, JB Lippincott Co.

11. Rosenbaum MB and others: Relevance of phase 3 and phase 4 block in clinical electrophysiology. In Befeler B, editor: Selected topics in cardiac arrhythmias, Mt Kisco, NY, 1980, Futura Publishing Co, Inc.

12. Marriott HJL: Differential diagnosis of supraventricular and ventricular tachycardia, Geriatrics 25:91, 1970.

13. Wellens HJJ and others: Medical treatment of ventricular tachycardia: considerations in the selection of patients for surgical treatment, Am J Cardiol 49:187, 1982.

14. Gulamhusein S and others: Electrocardiographic criteria for differentiating aberrancy and ventricular extrasystole in chronic atrial fibrillation: validation by intracardiac recordings, J Electrocardiol 18:41, 1985.

15. Kindwall E, Brown J, and Josephson ME: Electrocardiographic criteria for ventricular tachycardia in wide complex left bundle branch block morphology tachycardia, Am J Cardiol 61:1279, 1988.

16. Weilens HJJ and others: Initiation and termination of ventricular tachycardia by supraventricular stimuli, Am J Cardiol 46:576, 1980.

17. Wellens HJJ, Schuilenberg RM, and Durrer D: Electrical stimulation of the heart in patients with ventricular tachycardia, Circulation 46:216, 1972.

18. Guerot U and others: Tachycardie par re-entree de branch a branche, Arch Mal Coeur 67:1, 1974.

19. Wellens HJJ: Pathophysiology of ventricular tachycardia in man, Arch Intern Med 68:969, 1975.

20. Denes P and others: Electrophysiological studies in patients with chronic recurrent ventricular tachycardia, Circulation, 545D:229, 1976.

21. Wellens HJJ, Duren DR, and Lie KL: Observations on mechanisms of ventricular tachycardia in man, Circulation 54:237, 1976.

22. Myerburg RJ and others: Ventricular ectopic activity after premature atrial beats in acute myocardial infarction, Br Heart J 39:1033, 1977.

23. Zipes DP and others: Atrial induction of ventricular tachycardia: reentry versus triggered automaticity, Am J Cardiol 44:1, 1979.

24. Langendorf LR, Pick A, and Wintermitz M: Mechanisms of intermittent bigeminy. 1. Appearance of ectopic beats dependent upon the length of the ventricular cycle, the "rule of bigeminy," Circulation 11:422, 1955.

25. Vera Z and others: His bundle electrography for evaluation of criteria in differentiating ventricular ectopy from aberrancy in atrial fibrillation, Circulation 46(suppl II):90, 1972.

26. Rosenblueth A: Two processes for auriculoventricular and ventriculo-auricular propagation of impulses in the heart, Am J Physiol 194:495, 1958.

27. Marriott HJL and Bieza CF: Alarming ventricular acceleration after lidocaine administration, Chest 61:682, 1972.

CHAPTER 13

Differential diagnosis in the broad QRS tachycardia

Because new drugs for the treatment of supraventricular tachycardia (SVT) can be fatal to the patient with ventricular tachycardia (VT),[1] the differential diagnosis in broad QRS tachycardia has become extremely important.

The "lidocaine reflex"

In the early days of coronary care units, diagnostic errors were usually made because aberration was not recognized. Broad beats would often elicit the "lidocaine reflex" simply because they were broad, thus delaying initiation of appropriate therapy for SVT, severely compromising patients with poor left ventricular function who possibly could not tolerate SVT with rapid ventricular rates and, on occasion, resulting in enough slowing of the atrial rate to permit 1:1 conduction.[2]

Overdiagnosis of aberration

Today informed physicians and coronary care nurses are well acquainted with the mechanism of aberrant ventricular conduction. However, once the mechanism of aberration was learned, the pendulum quickly swung in the opposite direction to overdiagnosis of aberration.[1,3-5] The greatest number of errors in the diagnosis of broad QRS tachycardias are made because those responsible strive to prove aberration, often unaware of the morphological clues that identify VT. In many cases the only guideline applied to the broad QRS tachycardia is the 23-year-old morphological finding of rSR′ in V_1. Although it is true that this pattern usually indicates SVT with right bundle branch block (RBBB) aberration, many more important morphological rules provide strong evidence for VT.

New findings

Invasive studies have not only confirmed our present knowledge but have provided new clues as well, and they have established the surface ECG as a superior diagnostic tool.[6-9] Recently described electrocardiographical findings indicate that the same diagnostic results can be achieved in both narrow and broad QRS tachycardia using multichannel ECG recordings as with invasive, expensive techniques.[7-13] Since the introduction of His bundle electrograms, thousands of patients have been studied, providing firm surface ECG signs of VT and aberrant ventricular conduction.[10,14]

In the 1985 annual Bishop Lecture for the American College of Cardiology, Wellens[14] summarized the important ECG findings confirmed by electrophysiological studies. Because these new diagnostic clues have elevated the value of the ECG and because new ones are sure to emerge, he emphasized the importance of electrocardiography in the training and ongoing education of cardiologists and internists. He warned against unnecessary invasive cardiology in the differential diagnosis of arrhythmias and urged the use of multichannel ECGs. This chapter defines and illustrates new diagnostic clues on the surface ECG that, when applied to the regular tachycardia with a broad QRS complex, assure 90% accuracy in diagnosing the site of origin of the tachycardia.[9,10]

When in doubt

When a patient presents with a broad QRS tachycardia, diagnostic errors can be avoided by staying calm and following the rules.[10] If the patient is in poor hemodynamic condition, cardiovert; otherwise, systematically follow the diagnostic steps described below that will differentiate aberration from ectopy. Above all, when in doubt about the origin of the tachycardia, Wellens and associates[10] warn against the use of verapamil, suggesting the use of intravenous procainamide instead. One study observed a 44% incidence (11 out of 25 patients) of severe hemodynamic deterioration after intravenous verapamil (5 to 10 mg) was administered for sustained VT, necessitating immediate cardioversion.[15] Under less controlled conditions it is possible that hypotension may render the arrhythmia impossible to cardiovert. Procainamide has advantages in both VT and SVT: in addition to being antifibrillatory and terminating VT, it also slows conduction in accessory pathways and in the retrograde fast AV nodal pathway[16] and thus can terminate both circus movement tachycardia, which uses an accessory pathway, and the common form of AV nodal reentry, which uses a retrograde AV nodal fast pathway and anterograde slow pathway.

Hemodynamic status and age

In the differential diagnosis of broad QRS tachycardia, hemodynamic status and age *should not be used* since VT can occur at all ages and some patients are hemodynamically stable in spite of VT and are hemodynamically compromized during SVT.[17] More emphasis should be placed on ECG findings in broad QRS tachycardia than on the patient's age or hemodynamic status.

Steps in the differential diagnosis

The differential diagnosis of broad QRS tachycardia is made by evaluating QRS configuration, width, and axis and by recognition of AV dissociation. Precordial concordancy, capture beats, and fusion beats are signs of VT, although their occurrence is not frequent.

LEADS OF CHOICE. To make a diagnosis on the basis of morphology, it is first necessary to record the tachycardia in as many of the 12 leads as possible. If your system does not have the capability for recording concurrent leads, begin sequentially to record leads V_1, V_2, and V_6 for morphological clues and leads I and aVF for axis. If you are faced with the choice of only one lead because time is a factor, record V_1 (or MCL_1). If this is not done, morphology cannot be used, and, being left with the sometimes futile search for P waves to prove AV dissociation, your chances for a correct diagnosis plunge dramatically.

QRS CONFIGURATION. For the purpose of making a differential diagnosis on the basis of morphology, we have divided the broad QRS tachycardias into two groups: those that are mainly positive in V_1 and those that are mainly negative in V_1. (The references refer to the upright complex as "RBBB" type tachycardia and the negative complex as "LBBB" type tachycardia.[9,10])

In applying the morphological rules, it is important to understand that the clues specific for one type of tachycardia cannot be used for the other. For example, a q wave in lead V_6 could mean either VT or SVT, depending on the shape of the complex in V_1; if V_1 is upright, a little q in V_6 indicates SVT, but if V_1 is negative, it indicates VT.

QRS mainly positive in V_1. Fig. 13-1 illustrates the distinguishing features in VT and SVT when the QRS is mainly upright in V_1.

Ventricular tachycardia. When the QRS is mainly positive in V_1, a monophasic complex or diphasic complex[7,8,17-19] in V_1 and/or an R wave in V_6 that is deeper than the S wave is tall indicates VT. Gulamhusein and associates[19] gave the monophasic complex in V_1 42:1 odds.

Rabbit ear clue. In 1970 Marriott[17] reported on the studies conducted by Gozensky and Thorne, which were later published by them,[18] describing the now widely accepted "rabbit ear clue" as an aid in distinguishing ventricular ectopy from aberration: when there are two positive peaks in V_1, ectopy is indicated if the left peak is taller. When the right rabbit ear is the taller, it is not helpful in distinguishing ectopy from aberration because it is common to both. Gozensky and Thorne's findings were later confirmed by Wellens,[3] who found the taller left rabbit-ear configuration only in patients with ventricular tachycardia. Gulamhusein and others[20] found that the rabbit ear clue indicated ventricular ectopy 17:1.

Supraventricular tachycardia. Typical RBBB patterns (i.e., triphasic patterns in V_1 [rSR'] or in V_6 [qRs]) support a diagnosis of SVT with RBBB aberration.

QRS mainly negative in V_1

Ventricular tachycardia. Until the recent findings from Kindwall, Brown, and Josephson[9] in Philadelphia, there have been few morphological clues to distinguish aberration from ectopy when the QRS is mainly negative in V_1. Based on their findings, there are four morphological ECG signs found in leads V_1, V_2, and V_6 that are highly predictive of VT; they are as follows:

1. A broad R of 0.04 second or more in V_1 or V_2.[9,19-21]
2. A notched or slurred downstroke on the S or QS wave in V_1 or V_2.
3. A distance of 0.07 second or more from the onset of the ventricular complex to the nadir of the QS or S in V_1 or V_2.
4. Any Q in V_6, but ONLY if the complex is mainly negative in V_1; this clue cannot be applied to the tachycardia that is positive in V_1.

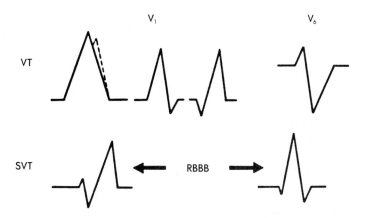

Fig. 13-1. When V_1 is positive, ventricular ectopy is indicated in that lead by a monophasic or diphasic complex or by the rabbit ear clue (left ear taller than the right). Supraventricular ectopy (RBBB aberration) is indicated by triphasic patterns, rSR' in V_1 and qRs in V_6. *VT,* Ventricular tachycardia; *SVT,* supraventricular tachycardia; *RBBB,* right bundle branch block. (From Conover M: Understanding electrocardiography, ed 5, St. Louis, 1988, The CV Mosby Co.)

Table 13-1 lists the specificity, sensitivity, and predictive accuracy of each of the four findings. Fig. 13-2 illustrates the distinguishing features between VT and SVT when V_1 is mainly negative. It is important to use both V_1 and V_2 since initial forces are often isoelectric in V_1, leading to misclassification of tracings. The criterion most susceptible to error, according to Kindwall, Brown and Josephson,[9] is measurement of the distance to the nadir of the S wave because this point is sometimes so deep that it goes off the graph paper and cannot be seen and because of the inherent limitation in measuring intervals at paper speeds used clinically (25 mm/sec).

Before Kindwall, Brown, and Josephson's recent studies,[9] the broad R wave with a mainly negative complex in V_1 as an indicator of ventricular ectopy was pointed out by Rosenbaum[20] in 1969 as part of an electrocardiographical trilogy, with the other two findings being right axis deviation and a monophasic R in V_6. In 1972 Swanick, La Camera, and Marriott[21] also pointed out the broad R with the mainly negative complex in V_1 as a sign of VT.

Limitations associated with this new criteria for the differential diagnosis when the broad QRS tachycardia is mainly negative in V_1 include the following[9]:

1. Left bundle branch block (LBBB) in sinus tachycardia or atrial flutter with the same morphology as VT (e.g., broad R and slurred downstroke in V_1 and/or V_2). In such a case the sinus rhythm tracing without the tachycardia would expose the problem.
2. Antidromic circus movement tachycardia (using an accessory pathway in the anterograde direction). This mechanism produces a tachycardia identical in morphology to VT.
3. Antiarrhythmic drugs that slow conduction, possibly producing a QRS that fits the morphological description for VT. These drugs may broaden the R wave and produce a delayed S nadir in V_1 or V_2, although a Q wave in V_6 would not be affected.

Table 13-1. ECG signs of VT when mainly negative in V_1 (using leads V_1, V_2, and V_6)

Criteria	Specificity (%)	Sensitivity (%)	Predictive accuracy (%)
R > 30 msec in V_1 or V_2	100	36	100
Any Q in V_6	96	55	98
>60 msec to S nadir in V_1 or V_2	96	63	98
Notched downstroke in S or QS in V_1 or V_2	96	36	97
Combined criteria	89	100	96

Modified from Kindwall E, Brown J, and Josephson ME: Am J Cardiol 61:1279, 1988.

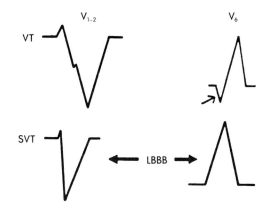

Fig. 13-2. When V_1 is negative, ventricular ectopy is indicated in V_1 and V_2 by a broad R, slurred or notched downstroke to the S, and/or a distance of >0.06 sec to the nadir of the S wave. Supraventricular ectopy (LBBB aberration) is indicated in V_1 and V_2 by a narrow, sharp r and a sleek, quick downstroke to the S or in V_6 by a monophasic R (as in the typical pattern of LBBB). The typical V_6 LBBB pattern shown here may also be seen in VT and by itself does not indicate SVT. *VT*, ventricular tachycardia; *SVT*, supraventricular tachycardia; *LBBB*, left bundle branch block. (From Conover M: Understanding electrocardiography, ed 5, St. Louis, 1988, The CV Mosby Co.)

Supraventricular tachycardia. In contrast, the pattern in V_1 and V_2 of SVT with LBBB aberration has a narrow r (if one is present) and a clean, swift downstroke of the S wave. This clean, sharp downstroke pattern is also seen in sinus rhythm with LBBB. In V_6 the typical LBBB pattern (monophasic R) is also seen and compliments the pattern in V_1 and V_2; however, the monophasic R in V_6 is also seen in conjunction with the typical VT pattern of a broad R or slurred downstroke in V_1 or V_2.

QRS WIDTH. A QRS of more than 0.14 second favors VT. Exceptions to this rule are some cases of preexisting bundle branch block, antidromic circus movement tachycardia, atrial fibrillation with conduction over an accessory pathway, and digitalis toxicity.

QRS AXIS. An axis in "no-man's-land" (−90 to −180 degrees) is a widely recognized strong indicator of VT. Otherwise, axis deviation is only helpful when the tachycardia is mainly upright in V_1, in which case both an abnormal left (>−30 degrees) axis and an abnormal right (>+120 degrees) axis favor VT.[14] When the pattern is mainly negative in V_1, left axis deviation has low specificity (41%) and is therefore of no value by itself.[9,22]

AV DISSOCIATION

Independent P waves. Half of all VTs have AV dissociation, a few of the other half have atrial fibrillation, and the rest have some form of retrograde conduction to the atria (usually 2:1 retrograde conduction or some form of retrograde Wenckebach period).[7,10] AV dissociation is recognized on the ECG when regular independent P waves are seen (Fig. 13-3).

In Fig. 13-4 there is 2:1 retrograde conduction and therefore VT. In Fig. 13-5, P waves are easily seen in leads II, III, and V_1; they do not have a constant relationship to the QRS. Therefore there is either AV dissociation or some type of retrograde conduction to the atria. When the RP intervals are measured, a Wenckebach pattern emerges. There is 4:3 retrograde Wenckebach conduction from the VT (i.e., the RP gets longer and longer for three cycles, and then the fourth P wave is dropped).

ADDITIONAL HELPFUL CLUES

Concordant precordial pattern, capture beats, and fusion beats. A concordant precordial pattern (all positive or all negative complexes in the chest leads) is a strong indicator of VT, as are capture beats and fusion beats. Capture beats and fusion beats occasionally occur during VT when a sinus impulse is conducted into the ventricles and either entirely captures the ventricles or collides with the ventricular ectopic impulse (fusion); each occurrence results in a beat that is narrower than those of the tachycardia (Fig. 13-6).

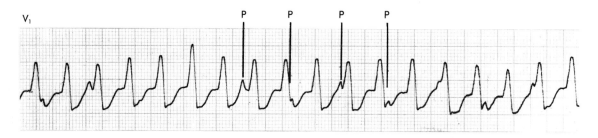

Fig. 13-3. Ventricular tachycardia with AV dissociation. Note the regular and independent P waves in this tracing. If only three complexes were available, one would be able to identify P waves and lack of 1:1 conduction. (From Conover M: Understanding electrocardiography, ed 5, St. Louis, The CV Mosby Co.)

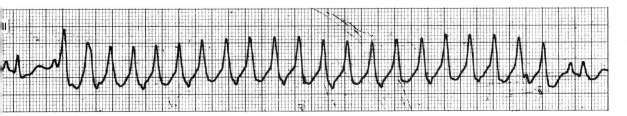

Fig. 13-4. Ventricular tachycardia with 2:1 retrograde conduction. The VA conduction ratio is very apparent when the whole tracing is viewed. When only two complexes are available, a P wave is seen associated with one QRS and not with another . . . lack of 1:1 conduction.

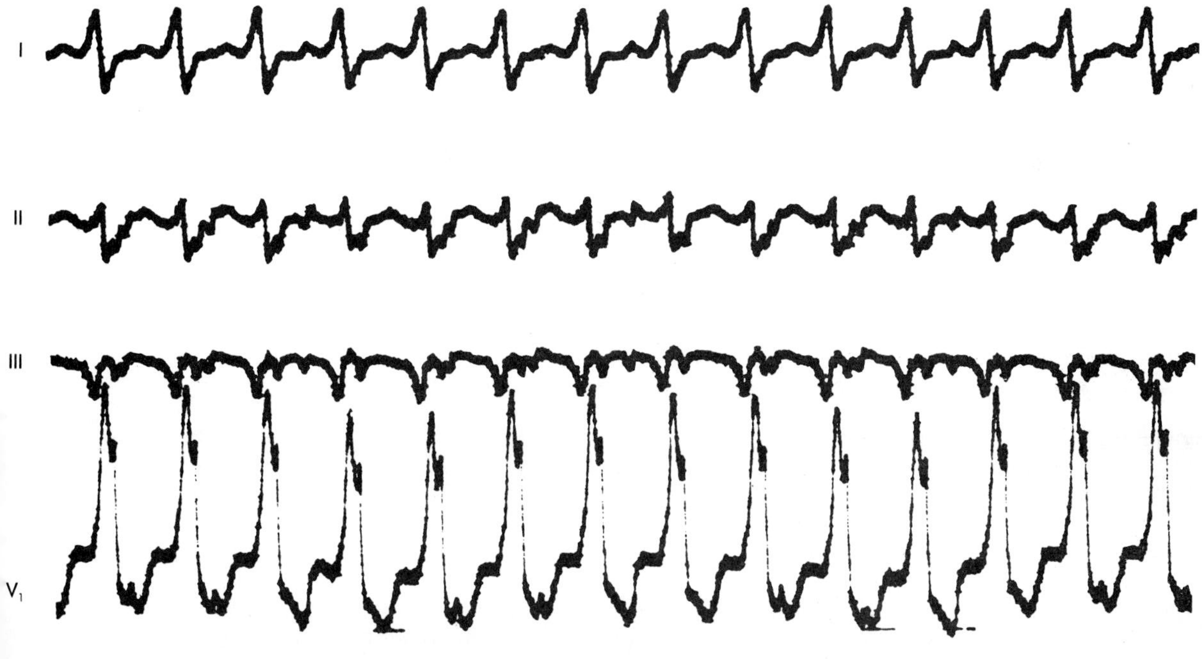

Fig. 13-5. Ventricular tachycardia with 4:3 retrograde Wenckebach period. The RP interval gets longer and longer until there is a dropped P wave. (Courtesy Hein JJ Wellens, MD.)

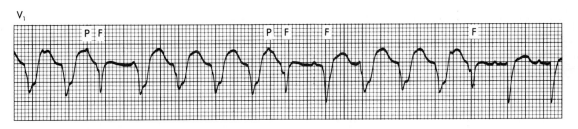

Fig. 13-6. Ventricular fusion *(F)* in ventricular tachycardia.

Negative QRS in lead I. Swanick, La Camera, and Marriott[22] observed that two thirds of the examples of right ventricular ectopic beats under investigation had a negative QRS in lead I, a polarity that was not found in any of the examined examples of LBBB. This observation would reflect one of Rosenbaum's three findings[21] in right ventricular ectopy (right axis deviation), or it could indicate an axis in "no-man's-land," another strong indicator of ventricular ectopy.

QRS deeper in V_4 than in V_1. Also in Swanick, La Camera, and Marriott's study,[22] more than half of the right ventricular ectopics had a more deeply negative QRS complex (QS or rS) in V_4 than in V_1, whereas only 7% of the examples of LBBB manifested a similar V_4/V_1 relationship.

BEDSIDE DIAGNOSIS OF VT

Physical signs. As well as evaluating the ECG, the clinician should inspect the patient for physical signs that are hallmarks of AV dissociation: irregular cannon A waves in the jugular pulse, varying intensity of S_1, and beat-to-beat changes in systolic blood pressure, indicated by changing Korotkoff sounds.[7,16,23] Although several cases of SVT with aberration and AV dissociation have been reported, AV dissociation remains a valid diagnostic clue that is highly suggestive of VT.[7]

History. Tchou and associates[24] found that the patient's history can be helpful in improving the clinical diagnosis of VT. Their study involved 31 consecutive patients referred for ECG documentation of sustained broad QRS tachycardia. Each patient was asked if he had had a prior myocardial infarction and if the symptoms of tachycardia started only after the infarction. A "yes" answer to both questions prompted a diagnosis of VT. Twenty-nine patients had VT, and 28 of them were correctly diagnosed through the history alone.

Clinical application

In Figs. 13-7 to 13-18 there are no legends so that you can try your skill in differentiating aberration from ectopy. Remember, follow the four rules: (1) morphology; (2) axis; (3) QRS width; and (4) AV dissociation or at least lack of 1:1 conduction. Look for P waves distorting ST segments, T waves, and QRS complexes. Observe the polarity of the QRS complexes in the precordial leads and look for fusion beats. Write down your conclusions and check them with the answers below.

QRS morphology. The QRS in Fig. 13-7 is V_1-negative, with a slurred down-stroke in V_1 and an interval of 0.13 second from the onset to the nadir of the QS complex. There is concordant precordial negativity—signs of VT.

Axis. The axis is beyond −30 degrees and is not helpful when the QRS is mainly negative in V_1.

QRS width. It is >0.14 second, a sign of VT.

AV dissociation. Independent P waves are seen in leads I, III, aVR, and aVF, and one P wave is seen in V_4, V_5, and V_6, a sign of VT.

Diagnosis. The diagnosis is VT.

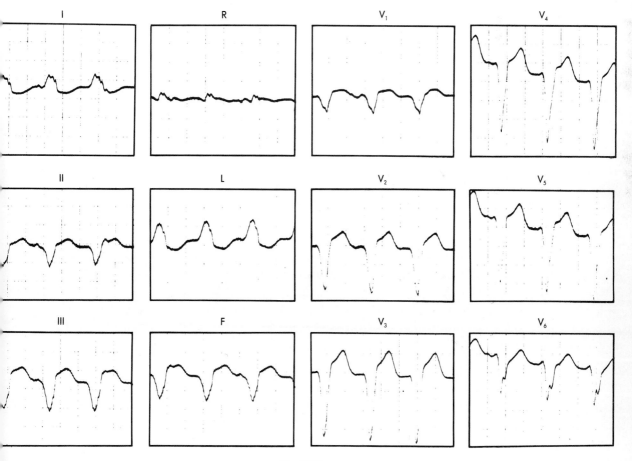

Fig. 13-7

QRS morphology. The QRS in Fig. 13-8 is V_1-negative, with a sharp, narrow r in V_1 and V_2 and a clean downstroke of the S wave until just before reaching its nadir. The distance from the onset of the QRS to the nadir of the S wave is at least 0.08 second; thus there are two signs of LBBB aberration (narrow R and clean downstroke) and one of VT (0.08 second to the nadir of the S).

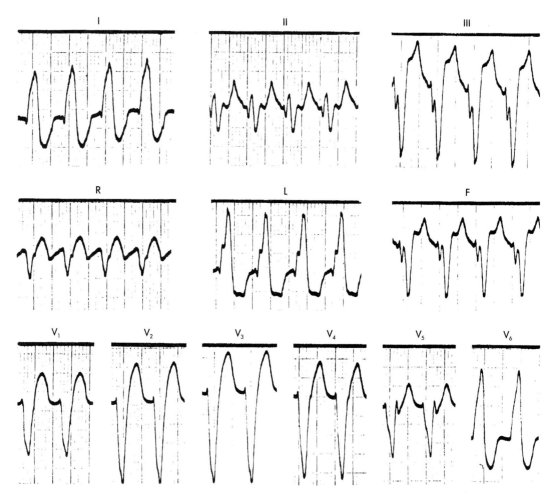

Fig. 13-8. (From Stein E: The electrocardiogram, Philadelphia, 1976, WB Saunders Co.)

Axis. The axis is beyond −30 degrees—not helpful when the QRS is mainly negative in V_1.

QRS width. It is >0.14 second, a sign of VT.

AV dissociation. P waves are not seen (unhelpful).

Diagnosis. The diagnosis is SVT with LBBB aberration because of the narrow r and clean downstroke of the S wave. Fig. 13-9 is lead III from the same patient after carotid sinus massage, revealing an underlying mechanism of atrial flutter.

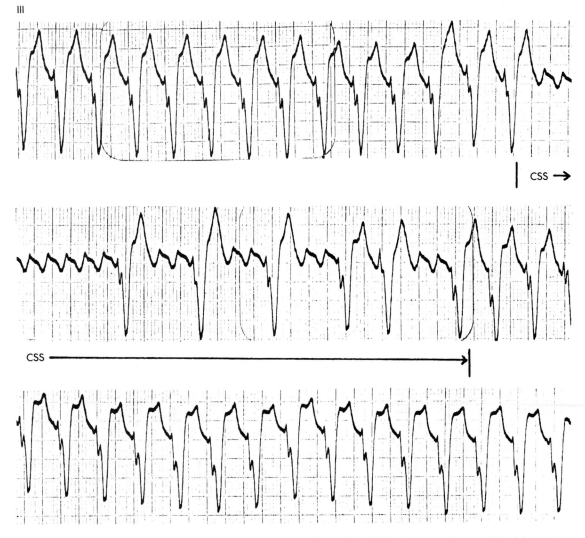

Fig. 13-9. Same patient after carotid sinus massage. (From Stein E: The electrocardiogram, Philadelphia, 1976, WB Saunders Co.)

QRS morphology. The QRS in Fig. 13-10 is V_1-positive, with a diphasic complex (Rs) in V_1 and an S wave in V_6 that is deeper than the R wave is tall—signs of VT.

Axis. The axis is right at approximately +125 degrees, a sign of VT.

QRS width. It is 0.18 second, a sign of VT.

AV dissociation. AV dissociation is present, a sign of VT. A P wave is plainly visible in lead II just before the first QRS complex. One is also distorting the third QRS. The P waves are independent of the ventricular rhythm. The P-like deflection in V_1 is really a negative T and illustrates the pitfalls associated with looking for P waves in broad QRS tachycardia.

Fusion beats. There are bonus clues in this ECG—fusion beats, which are indicative of VT. (See if you can locate them before reading further). They are the second beat in simultaneous leads I, II, and III and the last beat in simultaneous leads V_1, V_2, and V_3.

Diagnosis. The diagnosis is VT.

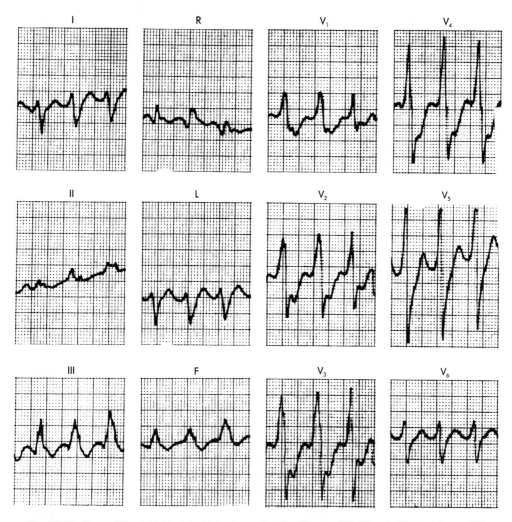

Fig. 13-10. (From Gilbert M: Ventricular tachycardias. In Wagner GS, Waugh RA, and Ramo BW, editors: Cardiac arrhythmias, New York, 1983, Churchill Livingstone Inc. By permission of Churchill Livingstone Inc.)

QRS morphology. The QRS in Fig. 13-11 is V_1-negative, with a narrow r and clean downstroke to the S in V_1 and V_2—a sign of SVT.

Axis. The axis is beyond -30 degrees, not helpful when the QRS is mainly negative in V_1.

QRS width. It is approximately 0.14 second.

AV dissociation. P waves are not seen (inconclusive).

Diagnosis. The diagnosis is SVT with LBBB aberration.

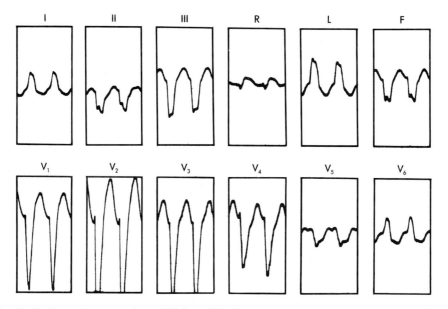

Fig. 13-11. (From Josephson M and Wellens HJJ: How to approach complex arrhythmias, Miami, 1987, Medtronic.)

QRS morphology. The QRS in Fig. 13-12 is V_1-negative, with a broad R, a slurred downstroke to the S, and a delay of 0.08 second from the onset of the R to the nadir of the S wave in V_1 and V_2. In V_6 there is a Q (remember to apply this clue only with the upright QRS in V_1). There are four signs of VT.

Axis. The axis is beyond −30 degrees, not helpful when the QRS is mainly negative in V_1.

QRS width. It is 0.18 second (in V_4) (supports VT).

AV dissociation. Yes—an independent P wave is in V_5 and it supports VT.

Diagnosis. The diagnosis is VT.

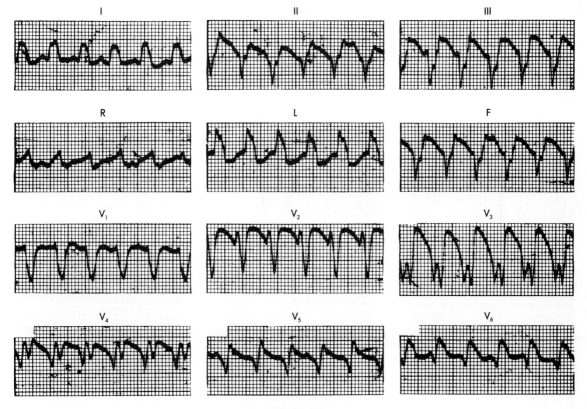

Fig. 13-12

QRS morphology. The QRS in Fig. 13-13 is V_1-negative, with a narrow r and clean downstroke to the S in V_1 and V_2—a sign of SVT.

Axis. The axis is normal (not helpful).

QRS width. It is approximately 0.18 second (supports VT).

AV dissociation. P waves are not seen (inconclusive).

Diagnosis. The diagnosis is SVT with LBBB aberration.

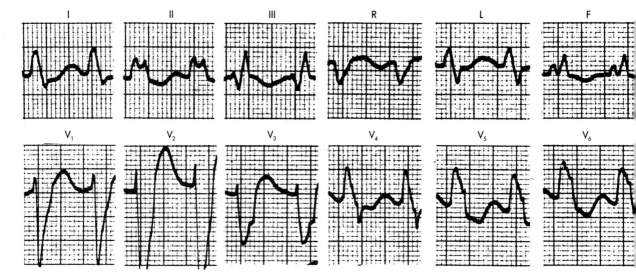

Fig. 13-13. (From Josephson M and Wellens HJJ: How to approach complex arrhythmias, Miami, 1987, Medtronic.)

QRS morphology. The QRS in Fig. 13-14 is V_1-negative, with a broad R and a delay of >0.06 second from the beginning of the R to the nadir of the S in V_1 and V_2—a sign of VT.

Axis. The axis is beyond -30 degrees—not helpful when the QRS is mainly negative in V_1.

QRS width. It is approximately 0.20 second (supports VT).

AV dissociation. A negative P wave is seen just before the second complex in aVR and is not found in the same place in neighboring complexes—a sign of absence of 1:1 conduction (favors VT).

Diagnosis. The diagnosis is VT.

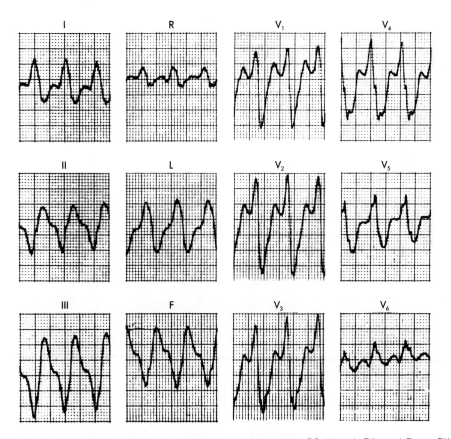

Fig. 13-14. (From Gilbert M: Ventricular tachycardias. In Wagner GS, Waugh RA, and Ramo BW, editors: Cardiac arrhythmias, New York, 1983, Churchill Livingstone Inc. By permission of Churchill Livingstone Inc.)

QRS morphology. The QRS in Fig. 13-15 is V_1-positive, with a diphasic (QR) complex in V_1 and a deep S in V_6—signs of VT.

Axis. The axis is beyond -30 degrees (supports VT).

QRS width. It is 0.16 second (supports VT).

AV dissociation. P waves are not identified (inconclusive).

Diagnosis. The diagnosis is VT.

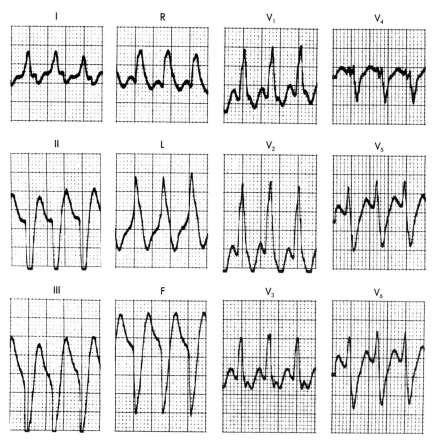

Fig. 13-15

QRS morphology. The QRS in Fig. 13-16 is V_1-positive, with a QS in V_6—a sign of VT. The pattern in V_1 is inconclusive.

Axis. The axis is beyond -30 degrees (supports VT).

QRS width. It is 0.16 second (supports VT).

AV dissociation. P waves not identified (inconclusive).

Diagnosis. The diagnosis is VT.

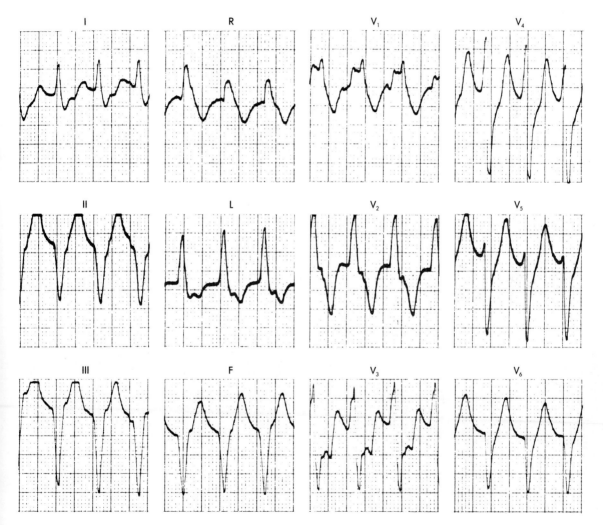

Fig. 13-16

QRS morphology. The QRS in Fig. 13-17 is V_1-positive, with a monophasic R in V_1 and concordance of the pattern in the precordial leads. Such a pattern strongly supports a diagnosis of VT.

Axis. The axis is to the right.

QRS width. It is 0.16 second (supports VT).

AV dissociation. P waves are not identified (inconclusive).

Diagnosis. The diagnosis is SVT. This is atrial fibrillation with conduction over an accessory pathway (Wolff-Parkinson-White syndrome). Whenever a broad QRS tachycardia is irregular and has a rate greater than 200 beats/min, this diagnosis is likely and must be ruled out. This condition produces an ECG that is indistinguishable from VT except that it is irregular; VT is regular 75% of the time.

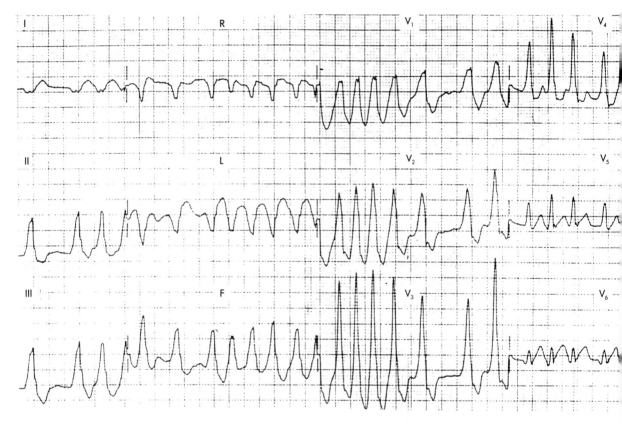

Fig. 13-17

QRS morphology. The QRS in Fig. 13-18 is V_1-positive, with a diphasic complex (QR) in V_1 and a deep S wave in V_6—signs of VT.

Axis. The axis is to the right.

QRS width. It is 0.16 second (supports VT).

AV dissociation. AV dissociation present. P waves are seen lead II in the second T, the fourth ST segment, just before the penultimate QRS, and in the last T wave (Fig. 13-18, *B*) (supports VT).

Diagnosis. The diagnosis is VT.

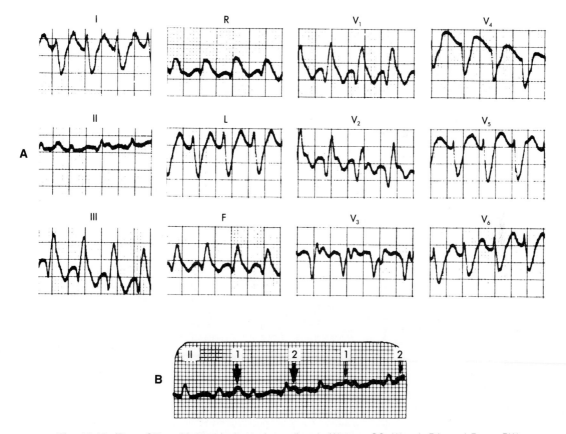

Fig. 13-18. (From Gilbert M: Ventricular tachycardias. In Wagner GS, Waugh RA, and Ramo BW, editors: Cardiac arrhythmias, New York, 1983, Churchill Livingstone Inc.)

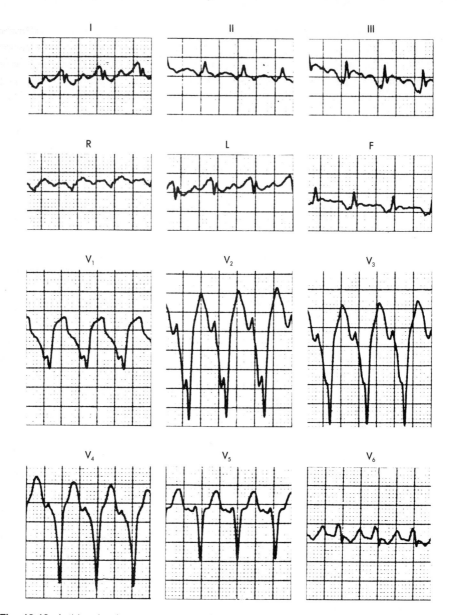

Fig. 13-19. Antidromic circus movement tachycardia. This is a supraventricular tachycardia that cannot be distinguished on the surface ECG from ventricular tachycardia because entry into the ventricles from the atria is through an accessory pathway outside of the intraventricular conduction system. (From Conover M: Understanding electrocardiography, ed 5, St. Louis, 1988, The CV Mosby Co.)

Exceptions to the rules

Exceptions to the rules outlined previously are antidromic circus movement tachycardia, atrial fibrillation with conduction over an accessory pathway, preexisting bundle branch block (BBB), and digitalis toxicity.

Antidromic circus movement tachycardia. This is the mechanism in a small percentage of SVTs in patients with Wolff-Parkinson-White (WPW) syndrome; the more common circus movement in this condition is orthodromic (anterograde conduction down the AV node). In antidromic circus movement, the current uses the accessory pathway in the anterograde direction and the AV node retrogradely. Because the entrance of the impulse into the ventricle is outside of the conduction system, the tachycardia is indistinguishable from VT on the ECG, although it may be slightly irregular because of retrograde block in one of the fascicles. Fig. 13-19 is an example of an antidromic circus movement.

Atrial fibrillation with conduction over an accessory pathway. A broad QRS tachycardia that is irregular with a ventricular rate of more than 200 beats/min should immediately arouse the suspicion of atrial fibrillation with conduction over an accessory pathway.[7] As well as being rapid, this arrhythmia is irregular, and the QRS complexes resemble those of VT in morphology. Such a rhythm is seen in Fig. 13-20.

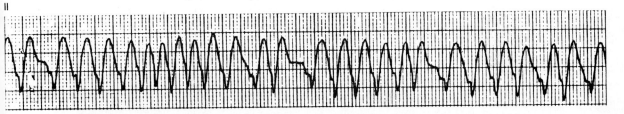

Fig. 13-20. Atrial fibrillation with conduction over an accessory pathway. This tachycardia resembles ventricular tachycardia except for its irregularity. It is identified because it is fast, broad, and irregular (FBI) and because of the patient's history. (From Conover M: Understanding electrocardiography, ed 5, St. Louis, 1988, The CV Mosby Co.)

Preexisting BBB. When preexisting BBB is present, the differential diagnosis of tachycardia may be difficult. However, if the sinus rhythm is available for comparison, an SVT will often have a QRS morphology identical to that of the sinus rhythm, whereas the morphology of VT will be different.[25] In the study done by Wellens,[3] the sinus rhythm was not made available to the investigators. Figs. 13-21 and 13-22 show that the differential diagnosis can often be made if the sinus rhythm is available for comparison. In Fig. 13-21 although there is RBBB during sinus rhythm, the tachycardia is clearly ventricular in origin. Note in Fig. 13-22 that the shape of the ventricular complex during the SVT is identical to that in sinus rhythm, whereas its shape during VT is different.

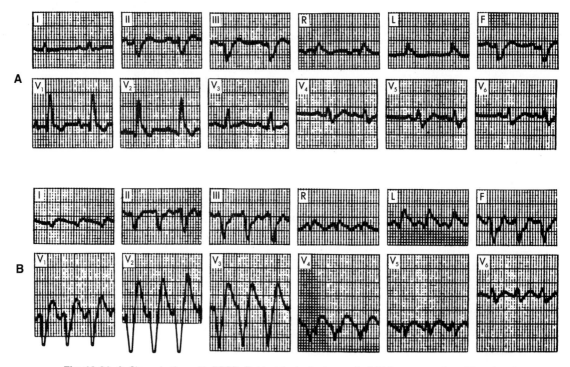

Fig. 13-21. A, Sinus rhythm with RBBB. **B,** Ventricular tachycardia (VT) in same patient. Note that the pattern in SVT is identical to that in sinus rhythm, whereas it is different in VT. (From Dongas J and others: Am J Cardiol 55:717, 1985.)

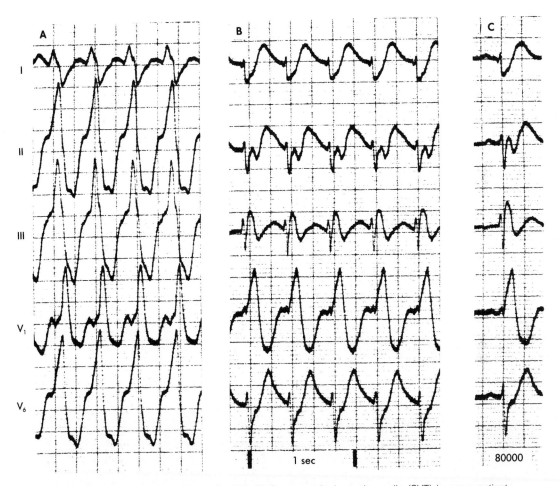

Fig. 13-22. A, Ventricular tachycardia (VT). **B,** Supraventricular tachycardia (SVT) in same patient. **C,** Sinus rhythm in same patient. Note that the pattern in SVT is identical to that in sinus rhythm, whereas it is different in VT. (From Wellens HJJ and others: Ventricular tachycardia—the clinical problem. In Josephson ME, editor: Ventricular tachycardia: mechanisms and management, Mt Kisco, NY, 1982, Futura Publishing Co, Inc.)

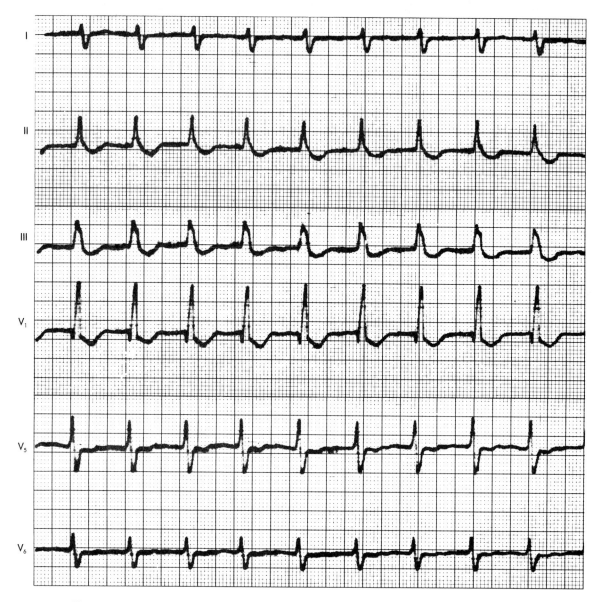

Fig. 13-23. Fasicular VT in digitalis toxicity. The mechanism is triggered activity, and the pattern is typical: incomplete RBBB and axis deviation. (From Josephson ME and Wellens HJJ: How to approach complex arrhythmias, Miami, 1987, Medtronic.)

Digitalis toxicity. Triggered activity is the common mechanism of VT in digitalis toxicity. As such, its focus is often in the fascicles. In fascicular VT the QRS is usually narrower than 0.14 second and has an incomplete RBBB shape, and there is often axis deviation.[26] Fig. 13-23 is an example of fascicular VT caused by digitalis toxicity. Note the RBBB pattern in V_1, the QRS width of <0.14 second, and the axis deviation, typical patterns in fascicular VT resulting from digitalis toxicity. Because there is right axis deviation, we know that the focus is in the anterior (superior) fascicle.

Summary

The experience gained from years of invasive cardiology has yielded firm guidelines in the differential diagnosis of broad QRS tachycardia, confirming well-established clues and providing new ones. Specific evaluations obtained by the informed investigator guarantee 90% diagnostic accuracy; they are QRS shape, QRS axis, and QRS width; AV dissociation and precordial concordancy; fusion beats; and capture beats. QRS morphology takes precedence when there are conflicting clues from QRS axis and width, especially in the light of new morphological clues in the tachycardia that is mainly negative in V_1 and V_2.

In broad QRS tachycardias that are V_1-positive, a triphasic pattern in V_1 indicates supraventricular tachycardia (SVT), whereas a monophasic pattern, diphasic pattern, or the rabbit ear clue indicates ventricular tachycardia (VT); in V_6 a triphasic qRs indicates SVT, whereas an S that is deeper than the R is tall indicates VT. In broad QRS tachycardias that are V_1-negative. A narrow r or a quick, clean downstroke to the S wave in V_1 and/or V_2 indicates SVT, whereas an R (if present) of 0.04 second or more, a slurred or notched downstroke of the S, or a distance of 0.07 second or more to the lowest point of the S indicates VT. A QRS width of more than 0.14 second suggests VT. An abnormal axis (>−30 degrees or >+120 degrees) favors VT in a V_1-positive pattern, but left axis deviation is not a useful clue in V_1-negative tachycardia.

AV dissociation is present in half of all VTs; the other half has some form of retrograde conduction to the atria. Thus the physical signs of AV dissociation should be looked for, and the ECG should be evaluated for AV dissociation or lack of 1:1 conduction.

REFERENCES

1. Stewart RB, Bardy GH, and Greene HL: Wide complex tachycardia: misdiagnosis and outcome after emergent therapy, Ann Intern Med 104:766, 1986.
2. Marriott HJL and Bieza CF: Alarming ventricular acceleration after lidocaine administration, Chest 61:682, 1962.
3. Wellens HJJ: The wide QRS tachycardia, Ann Intern Med 104:879, 1986.
4. Morady F and others: A prevalent misconception regarding wide-complex tachycardia, JAMA 254:2790, 1985.
5. Dancy M, Camm AJ, and Ward D: Misdiagnosis of chronic recurrent ventricular tachycardia, Lancet 2:320, 1985.
6. Vera Z and others: His bundle electrography for evaluation of criteria in differentiating ventricular ectopy from aberrancy in atrial fibrillation, Circulation 46(suppl II):90, 1972.
7. Wellens HJJ, Bar FWHM, and Lie KI: The value of the electrocardiogram in the differential diagnosis of a tachycardia with a widened QRS complex, Am J Med 64:27, 1978.
8. Wellens HJJ, and others: Medical treatment of ventricular tachycardia: considerations in the selection of patients for surgical treatment, Am J Cardiol 49:186, 1982.
9. Kindwall E, Brown J, and Josephson ME: Electrocardiographic criteria for ventricular tachycardia in wide complex left bundle branch block morphology tachycardia, Am J Cardiol 61:1279, 1988.
10. Wellens HJJ and others: The differentiation between ventricular tachycardia and supraventricular tachycardia with aberrant conduction: the value of the 12 lead electrocardiogram. In Wellens HJJ and Kulbertus HE, editors: What's new in electrocardiography? The Hague, 1981, Martinus Nijhoff, Publisher.
11. Bar FW and others: Differential diagnosis of tachycardia with narrow QRS complex (shorter than 0.12 sec), Am J Cardiol 54:555, 1984.
12. Morady F and Scheinman MM: Paroxysmal supraventricular tachycardia. II. Treatment. Mod Concepts Cardiovasc Dis 51:113, 1982.
13. Vera Z and others: His bundle electrography for evaluation of criteria in differentiating ventricular ectopy from aberrancy in atrial fibrillation. Circulation 46(suppl II):90, 1972.
14. Wellens HJJ: The electrocardiogram 80 years after Einthoven, J Am Coll Cardiol 7:484, 1986.
15. Buxton AE and others: Hazards of intravenous verapamil for sustained ventricular tachycardia, Am J Cardiol 59:1107, 1987.
16. Harvey WP and Ronan JA: Bedside diagnosis of arrhythmias, Prog Cardiovasc Dis 8:419, 1966.
17. Marriott HJL: Differential diagnosis of supraventricular and ventricular tachycardia, Geriatrics 25:91, 1970.
18. Gozensky C and Thorne D: Rabbit ears: an aid in distinguishing ventricular ectopy from aberration, Heart Lung 3:634, 1975.
19. Gulamhusein S and others: Electrocardiographic criteria for differentiating aberrancy and ventricular extrasystole in chronic atrial fibrillation: validation by intracardiac recordings, J Electrocardiol 18:41, 1985.
20. Rosenbaum MB: Classification of ventricular extrasystoles according to form, J Electrocardiol 2:269, 1969.
21. Swanick EJ, La Camera F, and Marriott HJL: Morphologic features of right ventricular ectopic beats, Am J Cardiol 30:888, 1972.
22. Wilson WS, Judge RD, and Siegel JK: A simple diagnostic sign in ventricular tachycardia, N Engl J Med 270:446, 1964.
23. Stewart RB, Bardy GH, and Greene HL: Wide complex tachycardia: misdiagnosis and outcome after emergent therapy, Ann Intern Med 104:766, 1986.
24. Tchou P and others: Useful clinical criteria for the diagnosis of ventricular tachycardia, Am J Med 84:53, 1988.
25. Dongas J and others: Value of preexisting bundle branch block in the electrocardiographic differentiation of supraventricular from ventricular origin of wide QRS tachycardia, J Am Coll Cardiol 55:717, 1985.
26. Vanagt EJ and Wellens HJJ: The electrocardiogram in digitalis intoxication. In Wellens HJJ and Kulbertus HE, editors: What's new in electrocardiography? The Hague, 1981, Martinus Nijhoff, Publisher.

CHAPTER 14

AV block

Everyone at all conversant with the terminology of cardiology is familiar with the conventional division of AV block into first, second, and third degrees. Few, however, appreciate what confusion, misunderstanding, and mismanagement this oversimplified classification has created. The situation has been compounded by deficient definitions and multiple misconceptions. It is with these unfortunate aspects of the subject that much of this chapter is concerned.

The PR interval

The normal PR interval, measured from the beginning of the P wave to the beginning of the QRS complex, ranges between 0.12 and 0.20 second. This is not to say that somewhat longer and shorter intervals necessarily indicate abnormality; in a study of normal youths between the ages of 15 and 23 years, 1.3% had PR intervals longer than 0.20 second, and the same percentage had intervals shorter than 0.12 second.[1] It may well be that these exceptions to the general rule represent merely the splayed extremities of a normal bell curve.

When all atrial impulses that should be conducted to the ventricles are so conducted, but with a PR interval of greater than 0.20 second, the term "first degree" AV block is generally applied.

Nonconducted beats

The term "second degree" block is applied when one or more (but not all) atrial impulses that should be conducted fail to reach the ventricles. It thus covers a great variety of conduction patterns of markedly variable significance.

When an atrial impulse fails to reach the ventricles, it is often referred to as a "dropped" beat. Usage of this term has been criticized, but it is difficult to find an adequate and appropriate substitute; it at least has the blessing of traditional use since Lewis.[2] Faute de mieux, we shall use it!

When an atrial impulse fails to reach the ventricles and a beat is "dropped," the individual circumstances must be taken into account. If it arrives at the AV junction early in the cycle when the junction is still normally refractory, it is not conducted; but neither is it "blocked," for block implies a *pathological* failure of conduction. Obviously one of the determinants of the prematurity with which an atrial impulse arrives at the junction is the atrial rate; and when the rate is exceedingly fast, as in atrial flutter, it is only proper that every other impulse should not be conducted. One of the normal functions of the AV node is to protect the ventricles from excessively rapid and therefore ineffective beating when the atria have gone berserk. Therefore 2:1 conduction resulting from normal refractoriness should not be called 2:1 *block*, which immediately places it in an abnormal category.

Before assessing the significance of a dropped beat, therefore, one must always consider the atrial rate and its inseparable partner, the RP interval. The failure of an atrial impulse to reach the ventricles can have a quite different significance if its P wave lands after the end of the T wave from what it will have if it is perched on the first part of the ST segment.

Type I and type II block

In 1899 Wenckebach,[3] without benefit of electrocardiograph and by simple observation of the pulses in the neck, described the form of AV block that bears his name, in which the AV conduction time progressively lengthens until a beat is dropped (Fig. 14-1).

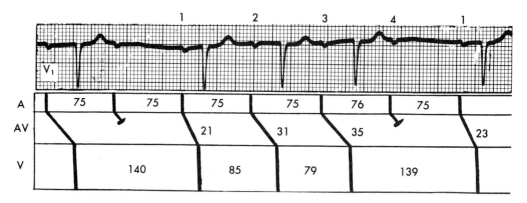

Fig. 14-1. Typical 4:3 Wenckebach period—of the four atrial impulses *(1, 2, 3, 4)*, only three reach the ventricles. Characteristic features include the following: the first PR is slightly prolonged (0.21 sec); the larger PR increment is between the first and second PR (from 0.21 to 0.31 sec); as the increment decreases, the ventricular cycle shortens (from 0.85 to 0.79 sec); the longest cycle (of the dropped beat—1.39 sec) is less than twice the shortest ventricular cycle (0.79 sec); and there is no BBB.

Seven years later Wenckebach in Vienna and Hay[5] in Scotland both described a second form of AV block in which there was no progressive lengthening of the conduction time before conduction failed (Fig. 14-2).

In 1924 Mobitz[6] correlated these earlier clinical findings with those in the electrocardiogram and suggested that the first type (1899) be called "type I" and the second type (1906) "type II." Hence they have since been frequently referred to as Mobitz type I and Mobitz type II block but are just as appropriately called Wenckebach type I and Wenckebach type II.[7,8] In later years His bundle recordings have repeatedly demonstrated that type I block is usually a manifestation of AV nodal block, whereas type II is always infranodal block and is usually a manifestation of bilateral bundle branch block (BBB).[9-12]

Useful as this classification has proved to be and widely as the terms type I and type II are used, most authorities fail to explain fully how they are using them, and the simple division into two types is beset with ambiguities.

If the terms are confined only to the basic patterns of block originally described, the terms are too restrictive, and their usefulness is decreased. For example, if a patient has an atrial rate of 80 beats/min with 3:2 Wenckebach periods, it is generally accepted as classical type I block. If the atrial rate increases to 100 beats/min, however, with the result that the conduction ratio changes to 2:1, it is still the same type of block (i.e., type I), although there no longer is the progressive increase in conduction times (PR intervals) before each dropped beat that is characteristic of the classical Wenckebach. Thus, if only examples with increasing PR intervals are included, important samples of type I block are excluded.

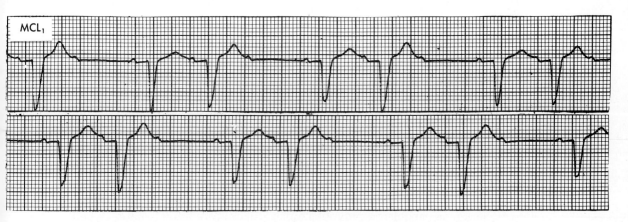

Fig. 14-2. Typical example of type II 3:2 AV block. Characteristic features include the following: consecutive atrial impulses are conducted with the same PR interval (0.18 sec) immediately before the dropped beat; the PR after the dropped beat is the same as the PR before it; the PR is of normal duration; and there is a bundle branch block.

Anatomy versus behavior

Two ingredients blend indefinably to produce the recipe for both type I and type II block: pathophysiological behavior and the anatomical level of the block. Unfortunately, there is an irreconcilable dichotomy between anatomy and behavior. Most authorities, correctly following traditional usage, use the terms type I and type II as behavioral descriptions.[13-16] Yet there is little doubt that the anatomical level of the lesion is clinically more important than its physiological behavior; for example, Wenckebach periodicity in a bundle branch, in the presence of contralateral bundle branch block, is behaviorally type I but clinically and prognostically is more appropriately considered type II.[8,17] Consequently, a division into nodal and infranodal, or proximal and distal,[17] has much to commend it.

It would therefore be ideal if we could infallibly distinguish between AV nodal block (and call it type I) and infranodal block (and call it type II) from the clinical tracing. Unfortunately we cannot; and in many situations intracardiac recordings — the only sure way of accurately localizing the level of the block — are neither available nor desirable. Fortunately, with a knowledge of the attributes of both types of block (Table 14-1), aided at times by the result of carotid sinus massage and/or atropine administration,[18] as well as exercise and catecholamines[18a] we can usually make an intelligent and correct guess. Table 14-2 lists the three noninvasive means of differentiating AV nodal from infranodal block.

Important exceptions to the usual findings are as follows.

1. Many Wenckebach periods are atypical[19] and fail to show all the classical features depicted in Fig. 14-1.
2. Rarely, the classical Wenckebach period can develop in the bundle of His, and then the ECG is indistinguishable from the nodal Wenckebach period.
3. The all-or-none conduction that characterizes the bundle branches may be found in the His bundle, and then type II block may be encountered with a narrow QRS complex.[8,20-23] This combination occurs almost exclusively in elderly women.[8]
4. In the presence of existing BBB, progressive lengthening of the PR interval before a dropped beat is caused in perhaps 25% of cases[17] by progressive delay in the contralateral bundle branch.[24,25]

Despite such significant exceptions, "in most instances, the differentiation can be made easily and reliably from the surface ECG."[15] What it all boils down to is that when we say type I, we mean "probably nodal and usually benign" and when we say type II, we mean "certainly infranodal and definitely malignant." Genuine type II block is an unequivocal indication for an artificial pacemaker, whereas type I block seldom is.

Table 14-1. Established characteristics of type I and type II block

	Type I	Type II
Clinical	Usually acute Inferior infarction Rheumatic fever Digitalis Propranolol	Usually chronic Anteroseptal infarction Lenegre's disease Lev's disease Cardiomyopathy
Anatomical	Usually AV nodal— sometimes His bundle	Always subnodal—usually bundle branches
Electrophysiological	Relative refractory period Decremental conduction	No relative refractory period All-or-none conduction
Electrocardiographical	RP/PR reciprocity Prolonged PR Normal QRS duration	Stable PR Normal PR Bundle branch block

Table 14-2. Noninvasive assessment of block level

	Type I (nodal)	Type II (infranodal)
Atropine	Improves	Worsens
Exercise and catecholamines	Improves	Worsens
Carotid sinus massage	Worsens	Improves

Wenckebach periodicity and RP/PR reciprocity

Although it may well prove an oversimplification, it is a convenient and practical concept to think of type I *behavior* as caused by an abnormally long relative refractory period (RRP) and type II as the result of little or no RRP.[16] In the prolonged RRP the rate of conduction depends on the moment of impulse arrival—the earlier it arrives at the AV node, the longer it takes to penetrate; the later it arrives, the shorter the penetration time (Fig. 14-3).

Thus it becomes obvious that the reason the Wenckebach type of conduction develops is that each successive impulse arrives earlier and earlier in the RRP of the AV node until, at last, one arrives during the absolute refractory period (ARP) and the impulse fails to get through.

A clinically practical concept results from translating this earlier and earlier arrival into terms of the surface tracing. Other things being equal, the earlier the impulse sets out from the sinus node, the earlier it will reach the AV node, and therefore the RP interval (measured from beginning of the QRS to beginning of the next P wave) gives us an approximate—and in practice highly satisfactory—indication of the relative earliness of arrival at the AV node. In terms of the clinical tracing the shorter the RP is, the longer the PR, and the longer the RP is, the shorter the PR; and so we can think and talk of "RP/PR reciprocity" and of "RP-dependent" PR intervals. If such reciprocity in the clinical tracing can be demonstrated, you can be sure that some part of the AV junction is exhibiting Wenckebach (type I) behavior.

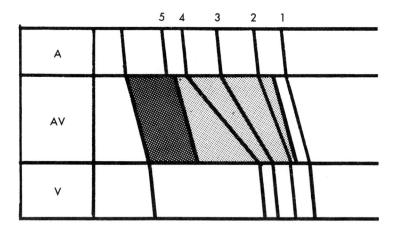

Fig. 14-3. Diagrammatic behavior of AV conduction during type I AV block. Dark stippling in the AV junction represents the absolute refractory period (ARP); light stippling represents the relative refractory period (RRP). If an atrial impulse *(1)* arrives at the AV node after the RRP is over, it is conducted normally. If it arrives a little earlier *(2)*, there will be some delay in AV conduction; and as it arrives earlier and earlier *(3* and *4)*, conduction time becomes longer and longer. Finally, the impulse arrives in the ARP *(5)* and is not conducted.

In Fig. 14-4 the reciprocal relationship between RP and its associated PR is nicely demonstrated. After the first three beats, which are conducted normally with a PR of 0.17 sec complementing an RP of 0.48 second, the last four beats are all conducted with progressively shortening PR intervals (exactly the converse of what happens in a Wenckebach sequence) because they complement progressively lengthening RP intervals (again, exactly the converse of what happens in a Wenckebach sequence).

In the classical Wenckebach period (see Fig. 14-1) the dropped beat fails to penetrate the diseased stratum of the AV node, which therefore enjoys a relatively long rest (RP interval equals 1.13 sec) with consequent optimal AV conduction (PR equals 0.21 sec). Now, suddenly, the RP dramatically shortens—from 1.13 to 0.52 sec—and the PR in consequence lengthens as dramatically—from 0.21 to 0.31 sec. This explains why the second PR in the Wenckebach sequence almost always shows the largest increment over the preceding PR—because it follows the most dramatic shortening of the RP; that is, it arrives much earlier in the RRP of the sick AV node.

On the other hand, if there is virtually no RRP, it follows that beats are conducted with the same facility, that is, with the same PR interval, whether early or late in diastole, provided they arrive after the ARP is finished (see Fig. 14-2); the PR is the same, regardless of the preceding RP, and RP/PR reciprocity is lacking.

It follows, in turn, from all this information that when *consecutive* atrial impulses are conducted, type I block is characterized by progressive lengthening of the PR before conduction fails altogether, whereas type II block has constant PR intervals when *consecutive* impulses are conducted before the dropped beat.

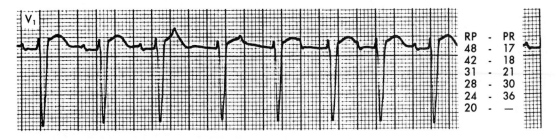

Fig. 14-4. Illustration of the reciprocal relationship between the RP interval and its complementing PR (see table at end of tracing). The last four conducted beats demonstrate the converse of what happens in Wenckebach conduction: as the RP gets longer with each successive beat, its complementary PR gets progressively shorter, whereas in Wenckebach conduction the PR progressively lengthens in response to a progressively shortening RP.

2 to 1 AV block

What of the situation, however, when only alternate beats are conducted with a resulting 2:1 ratio? With this ratio in both type I (see Fig. 14-5) and type II (see Fig. 14-6), the PR interval is, of course, constant in the beats that are conducted. This is true for type II since all PRs are constant in this type of block; but it is also true of type I block since, provided the atrial rhythm is regular, the RP intervals will be constant and so therefore will the PRs (recall that in type I block the PR is RP dependent). This fact has been the source of much misunderstanding, with consequent misdiagnosis and mistreatment.

Although it no longer qualifies as the Wenckebach phenomenon, when the classical form of Wenckebach conduction alternates with 2:1 conduction—such as in

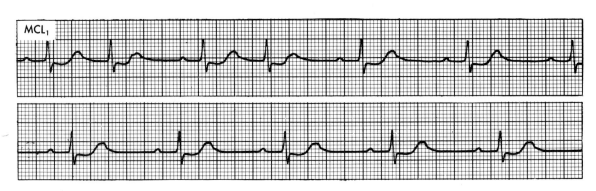

Fig. 14-5. From a patient with acute true posterior infarction. Note the prominent initial R wave with reciprocal ST depression. Strips are continuous; atrial rate throughout is 103 beats/min. At the beginning of the top strip there are two 3:2 Wenckebach periods; then through the bottom strip the conduction ratio changes to 2:1. Note that the PR interval is prolonged during the 2:1 conduction (0.25 sec).

Fig. 14-5—the type of block has not changed. Sometimes changes in the atrial rate produce changes in conduction ratios; sometimes the conduction ratios change spontaneously; but in these cases there can be no doubt that the type of block is unchanged. When the conduction ratio in Wenckebach periods changes from 5:4 to 4:3 or from 4:3 to 3:2, there is no doubt that the type of block is unchanged; why, when it goes one stage further and becomes 2:1, should there be an immediate flurry to change the type and its prognostic significance?

In Figs. 14-5 and 14-6 are two other features that are highly characteristic of the two types of second degree AV block and that can be of assistance in differentiating types when only 2:1 conduction is present. The prolonged PR and the absence of BBB are typical of pure type I block, whereas the normal PR and the presence of BBB are characteristic of type II.

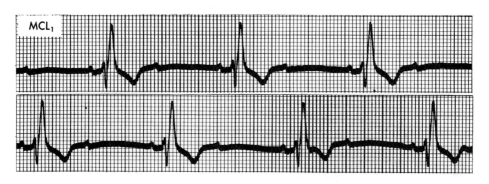

Fig. 14-6. Strips are continuous and show 2:1 AV block with RBBB. The atrial rate is 82 beats/min, and the combination of a normal PR interval (0.15 sec) with BBB makes it likely that this is type II AV block.

"Skipped" P waves

Another point that is not well appreciated and that leads to faulty diagnosis is that the atrial impulse that is conducted to the ventricles is not always represented by the P wave that immediately precedes the QRS. In Fig. 14-7 the group beating and the other "footprints" clearly identify a Wenckebach period.

Moreover, the increasing PR intervals in each group of beats are evident. However, in each group the first and second PR intervals are clearly too short for conduction, and therefore conduction must come from the preceding P wave (see ladder-gram).

Furthermore, these rather long PR intervals—reaching 0.69 second—bring to mind the oft asked question: "How long can a PR be and still represent conduction?" There is no established answer to this; but at least it can be said that a PR of 0.60 second is not uncommon, one of 0.70 second is sometimes seen, and one of 0.80 to 0.90 second is rare. Reports of PR intervals of more than 1 second have been published, but the validity of some of them is doubtful.

High-grade (or advanced) AV block

High-grade block represents a stage between the occasionally, or even alternately, dropped beats and complete block. High-grade block may be diagnosed when, *at a reasonable atrial rate* (say, 135 beats/min or less), two or more than two consecutive atrial impulses fail to be conducted; and this failure of conduction must happen *because of the existing block itself,* not because an escaping junctional or ventricular pacemaker anticipates and prevents conduction. Fig. 14-8 presents two examples of high-grade AV block—the one probably type I because of the inferior infarction and absence of BBB, and the other type II because there is BBB as well as a normal PR interval in the conducted beats.

The two conditions italicized above are necessary ingredients in the definition because, for example, if the fluttering atria are beating at a frantic rate of 300 beats/min, it would be absurd to call 4:1 block (in which three consecutive impulses are not conducted) high grade since a 4:1 ratio, producing a ventricular rate of 75, is exactly what the heart of both the therapist and the patient desires. Furthermore, the ventricular escape rate, quite apart from the block, can be a major determinant of nonconduction and cause of overdiagnosis, as we discuss later in this chapter.

Complete AV block

The AV block should be called complete when, and only when, the opportunity for conduction is optimal and yet none occurs. The key word here is opportunity since it is obvious that if there is no opportunity to do something, one cannot be blamed for not doing it. If there is less than optimal opportunity for the AV conduction sys-

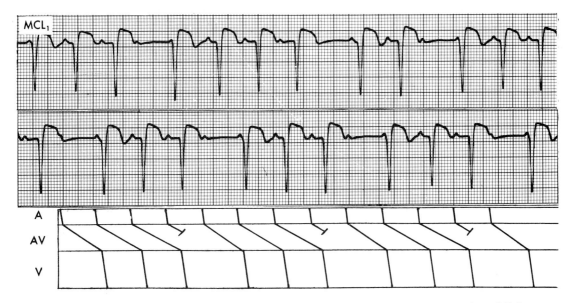

Fig. 14-7. Strips are continuous. Sinus tachycardia (rate, 125 beats/min) with 3:2, 4:3, and 5:4 Wenckebach periods. Note that the PR intervals are longer than the PP intervals.

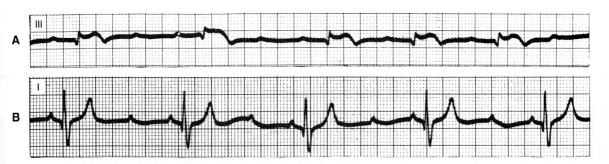

Fig. 14-8. High-grade (advanced) AV block. **A,** From a patient with acute inferior infarction, sinus tachycardia, and 3:1 and 2:1 AV block—presumably type I. **B,** From a 47-year-old patient, with no history of heart disease, initially seen with Adams-Stokes attacks. There is sinus tachycardia (rate, 122 beats/min) with 3:1 AV block. In this clinical context the normal PR (0.16 sec) with RBBB makes this likely to be type II block caused by sclerodegenerative disease of the conduction system.

tem to conduct, it cannot be regarded as a failure if it does not conduct; on the other hand, if it has every conceivable opportunity to conduct and invariably fails, it may well be blamed as a total failure. What then determines the presence or absence of opportunity for conduction? The several factors involved are listed on p. 265.

To make the diagnosis of complete block, there should be no conduction—recognized by the changing P-to-R relationship in the presence of a regular ventricular rhythm—but that absence of conduction must be in the presence of a slow enough ventricular rate (less than 45 beats/min, although some[26,27] require a ventricular rate of less than 40 beats/min), with P waves fully deployed across the RR intervals landing at every conceivable RP interval. Only then can one be satisfied that the opportunity for conduction is optimal and that the diagnosis of complete block is justified. These features require repeated emphasis because there is probably no entity in cardiology that is so often overdiagnosed and then overtreated.

Fig. 14-9 illustrates complete AV block: the ventricular rate is less than 45 beats/min, the ventricular rhythm is absolutely regular, and the P-to-R relationship is constantly changing as the P waves march resolutely through all phases of the ventricular cycle. Every possible chance for conduction is afforded, but none occurs; and so the diagnosis of the ultimate in block (complete) is warranted.

Acute complete block is usually caused by a lesion in the AV node such as in acute inferior infarction and less often in severe digitalis intoxication. In acute anterior infarction complete block is more devastating and is almost always caused by a simultaneous block in both bundle branches. Approximately 90% of chronic complete block is caused by bilateral BBB, with the remaining 10% caused by blockade at the level of the His bundle.

Ventricular asystole

As a rule, when AV conduction fails, an escaping pacemaker, junctional or ventricular, comes to the rescue. However, if the failure of conduction is associated with reluctant subsidiary pacemakers, ventricular asystole results. This sinister situation, if unrelieved, is obviously and rapidly fatal. The most common context for this occurrence is as an ominous and usually fatal climax of type II block; that is, it develops spontaneously against a background of existing BBB, presumably because the other bundle branch is suddenly blocked (Fig. 14-10, A).

Ventricular asystole is not always so sinister. If it develops as a result of a vagal storm such as with vomiting (Fig. 14-10, C), the level of block is in the AV node and the disturbance may be relatively mild and transient. A third mechanism of asystole (Fig. 14-10, B) is tentatively assumed caused by a phase 4 phenomenon since the block and the consequent asystole develop only after a lengthening of the atrial cycle, suggesting that the AV node may have spontaneously depolarized to an unresponsive level (p. 194).

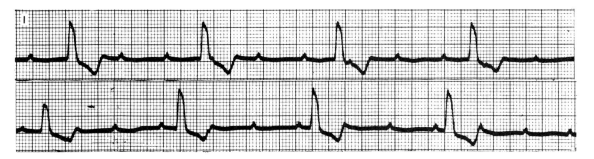

Fig. 14-9. Complete AV block. Strips are continuous. In the presence of sinus tachycardia (rate, 108 beats/min) there is an independent idioventricular rhythm (rate, 36 beats/min). Note that the ventricular rhythm is absolutely regular, whereas the P to R relationship is constantly changing.

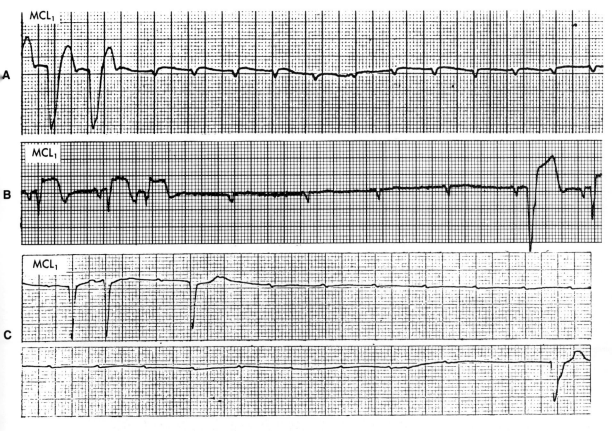

Fig. 14-10. Three examples of transient ventricular asystole caused by sudden failure of AV conduction in the absence of an escaping pacemaker. **A,** *Spontaneous* asystole in the presence of LBBB, probably representing end-stage type II block. **B,** From a patient with acute anteroseptal infarction. Asystole is precipitated by an atrial premature beat (as were many repeated periods of asystole); the atrial premature beat lengthens the ensuing sinus cycle, suggesting that the failure of conduction might be caused by a *phase 4 phenomenon*. **C,** Strips are continuous. *Vagal* asystole, precipitated by vomiting, in a patient with acute inferior infarction.

Need to reclassify

There are several reasons the diagnosis and management of the AV blocks are in a state of confusion.

Definitions wanting. The first reason is that most authors seem not to realize that there is any uncertainty in the current situation. In fact, in more than 50 articles dealing with the subject of complete AV block published in English since the advent of coronary care in 1962, not a single author considered it necessary to define AV block—presumably because it is tacitly, but erroneously, assumed that the term is uniformly used by and means the same to all. How far this is from the truth will become apparent.

Not only is complete block almost never defined, but on the rare occasions when it is, the definition is usually found wanting. Much the same is true of the usage and definition of other important categories of block such as "type II block" and "high-grade block."

Nondegrees of block. The second source of inconsistency resides in the usage of "degrees." The word, by definition, should indicate a measure of the severity of the AV conduction disturbance. However, this is not necessarily the case. Consider, for example, the rhythm strips in Fig. 14-11. By any criterion the top strip (Fig. 14-11, *A*) is an example of 2:1 AV block, a ratio that some regard as "high-grade" block (see below),[8,28,29] whereas the second strip (Fig. 14-11, *B*) shows no sign of any block. In fact, the owner of strip *B* has worse block than the patient in strip *A* because patient B develops 2:1 block when the atrial rate accelerates to only 84 beats/min (Fig. 14-11, *D*), whereas patient A is able to conduct 1:1 at a rate of 100 beats/min (Fig. 14-11, *C*). Obviously a patient who develops 2:1 conduction at a rate of 84 has worse block than one who can conduct every beat at a rate of 100 beats/min. In evaluating the severity of AV block, *rate* is far more important than *ratio;* yet, unfortunately, our definitions of "degrees" have for decades been partially predicated on ratios to the neglect of rate. Indeed, when the conduction ratio changes with an increase in rate, it may be described as a change for the worse in the degree of block[30] rather than being recognized for what it is: a change in *rate* with a secondary and consequent change in the conduction *ratio*, not in the degree of block.

Let us hammer this point home with a diagram. In Fig. 14-12 each conducted beat is followed by an identical prolonged refractory period (shaded area); that is, the "degree" of severity of block is the same throughout the diagram. At the beginning of the strip the atrial cycle length is 100 (rate, 60 beats/min), but after three beats the atrial cycle shortens to 76 (rate, 79 beats/min), and 2:1 conduction develops; yet it is obvious that the severity (i.e., "degree") of block has not changed. The primary change is the atrial rate, and the secondary change is the conduction ratio. The message is that we should not assess the seriousness of any AV block from the conduction ratio alone without taking the associated rate into consideration.

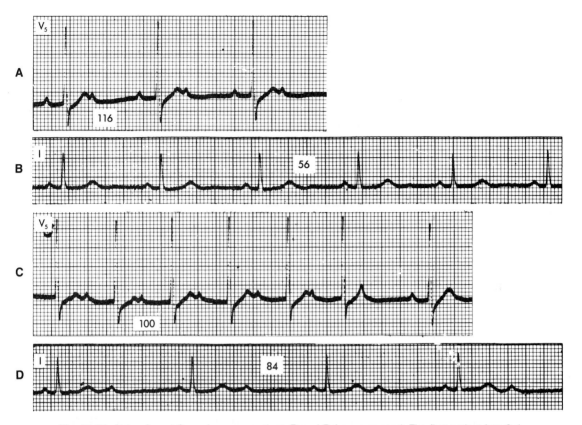

Fig. 14-11. Strips **A** and **C** are from one patient, **B** and **D** from a second. The first patient has 2:1 block at an atrial rate of 116 beats/min, **A,** but can conduct 1:1 at an atrial rate of 100 beats/min, **C,** whereas the second patient, although he conducts normally at 56 beats/min, **B,** develops 2:1 block at a rate of only 84 beats/min, **D.**

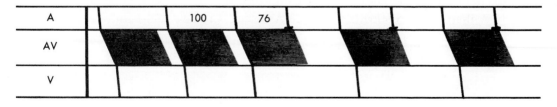

Fig. 14-12. Diagram illustrating the effect of atrial rate on the AV conduction ratio. Note that the abnormally long refractory period is identical throughout; that is, there is no worsening of the block, yet if the atrial cycle shortens from 100 (rate, 60 beats/min) to 76 (rate, 79 beats/min), the conduction ratio changes from 1:1 to 2:1.

Misconceptions rife. The third circumstance that fosters confusion is the prevalence of certain important misconceptions, some of which have been hinted at earlier in this chapter.

First, some authorities[8,28,29] regard 2:1 AV block as high grade or advanced. The absurdity of using the conduction ratio as an index of severity is obvious when one stops to realize that 2:1 block can be anything from a disaster to a boon. At an atrial rate of 70, 2:1 block may be a disaster; at an atrial rate of 130, 2:1 block may prove a blessing. Clearly the ratio alone, when used while in ignorance of the prevailing atrial and therefore ventricular rate, cannot give even an approximate idea of the block's severity.

A second misapprehension is the rather commonly encountered one that all 2:1 block is type II block, mainly owing to the fact that the PR intervals are constant and that one does not have to look far to find defective definitions of type II block such as "AV block with constant PR intervals"[31] and "constant PR intervals for conducted sinus beats irrespective of the ratio of atrial to ventricular depolarizations."[32] Faulty definitions such as these very often omit the key word *consecutive*—which we carefully emphasized earlier in this chapter. It is only when *consecutive*—repeat, CONSECUTIVE!—atrial impulses are conducted with identical PR intervals immediately before the beat is dropped that the constant PR criterion can be applied. Another common, and appropriate, way of stating the constant PR rule is to say that the PR after the dropped beat is the same as the PR before it. In the classical example of type II block in Fig. 14-2 the two consecutive PRs before the dropped beat are identical, and the PR immediately before the dropped beat is the same as the returning PR after it. What these variations of the rule are stating is simply that the PR is independent of the RP: it is the same after a short RP (before the dropped beat) as after a long RP (after the dropped beat); and, of course, the hallmark of type I block is RP/PR reciprocity.[33] Notice again the additional characteristic—but not invariable—features of type II block: the normal PR and the BBB.

In the acute setting of myocardial infarction, type I 2:1 block is, in fact, 20 or 30 times more common than type II 2:1 block—an important point to remember when temporary pacemakers are being brandished.

A third misconception is that when AV block is evident and most of the atrial impulses are not conducted, the block is "high grade" or "advanced."

Fig. 14-13 shows an example of AV block in which there are 21 atrial impulses, only one of which is completely conducted (there are possibly one or two fusion beats); yet, with so little conduction, the block is comparatively mild. The way to avoid the error of overdiagnosis in such cases is to focus on the conducted beat rather than on the numerous nonconducted ones because the beat that is conducted tells far more about the patient's conduction capability than do all the nonconducted beats together. It shows quite specifically the patient's current requirements for conduction. Concentrate on the solitary capture beat (fifth beat in top strip). We recognize that when the RP interval reaches a length of 0.60 second, the patient is able to conduct with a PR interval of 0.32 second. Thus we can deduce that at that time the patient had a 1:1 conduction capability if the atrial cycle equaled the cycle of the capture beat (i.e., cycle length equals 0.92 sec equals 64 beats/min). Furthermore, a person capable of conducting every beat at a rate of 64 beats/min with but a prolonged PR interval certainly does not have an advanced degree of AV block. Add to this reasoning the fact that the patient has an inferior wall infarction and that the capture beat manifests no BBB and you know that the block is almost certainly in the AV node.

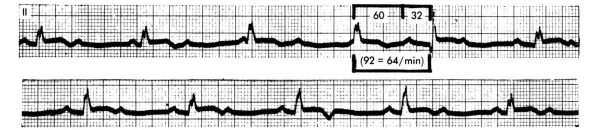

Fig. 14-13. Strips are continuous. From a patient with acute inferior myocardial infarction. Some (undetermined) degree of AV block (presumably type I), combined with an atrial rate of 88 beats/min and a ventricular escape rate of 47 beats/min, precludes conduction except for the one capture beat (fifth beat in the top strip) and two or three possible fusion beats in the bottom strip. The capture beat reveals that the patient is capable of conducting 1:1, with prolonged PR, at an atrial rate of 64 beats/min (see text).

A fourth misconception is that when AV block is clearly present and *none* of the atrial impulses is conducted, the block is necessarily complete.

In a tracing like that in Fig. 14-14, *A*, there is an obvious block since P waves are seen in situations where conduction should occur and does not. In fact, there is no AV conduction since the junctional rhythm is absolutely regular. Thus we have AV block and complete AV dissociation, but this is by no means the same as complete AV block.[13] These tracings should be diagnosed as "*some* (undetermined) degree of AV block that, combined with an accelerated junctional rhythm, produces complete AV dissociation." Yet more than half of 550 respondents to a questionnaire mailed to directors of cardiology departments and coronary care units asking how such an arrhythmia should be described called it complete AV block[34]; and published examples of the same interpretative error are abundant.

The argument here is that, although one cannot be sure that the block is not complete, there is a real possibility that it is relatively mild; therefore it is a mistake to assume the worst, label it the ultimate in block, and run the attendant risks of overdiagnosis—especially since we know that patients with acute myocardial infarction who show this arrhythmia as their worst manifestation of block usually have an excellent prognosis.

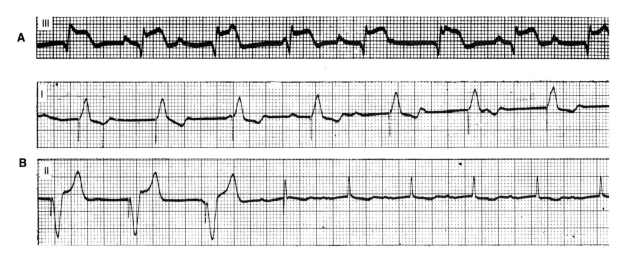

Fig. 14-14. A, Block/acceleration dissociation. Some (undetermined) degree of AV block (presumably type I), combined with an accelerated junctional rhythm at a rate of 68 beats/min, produces complete AV dissociation. **B,** Illustration of how mild a degree of AV block, when combined with an accelerated ventricular rate, can produce complete dissociation. In lead I there is obvious AV block, the paced rhythm has a rate of 62 beats/min, and there is complete AV dissociation. However, in lead II, a few seconds later, an atrial impulse—represented by a P wave landing at a critical RP interval—captures the ventricles and reveals the mildness of the underlying conduction disturbance.

Fig. 14-14, *B*, shows how mild such a block may prove to be. In lead I there is a paced ventricular rhythm of 62 beats/min. The P wave emerges from the QRS and marches backward across the RR interval without effecting capture—complete dissociation. However, in lead II, after the third beat, the P wave happens to land at exactly the right RP interval, and the atrial impulse captures the ventricles with a long PR interval. Once capture is effected, the atria remain in control for the rest of the strip, with gradually lengthening PR intervals indicating that, at the prevailing atrial rate, the underlying block, far from being complete, is a mild form of type I block. The fundamental truth so poorly appreciated is that *the combination of quite mild block with a ventricular rate in the 50s or 60s can produce periods of complete AV dissociation.* Absence of conduction is not necessarily the same as block. Pick and Langendorf[35] demonstrated years ago that complete AV dissociation could be produced in a patient with only first degree AV block by pacing his ventricle two or three beats faster than his sinus rate.

Therefore, when faced with a sample of AV block in which all or a significant majority of beats are not conducted, it is important to rehearse in one's mind the many influences that determine AV conduction and to assess the relative contribution of each:

1. State of AV junction and bundle branches
    a. Physiological refractoriness
    b. Pathological refractoriness
    c. Concealed conduction
2. Autonomic influences
3. Atrial rate
4. R/P relationships
5. Ventricular rate
6. Level of ventricular pacemaker

Dysrhythmias, such as that in Fig. 14-14, *A*, caused by the conspiracy of an undetermined degree of block with a subsidiary pacemaker beating at a rate faster than usual, clearly require a separate designation; and Marriott[31] has therefore suggested the term "block/acceleration dissociation."

Remedial measures

To introduce some semblance of order from the current chaos, three modifications commend themselves: (1) disturbances of AV conduction must be classified into many more categories than the oversimplification into three misleading "degrees"; (2) "degrees" of AV block as presently defined (or not defined!) should be abandoned, or at least deemphasized, since they have caused more confusion than they have contributed precision; and (3) rates, both atrial and ventricular, in view of the major role they play in determining the frequency and ratio of AV conduction, must be included in all definitions and diagnostic categorizations of block.

With the above considerations in mind, we should divide the AV blocks into more meaningful categories—meaningful from the viewpoint of placing the site of the lesion, assessing the prognosis, and deciding on the appropriate management. This division can, as we have emphasized, usually be done from the surface tracing, together with an informed appraisal of the clinical setting. As a short step in the right direction, we suggest that the disturbances of AV conduction be categorized and considered under at least the number of subdivisions listed below.

1. Prolonged PR interval
2. Block/acceleration dissociation
3. Occasional "dropped" beats
   a. Type I (Wenckebach periodicity)
   b. Type II
4. 2:1 AV block
   a. Type I
   b. Type II
5. High-grade block
   a. Type I
   b. Type II
6. Complete block
   a. Junctional escape
   b. Ventricular escape
7. Transient ventricular asystole
   a. Spontaneous
   b. Phase 4 (?)
   c. Vagal

REFERENCES

1. Van Hemel MM and Robles de Medina EO: Electrocardiographic findings in 781 males between the ages of 15 and 23 years. I. Arrhythmias and conduction disorders, Excerpta Medica Cardiovasc Dis Cardiovasc Surg, 23:981, 1975 (abstract).
2. Lewis T: The mechanism and graphic registration of the heart beat, London, 1925, Shaw & Sons.
3. Wenckebach KF: Zur Analyse des unregelmässigen Pulses. II. Ueber den regelmässig intermittirenden Puls, Z Klin Med 37:475, 1899.
4. Wenckebach KF: Beiträge zur Kenntnis der Menschlichen Herztätigkeit, Arch Anat Physiol, p 297, 1906.
5. Hay J: Bradycardia and cardiac arrhythmia produced by depression of certain functions of the heart, Lancet 1:139, 1906.
6. Mobitz W: Ueber die unvollständige Störung der Erregungsüberleitung zwischen Vorhof und Kamme des menschlichen Herzens, Z Ges Exp Med 41:180, 1924.
7. Knoebel SB, Parsons MN, and Fisch C: The role of transvenous pacing in acute myocardial infarction, Heart Lung 1:56, 1972.
8. Narula OS: His bundle electrocardiography and clinical electrophysiology, Philadelphia, 1975, FA Davis Co.
9. Damato AN and Lau SH: Clinical value of the electrogram of the conducting system, Prog Cardiovasc Dis 12:119, 1970.
10. Rosen KM: The contribution of His bundle recording to the understanding of cardiac conduction in man, Circulation 43:961, 1971.
11. Rosen KM, Gunnar RM, and Rahimtoola SH: Site and type of second degree AV block, Chest 61:99, 1972.

12. Haft JI, Weinstock M, and DeGuia R: Electrophysiologic studies in Mobitz type II second degree heart block, Am J Cardiol 27:682, 1971.

13. Langendorf R and Pick A: Atrioventricular block, type II (Mobitz)—its nature and clinical significance, Circulation 38:819, 1968.

14. Barold SS and Friedberg HD: Second degree atrioventricular block: a matter of definition, Am J Cardiol 33:311, 1974.

15. Zipe DP: Second-degree atrioventricular block, Circulation 60:465, 1979.

16. Pick A and Langendorf R: Interpretation of complex arrhythmias, Philadelphia, 1979, Lea & Febiger.

17. Del Negro AA and Fletcher RD: Indications for and use of artificial cardiac pacemakers, Curr Probl Cardiol 3(7):9, 1978.

18. Mangardi LM and others: Bedside evaluation of atrioventricular block with narrow QRS complexes; usefulness of carotid sinus massage and atropine administration, Am J Cardiol 49:1136, 1982.

18a. Bär FW, Den Bulk K, and Wellens HJJ: Atrioventricular dissociation. In MacFarlane PW and Veitch Lawrie T: Comprehensive electrocardiology, New York, 1989, Pergamon Press, Inc.

19. Denes P and others: The incidence of typical and atypical AV Wenckebach periodicity, Am Heart J 89:26, 1975.

20. Rosen KM and others: Mobitz type II block without bundle branch block, Circulation 44:1111, 1971.

21. Gupta PK, Lichstein E, and Chadda KD: Electrophysiological features of Mobitz type II A-V block occurring within the His bundle, Br Heart J 34:1232, 1972.

22. Rosen KM, Loeb HS, and Rahimtoola SH: Mobitz type II block with narrow QRS complex and Stokes-Adams attacks, Arch Intern Med. 1342:595, 1973.

23. Puech P, Grolleau R, and Guimond C: Incidence of different types of AV block and their localization by His bundle recordings. In Wellens HJJ, Lie KI, and Janse MJ, editors:

The conduction system of the heart: structure, function, and clinical implications, Philadelphia, 1976, Lea & Febiger.

24. Rosenbaum MB and others: Wenckebach periods in the bundle branches, Circulation 40:79, 1969.

25. Friedberg HD and Schamroth L: The Wenckebach phenomenon in left bundle branch block, Am J Cardiol 24:591, 1969.

26. Schamroth L: The disorders of cardiac rhythm, Oxford, 1980, Blackwell Scientific Publications, Ltd.

27. Pritchett ELC: Office management of arrhyth-rhythmias, Philadelphia, 1982, WB Saunders Co.

28. WHO/ISC Task Force: Definition of terms related to cardiac rhythm, Am Heart J 95:796, 1978.

29. Josephson ME and Seides SF: Clinical cardiac electrophysiology. Techniques and interpretations, Philadelphia, 1979, Lea & Febiger.

30. Danzig R, Alpern H, and Swan and HJC: The significance of atrial rate in patients with atrioventricular conduction abnormalities complicating acute myocardial infarction, Am J Cardiol 24:707, 1969.

31. Stock RJ and Macken DL: Observations on heart block during continuous electrocardiographic monitoring in myocardial infarction, Circulation 38:993, 1968.

32. Scheinman M and Brenman B: Clinical and anatomic implications of intraventricular conduction blocks in acute myocardial infarction, Circulation 46:753, 1972.

33. Langendorf R, Cohen H, and Gozo EG: Observations on second degree atrioventricular block, including new criteria for the differential diagnosis between type I and type II block, Am J Cardiol 29:111, 1972.

34. Marriott HJL: AV block: an overdue overhaul, Emerg Med 13(6):85, 1981.

35. Langendorf R and Pick A: Artificial pacing of the human heart: its contribution to the understanding of the arrhythmias, Am J Cardiol 28:516, 1971.

CHAPTER 15

Fusion

A fusion beat is the complex (ventricular or atrial) that results when two impulses simultaneously activate parts of the same myocardial territory (ventricular or atrial myocardium). The simultaneously spreading impulses produce a hybrid complex usually possessing recognizable features of the patterns produced by each alone. The fusion beat is unrecognizable clinically and is a purely electrocardiographical diagnosis.

Three of the more common mechanisms for fusion are diagrammatically represented in Fig. 15-1. They are as follows:

1. Ventricular fusion resulting from the simultaneous spread of a descending sinus impulse and an ectopic ventricular one in any of the following forms—ventricular extrasystole or escape, ventricular tachycardia in the absence of retrograde conduction to the atria, accelerated idioventricular rhythm (AIVR), parasystole, or a paced ventricular beat. Ventricular fusion involving a sinus impulse is likely to occur only with end-diastolic ectopic beats.
2. Ventricular fusion resulting from the simultaneous spread of two supraventricular impulses, one of them through an accessory pathway and the other through the normal route (preexcitation syndrome).
3. Atrial fusion resulting from the simultaneous spread of a sinus impulse and a retrograde one from either the AV junction or the ventricles.

Less often ventricular fusion can also result from the simultaneous spread of two ectopic ventricular impulses such as when two idioventricular pacemakers, one in each ventricle, are competing for control. All the potential fusion partners are shown in Table 15-1.

The ventricular fusion beat is of considerable value in recognizing ectopic ventricular rhythms. Most authorities believe that the presence of fusion favors ectopy with 85% to 90% odds. The argument runs as follows: if a supraventricular impulse enters the ventricles and merges with another impulse, that second impulse must have arisen within the ventricles since the AV junction would be rendered refractory by one descending supraventricular impulse, negating the possibility that a second supraventricular impulse could invade the ventricles in time to fuse with the first one.

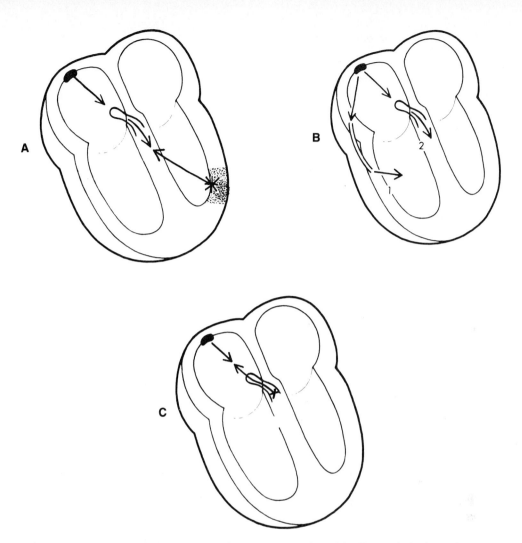

Fig. 15-1. A, Ventricular fusion because of ventricular ectopic activity. **B,** Ventricular fusion because of preexcitation. **C,** Atrial fusion.

Table 15-1. Potential partners in fusion (any impulse in **A** can fuse with any in **B**)

A	B
Sinus	Ectopic ventricular
Ectopic atrial	Extrasystole
Junctional	Tachycardia
Ectopic ventricular	Accelerated idioventricular
	Parasystole
	Escape
	Pacemaker
	Junctional conducted preferentially
	Sinus or ectopic atrial conducted by Kent bundle

Most of the time this argument is probably true; but Kistin[1] demonstrated that it was possible for a descending sinus impulse to fuse in the ventricles with an aberrantly conducted junctional beat. One explanation for this is that the junctional impulse spreads through Mahaim fibers to the ventricle, leaving the AV junction clear for passage of the simultaneous sinus impulse.

Ventricular fusion

CLINICAL SIGNIFICANCE. The clinical significance of ventricular fusion is simply that of the ventricular ectopic beat that contributes to it. Evaluation is in the light of the total clinical picture, and its significance is not altered because the ectopic beat happens to collide with a supraventricular impulse. The fact that there is fusion is purely circumstantial and relevant only to the extent that the ventricular ectopic beat itself is relevant.

There is some evidence that end-diastolic ectopic beats can be the result of excessive stretch of the conductive fibers within the ventricles such as would occur with an elevated left ventricular end-diastolic pressure secondary to congestive heart failure.

DIAGNOSIS. There are three main principles in the diagnosis of ventricular fusion[2]:

1. It should be diagnosed only if there is cogent reason to believe that two impulses were due at that moment. This principle is so self-evident that it seems unnecessary to say it, but there is an observed tendency for interpreters to hastily invoke fusion when an offbeat complex is not readily explained—and there is no doubt that "fusion beats" are plucked out of insubstantial air more than any other electrocardiographical phenomenon.
2. Ventricular fusion beats generally show a contour and a duration that are intermediate between the contour and duration of complexes of the fusing impulses (see "Exception to Rule 2" below).
3. The PR interval of a ventricular fusion beat may be the same as that of the sinus rhythm, or it may be shorter; but if it is shorter, it is not more than approximately 0.06 second shorter than the sinus PR. This is because virtually any ectopic impulse can reach the AV junction within 0.06 second and, once it has reached the junction, the way is barred for a descending impulse to enter the ventricles and fuse.

Exception to rule 2. When fusion occurs between a supraventricular impulse in the presence of bundle branch block (BBB) and an ectopic impulse arising in the ventricle on the same side as the BBB, the resulting fusion complex may be narrower than either the ectopic or the BBB pattern (see p. 298); similarly, if fusion develops between two ectopic ventricular impulses simultaneously arising from each ventricle, the resulting complex may be narrower than either ectopic beat.

In Fig. 15-2, *A*, the end-diastolic ventricular premature beat (VPB) is preceded by a PR interval of only 0.06 second; clearly the sinus impulse has not been conducted to the ventricles, and there is therefore no chance of fusion. In the same patient Fig. 15-2, *B*, shows another end-diastolic VPB. This time the PR interval is 0.16 second instead of the underlying 0.22, and the complex is a fusion beat. If a similar ventricular ectopic beat occurred after an even longer PR interval (e.g., 0.18 second), it is easy to visualize that the morphology of the ventricular complex would be quite different again from the fusion beat seen in *B*, looking more like the sinus impulse and less like the ectopic beat. Going one step further, if the ectopic ventricular focus did not discharge until after the sinus impulse actually entered the ventricles, the complex would be different still and would have the same PR interval as the conducted sinus beats (0.22 sec). Even if the ventricular ectopic focus were discharging with the same PR interval each time, the morphology of the fusion complexes might vary because of slight variation in the amount of myocardial tissue activated each time by the two fusing impulses and because the ectopic focus could discharge at any time from the beginning of the normal QRS until it was itself activated by the normal impulse, thus producing the same PR each time but with varying shapes to the fusion beat. Likewise, even with the same coupling interval (normal QRS to ectopic beat), each time the sinus cycle may vary slightly, resulting in different fusion complexes.

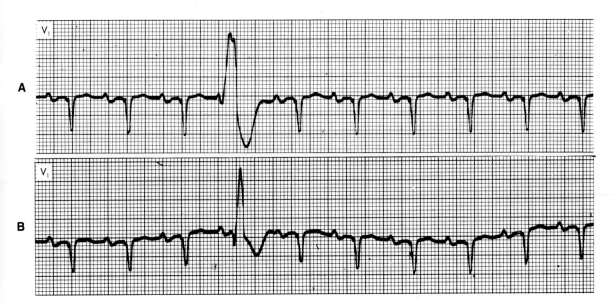

Fig. 15-2. End-diastolic ventricular extrasystoles. In **A** there is no chance for fusion because the PR interval is only 0.06 second. In **B** the ventricular extrasystole begins 0.14 second after onset of the P wave; thus fusion is possible.

Fig. 15-3 shows ventricular bigeminy in which the coupling intervals are long enough to deposit the extrasystoles after every other sinus P wave. Ventricular fusion beats (labeled 1, 2, 3, and 4) result from the gradually lengthening coupling interval. The first two extrasystoles capture the whole ventricular myocardium; but beginning with the third extrasystole, there is time for the sinus impulse to enter the ventricles before they have been completely activated from the ectopic center. As the coupling interval and, with it, the PR interval lengthen, the sinus contribution to the ventricular fusion complex increases (see laddergram).

Occasionally the coincidence of a more or less simultaneous atrial and ventricular extrasystole produces ventricular fusion, which may simulate an atrial premature beat (APB) with aberration. An example of this coincidence is illustrated in Fig.

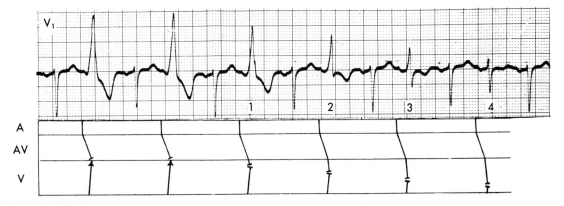

Fig. 15-3. End-diastolic ventricular extrasystoles landing after every other P wave. After the first two extrasystoles their coupling intervals progressively lengthen so that fusion occurs (beats *1, 2, 3,* and *4*) at progressively "lower" levels in the ventricles with more and more contribution from the sinus impulse. The PR interval of beat 4 is as long as that of the sinus beats.

15-4. The third beat (A) is an APB, the fifth and last beats (V) are VPBs, and the eighth beat (F) is a fusion beat between atrial and ventricular extrasystoles. If the fusion beat is taken out of context without the evidence of the surrounding beats, it is seen as a bizarre QRS-T preceded by a premature P wave and is therefore diagnosed as an APB with aberration. Since a fusion beat is partly an ectopic ventricular beat, it carries clinical and therapeutic implications different from those of an APB.

Fig. 15-5 is an accelerated idioventricular rhythm with a rate almost the same as the sinus rhythm. Thus when the sinus rhythm slows just a little, the ventricular ectopic focus discharges. In such a situation ventricular fusion is common (the second to sixth beats). The last three are pure ventricular ectopic beats, but they are somewhat distorted by the simultaneous occurrence of sinus P waves.

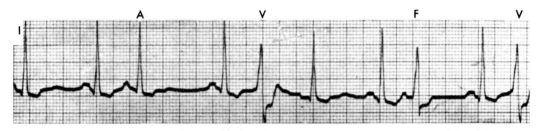

Fig. 15-4. *A*, Atrial extrasystole; *V*, ventricular extrasystole; *F*, fusion between simultaneous atrial and ventricular extrasystoles.

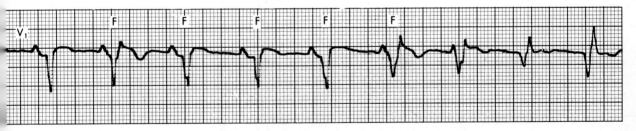

Fig. 15-5. Ventricular fusion beats *(F)* caused by an accelerated idioventricular rhythm.

15-6 note the changing shapes of the fusion beats, a phenomenon that
to diagnostic confusion when the mechanism is poorly understood. This
interval is 0.18 second; with the VPBs the PR shortens by 0.2 to 0.6
ulting in varying degrees of fusion. The shorter the PR, the greater is
the contribution from the ectopic impulse to the fusion beat.

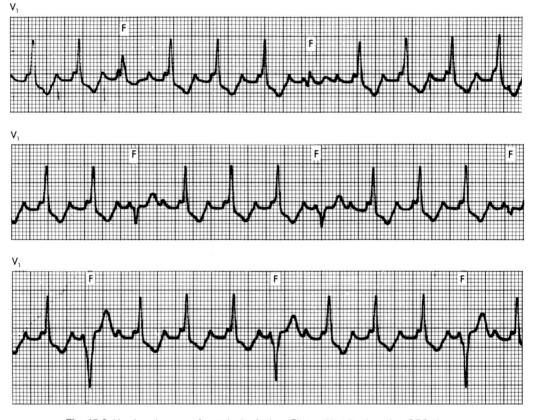

Fig. 15-6. Varying degrees of ventricular fusion *(F)*, resulting in changing QRS shapes.

Fig. 15-7 again shows the confusing face of bigeminal end-diastolic ventricular ectopy. The sinus beats are conducted with right bundle branch block (RBBB). In the top tracing (A) supernormal AV and intraventricular conduction might be suspected since P waves with shorter PR intervals precede the narrower normal-looking beats. However, a second tracing (B) clearly indicates that *the narrower complexes are really fusion beats* and that the shortening of the PR interval is the result of the premature ventricular ectopic beat and not a true reflection of AV conduction time. Since the *right* BBB complex is normalized by fusion with a ventricular beat, the ectopic focus must be in the *right* ventricle.

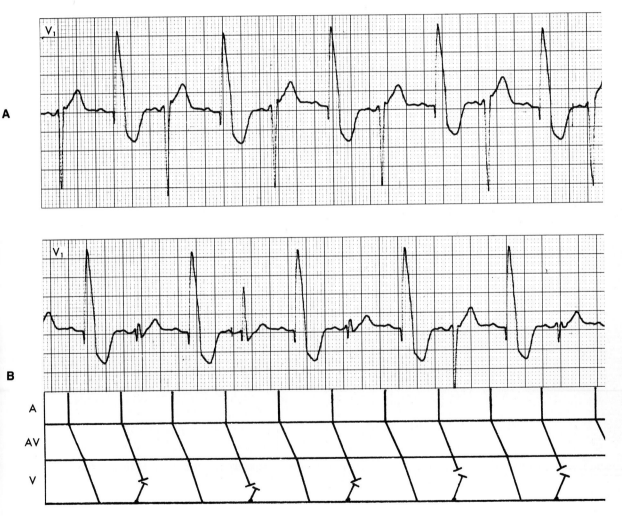

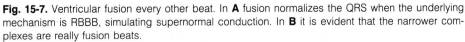

Fig. 15-7. Ventricular fusion every other beat. In **A** fusion normalizes the QRS when the underlying mechanism is RBBB, simulating supernormal conduction. In **B** it is evident that the narrower complexes are really fusion beats.

Fig. 15-8 shows the same arrhythmia, bigeminal end-diastolic VPBs, all of which produce multiform fusion beats.

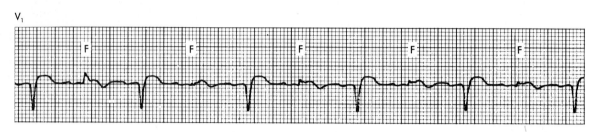

Fig. 15-8. Bigeminal end-diastolic ventricular extrasystoles producing multiform fusion beats *(F)*.

Fusion in parasystole

Fig. 15-9 is a parasystolic rhythm with one fusion beat. Note that even though the first ventricular ectopic is end-diastolic, it is not a fusion beat. This is because the underlying PR interval is 0.14 second and the ventricular complex begins only 0.04 second after the onset of the P wave, giving the ectopic impulse 0.10 second to activate the ventricles before the sinus impulse is expected.

Take a good look at Fig. 15-10 and use your calipers before you read on! The intervals between the negative deflections are approximately the same, but we hope you did not mistake the artifact for ventricular parasystole with fusion. Note that the deep negative deflections do not interrupt or disturb the cardiac cycle. They are therefore clearly artifacts.

Fusion during accelerated idioventricular rhythm

Accelerated idioventricular rhythm (AIVR) is a common source of fusion because its rate is often closely similar to the competing sinus rate. The ectopic focus therefore asserts itself just as soon as the sinus rate slows slightly. This occurrence is illustrated in Fig. 15-11. When the sinus cycle lengthens by as little as 0.04 second, a fusion beat occurs. The ectopic ventricular focus is firing at a rate of 88 beats/min; as long as the sinus rhythm remains at 90 beats/min or faster such as at the beginning of the strip, the enhanced ventricular automaticity is not manifest. In this tracing the sinus rhythm slows slightly after the third beat, permitting fusion until, at the seventh beat, the ectopic focus assumes complete control of the ventricles with no contribution from the sinus impulse.

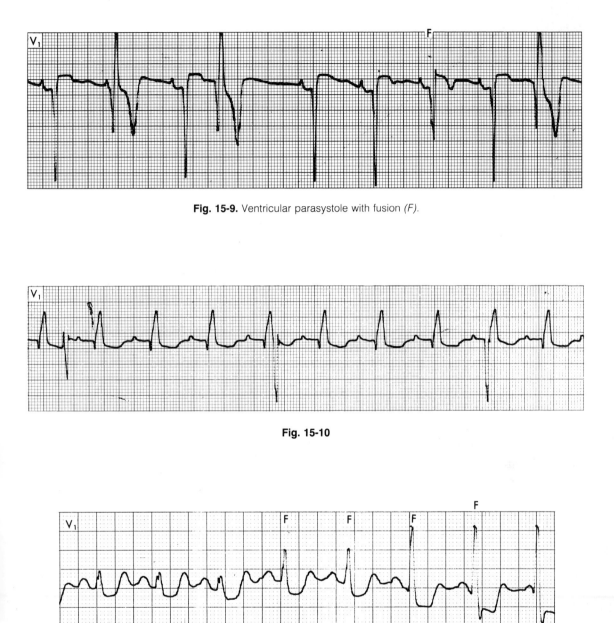

Fig. 15-9. Ventricular parasystole with fusion *(F)*.

Fig. 15-10

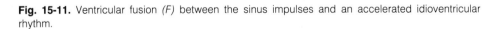

Fig. 15-11. Ventricular fusion *(F)* between the sinus impulses and an accelerated idioventricular rhythm.

Fig. 15-12 is a champion tracing, boasting no less than 37 consecutive fusion beats! At the beginning of the tracing are pure ectopic beats; at the end are pure sinus beats. Between the two Xs all are fusion beats, with the varying contributions from the isorhythmic sinus and ventricular impulses producing a kaleidoscope of configurations.

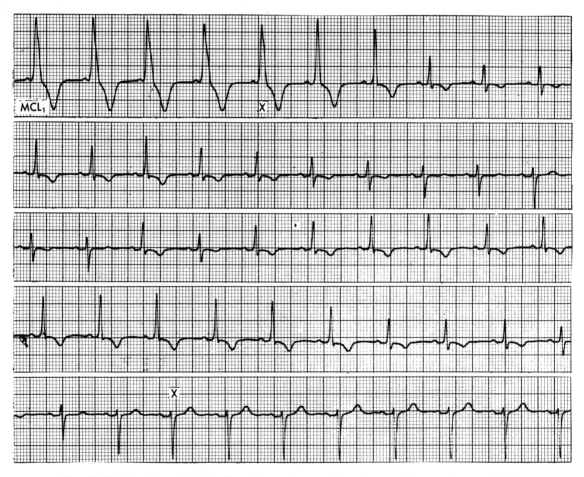

Fig. 15-12. Fusion in profusion! In these five continuous strips, between the complexes marked X, there are 37 consecutive fusion beats between the sinus impulses and a competing accelerated idioventricular rhythm.

Fig. 15-13 illustrates a similar mechanism but looks completely different because of the underlying left bundle branch block (LBBB). Note the three fusion beats in the middle of the tracing, the last of which actually normalizes the complex, presumably because the ectopic focus is in the left ventricle. The ectopic rhythm takes over by usurpation (the first fusion beat ends a measurably shorter cycle than the preceding sinus cycles); but it promptly slows again and, after the third fusion beat, surrenders control to the sinus pacemaker.

V₁

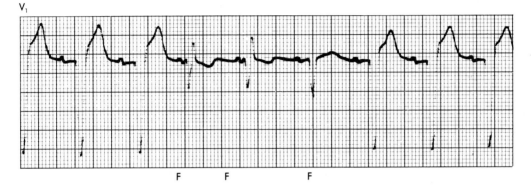

Fig. 15-13. An underlying LBBB with three fusion beats *(F)* caused by an ectopic focus in the left ventricle.

Fusion beats in the diagnosis of ventricular tachycardia

The value of fusion beats in the diagnosis of ventricular tachycardia was emphasized by Dressler and Roesler[3]; these beats are therefore often referred to as "Dressler beats." Their presence is considered excellent evidence in favor of ventricular tachycardia since fusion almost always reflects ventricular ectopy. However, their value is limited because they are seldom seen if the rate is much greater than 150 beats/min. All the examples published by Dressler and Roesler had rates less than this one. Another limiting factor is the fact that it is also possible for a junctional tachycardia with BBB (mimicking ventricular tachycardia) to produce fusion beats.[4]

In Fig. 15-14 there is a tachycardia of 150 beats/min and fusion beats. The fusion beats occur when the sinus P wave is so placed that conduction takes place before the ventricular ectopic focus can completely activate the ventricles.

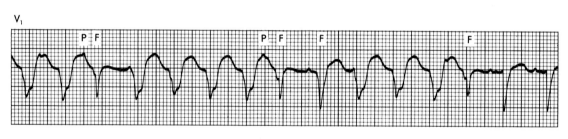

Fig. 15-14. Ventricular tachycardia (rate, 150 beats/min) with fusion beats *(F)*.

Fig. 15-15, *A*, is a tracing that was erroneously diagnosed as ventricular tachycardia because of the fusion beat in the middle of the tracing; and it is indeed a tachycardia at 132 beats/min with one fusion beat. The ventricular complexes are broad and resemble ventricular tachycardia; but, if you examine Fig. 15-15, *B*, from the same patient, you see two consecutive VPBs. The compensatory pause gives the P wave a chance to show up and identify the tachycardia as sinus, with BBB and ventricular extrasystoles occasionally producing fusion.

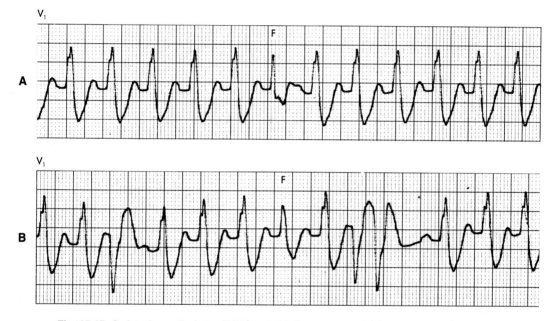

Fig. 15-15. A, A tachycardia (rate, 132 beats/min) that was wrongly diagnosed as ventricular tachycardia because of the fusion beat *(F)*. **B,** This tracing from the same patient establishes the tachycardia as sinus with BBB and frequent VPBs. A fusion beat *(F)* can also be seen.

Fusion with ventricular escape beats

Fig. 15-16, *A*, in both leads shows progressive slowing of the sinus rate until, by the fourth complex, a ventricular escape focus asserts itself at a rate of 48 beats/min for three beats only. Then the SA node accelerates enough to recapture the ventricles. The first and third ectopic beats produce fusion complexes.

Fig. 15-16, *B*, begins with 2:1 AV block and ends with two idioventricular beats. The fourth beat in the strip is somewhat narrower than the idioventricular beats, is preceded by a P wave at a conductible interval, and is therefore a fusion beat.

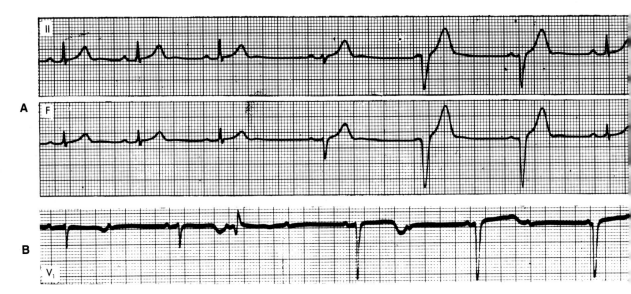

Fig. 15-16. Fusion with ventricular escape beats. **A,** In each strip the sinus rhythm slows and allows an idioventricular center to escape for three beats. The first and third of these escapes in each strip form fusion beats. **B,** The strip begins with 2:1 AV block (note the different PR intervals of the conducted beats—presumably type I block with RP-dependent PR intervals); then a ventricular extrasystole is followed by a longer cycle that enables an idioventricular pacemaker to escape. The first of the three escape beats is narrower than the last two, is preceded by a P wave at a conductible interval, and is clearly a fusion beat *(F)*.

In Fig. 15-17 an idioventricular rhythm momentarily takes over because of a profound bradycardia secondary to 2:1 AV block. Note that the third and fourth beats in the top strip are fusion beats. Although the conducted pattern is LBBB, the fourth complex is actually normalized by the fusion—because the ectopic focus is on the same side as the BBB (see also Fig. 15-8).

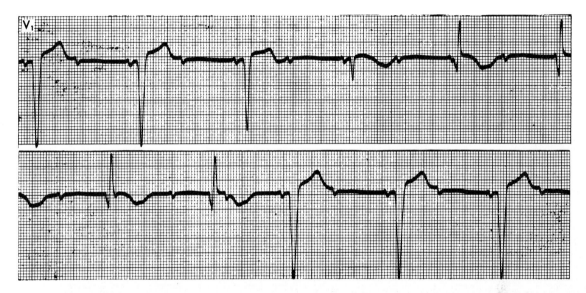

Fig. 15-17. Strips are continuous. The basic rhythm is sinus with AV block, probably type II, with 2:1 AV conduction and LBBB seen at the beginning of the top strip and in the second half of the bottom strip. The last two beats in the top strip and the first two in the bottom strip represent an idioventricular rhythm from the left ventricle. The third and fourth beats in the top strip are fusion beats (note the normalization of beat 4).

Fusion with paced beats

Artificial pacemakers are prolific factories of fusion beats, which can occur with both demand and fixed-rate pacemakers.

Fig. 15-18 shows a demand pacemaker producing fusion beats (F) as the sinus rhythm accelerates and takes control. When the sinus P wave emerges in front of the pacemaker spike, partial conduction occurs, and fusion results.

Fig. 15-19 shows a fixed-rate pacemaker ignoring and competing with the conducted sinus beats in the top strip; but toward the end of the bottom strip, fusion (F) finally occurs.

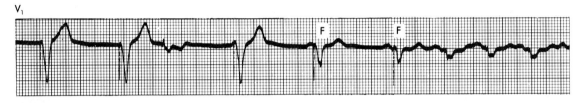

Fig. 15-18. Fusion between paced and sinus beats. In the second half of the strip a demand right ventricular pacemaker produces fusion *(F)* with an accelerating sinus rhythm.

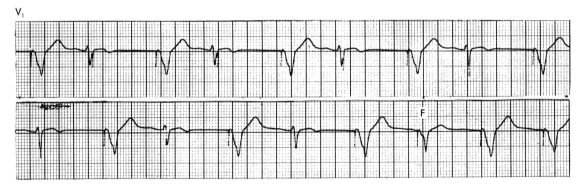

Fig. 15-19. Strips are continuous. A fixed-rate right ventricular pacemaker beats relentlessly in competition with the sinus rhythm to produce a form of "escape-capture" bigeminy in the top strip. Toward the end of the bottom strip it at last achieves fusion *(F)*.

Ventricular fusion in preexcitation

Although fusion is useful in the diagnosis of ventricular ectopy, it can also occur between two supraventricular impulses. In the presence of an accessory pathway (preexcitation), provided the orthodoxly conducted impulse reaches the ventricles before the accessory impulse has had time to activate the entire ventricular myocardium, the ventricular complexes will all be fusion beats.

In the bottom strip of Fig. 15-20 note the progressively widening QRS interval of the sinus beats, reflecting increasing degrees of preexcitation and resulting from changing contributions from each of the two wave fronts, both emanating from the SA node and reaching the ventricle through different pathways. Note that as the QRS broadens, the PR shortens ("concertina" effect).

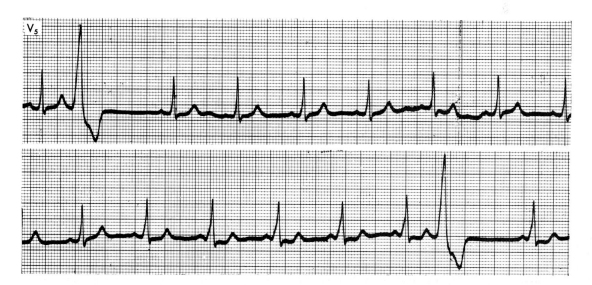

Fig. 15-20. Strips are continuous. Preexcitation syndrome interrupted by two ventricular extrasystoles. The "concertina" effect is seen at the beginning of the bottom strip, where the first three or four beats manifest progressive widening of the QRS with corresponding shortening of the PR.

Atrial fusion

When two impulses simultaneously invade the atria, atrial fusion results. This fusion is most often seen when an accelerated junctional focus competes with the sinus rhythm. In such a case, if the junctional pacemaker sends its retrograde impulse into the atrium at the same time that the sinus impulse is also activating atrial muscle, an atrial fusion beat results (Figs. 15-21 and 15-22).

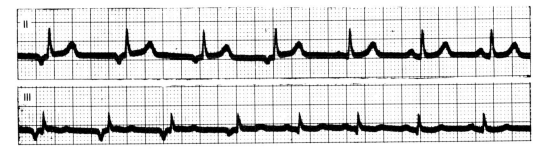

Fig. 15-21. In each lead a junctional rhythm with retrograde conduction shifts to sinus rhythm. In lead II the third, fourth, and fifth P waves are intermediate in form between retrograde and sinus Ps and presumably represent atrial fusion. In lead III only the fourth P wave is caused by fusion.

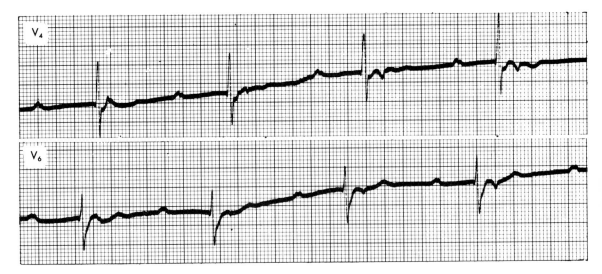

Fig. 15-22. Complete AV block, yet retrograde VA conduction occurs after the third and fourth beats in lead V_4 and after the fourth beat in V_6. Following the second QRS in V_4 and the second and third QRSs in V_6, sinus and retrograde P waves coincide to produce atrial fusion.

Atrial fusion may also be seen when an ectopic ventricular beat is followed by retrograde conduction to the atria at a time when the SA node has just discharged.

With an esophageal lead Kistin and Landowne[5] demonstrated that retrograde conduction to the atria was a common event after a ventricular extrasystole. They suggested that this event is often missed in the clinical tracing because fusion produces a relatively isoelectric P wave.

Summary

Fusion beats can be either atrial or ventricular and result from the collision of electrical impulses from different sources. A ventricular fusion beat results when a supraventricular impulse (usually sinus) meets with a ventricular impulse within the ventricles. An atrial fusion beat results when the sinus impulse meets with an atrial ectopic impulse within the atria. The atrial ectopic impulse could have originated within the atria or could have been conducted retrogradely from a ventricular beat. If the two forces within the one chamber are at their peak simultaneously, they cancel each other, resulting in a narrow, low-amplitude ECG complex. However, a fusion beat can be changed only slightly if, for example, the ventricular ectopic beat is located so that it can discharge toward the end of normal ventricular activation. Thus a fusion beat can be slightly premature, can occur slightly after the onset of the complex of the underlying rhythm, or can be initiated anywhere in between these two extremes. If the ectopic beat is too premature, it will capture the entire ventricles, negating any possibility of fusion; if it is too late, the focus remains dormant since the ventricles will already have been activated by the normal beat.

REFERENCES

1. Kistin AD: Problems in the differentiation of ventricular arrhythmia from supraventricular arrhythmia with abnormal QRS, Prog Cardiovasc Dis 9:1, 1966.
2. Marriott HJL and others: Ventricular fusion beats, Circulation 26:880, 1962.
3. Dressler W and Roesler H: The occurrence in paroxysmal ventricular tachycardia of ventricular complexes transitional in shape to sinoauricular beats. Am Heart J 44:485, 1952.
4. Conover MB: Understanding electrocardiography, ed 5, St. Louis, 1988, The CV Mosby Co.
5. Kistin AD and Landowne M: Retrograde conduction from premature ventricular contractions, a common occurrence in the human heart, Circulation 3:738, 1951.

CHAPTER 16

Parasystole

Parasystole is a form of altered automaticity (either normal enhanced automaticity or abnormal automaticity) that can occur in the atria, AV junction, ventricles, or even in the sinus node[1]; the automatic beats are independent in that (1) the focus is surrounded by an abnormal (depressed) area that shields it from being discharged or reset by extraneous impulses and (2) the automatic activity of the parasystolic focus does not require an initiating or triggering impulse.[2-11] Protection by the surrounding shield may be absolute, intermittent, or modulated. Whatever form the zone of protection assumes, when it is effective, the underlying rhythm (usually sinus) in no way determines whether or not the parasystolic focus fires, although in the modulated form it may have some influence on its timing. Thus parasystolic beats have a random relationship to the underlying rhythm on the surface ECG. For the same reason the interectopic intervals in classical parasystole (absolute protection) are simple multiples of a common denominator, reflecting the rate and the undisturbed rhythm of the parasystolic focus, although the impulses themselves need not appear regularly.

In its modulated form the parasystolic focus is protected from being reset but does not necessarily maintain fixed cycle lengths. This modulation has been demonstrated by sophisticated electrophysiological technics in Moe's laboratory,[3-5,9,12-14] expanding the knowledge of the mechanism of parasystole. Other forms of parasystole are intermittent parasystole and parasystole with exit block from the ectopic focus; a mimic of parasystole is reentry with varying degrees of conduction delay. This chapter describes and illustrates the various types of parasystole in the light of recent studies.

Mechanism of impulse formation

Microelectrode techniques[2-11] demonstrate that (1) the appearance of automatic activity does not require an initiating event, (2) parasystole originates in a relatively small group of cells, and (3) parasystole may be generated either because of enhanced normal automaticity (membrane potentials from -90 to -70 mV), abnormal automaticity (membrane potentials from −60 to −40 mV), or triggered activity resulting from afterdepolarizations in a protected focus. El-Sherif[15] reported a triggered rhythm in the dog caused by delayed afterdepolarizations in an ischemic postinfarction endocardial preparation that demonstrated the characteristic entrance block of the parasystolic rhythm.

Rate of discharge

According to Watanabe,[16] the common range of discharge rates in ventricular parasystole is 38 to 60/beats/min. However, Scherf and others[17,18] report that experimental ventricular parasystolic rates often reach 150 to 300 beats/min. Clinically, supraventricular parasystole exhibits slower rates than those of ventricular parasystole, with the atrial variety even slower than the junctional one.[18-20]

Entrance block through the years

Experiments using microelectrode techniques have established that entrance block prevents extraneous impulses from traversing an area of depressed conduction to discharge (reset) the ectopic focus,[21] although it is now known that they may modulate its rhythm.[2-8,12] Parasystole requires such a circumstance (i.e., the dominant pacemaker [usually sinus] coexists with, but never discharges, the ectopic pacemaker). The mechanism by which entrance block is achieved has been the source of debate and speculation for more than half a century. Some of the theories advanced are reviewed.

1912. The concept of entrance block in parasystole was introduced by Fleming[22] in 1912 and by Kaufmann and Rothberger[23] who first defined parasystole and described its classical ECG criteria as they are known today. At this time a zone of unidirectional block surrounding the parasystolic focus was described and referred to as *schutzblockierung*—protective block. The assumption of these authors that a parasystolic pacemaker is completely autonomous is no longer tenable. These same authors also postulated the possibility of a temporary loss of protection, thus implying what is known today as intermittent parasystole.[24-27]

1944 to 1967. These years saw the advancement of a multiplicity of theories to explain the protection enjoyed by a parasystolic focus.

In 1944, Vedoya[28] envisaged the protection of parasystole in terms of two spherical zones, each having a different refractory period.

Scherf and Schott[29] disagreed with the concept of a zone of unidirectional block completely surrounding the ectopic focus; they suggested that entrance block may be the result of disproportion between the excitability of the tissue surrounding the parasystolic focus and the strength of the sinus impulse. The same authors also suggested that if the automatic focus had a rapid rate, the refractoriness secondary to the rate would offer protection of the focus. Early studies by Scherf and Chick[30] suggested that the rapid rate of some parasystolic centers left the tissue surrounding it refractory. In these studies experimental parasystolic rates were as high as 300 beats/min.

Schamroth[31] similarly claimed that the protection enjoyed by a parasystolic focus resulted from its own rapid discharge, with its slow manifest rate accounted for by a high ratio (up to 9:1) exit block.

Hoffman's groups[32-35] reported the theory that the mechanism responsible both for the activity of the ectopic focus and for its protection is phase 4 depolarization. The level of membrane potential at the time of excitation is among the variables that determine conduction velocity. Reduced membrane potentials exist during both phase 3 and phase 4. If stimulation occurs during phase 4 in conjunction with a shift in the threshold potential toward zero and/or an impairment of membrane responsiveness, conduction disturbances can be expected. For example, if the threshold potential at the time of excitation is −60 mV instead of −70 mV, conduction is impaired or blocked altogether. Thus the ectopic focus would be surrounded with tissue in which there is an exit block that could become a two-way block. These facts could explain the intermittent nature of some parasystoles in that any further enhancement of phase 4 depolarization (along with the shift in threshold potential and/or impairment of membrane responsiveness) could prevent propagation altogether; and by the same token any reduction in phase 4 depolarization might permit the parasystolic beats to reappear because of a decrease in the degree of exit block.[32-35]

When phase 4 depolarization is not accompanied by this shift in threshold potential and/or an impairment of membrane responsiveness such as would result from bradycardia, there is no significant conduction disturbance because the membrane potential at the time of excitation is normal.

If phase 4 depolarization exists in conjunction with impaired membrane responsiveness, irrespective of the threshold potential, the resulting action potential is reduced in V_{max} and dV/dt (the height and speed of the rise of phase 0). This reduction results in decremental conduction, which may be enough to provide entrance or exit block.

1973. Finally, Cranefield, Wit, and Hoffman[21] confirmed through microelectrode studies that entrance block was caused by one-way block in depressed tissue. Thus the protection associated with a parasystolic focus is an abnormal mechanism and cannot be equated with the normal refractory period that occupies the entire cycle during a tachycardia.[36]

1976. From 1976 until 1983, data was published from biological and mathematical models that have established that variations in the parasystolic cycle length can result from an electrotonic influence on the parasystolic center through extraneous impulses across the region of protection.[2-8,12] Electrotonic modulation is discussed in the section "Modulated ventricular parasystole (p. 301)."

Rosenbaum and others[37] invoked both phase 3 and phase 4 block as the mechanism of protection for the parasystolic focus—"perfect parasystole" having absolute protection and intermittent parasystole having a "window" of normal conduction through which the parasystolic focus could be invaded and reset. Rosenbaum and associates believe that the parasystolic focus comprises a small group of moderately injured Purkinje fibers, or even a single fiber, in which phase 3 block and phase 4 block consecutively provide an entrance block through which no extraneous impulse can enter as long as there is no gap of normal conduction between the two phases. According to their tenet, the critical factor determining the presence of parasystole is the duration of the period during which normal conduction can occur. If it is long, sinus impulses will repeatedly penetrate to discharge and reset the ectopic focus, and the periods of protection will be limited (to the beginning and end of the parasystolic cycle). In such cases it would not be possible to document a parasytolic cycle. With a greater degree of injury, protection of the focus can be absolute, producing two-way instead of one-way block (concealed parasystole).

To help visualize the parasystolic mechanism involving phase 3, phase 4, and a potential intermediate normal conduction range, Rosenbaum and associates[37] have constructed an artificial parasystole that illustrates two types of parasystole that deviate from the classical criteria.

Fig. 16-1 illustrates a parasystole in which the calculated ectopic cycles are not maintained with the expected regularity. In the top panel P represents the discharge rate of the parasystolic focus; at X the sinus impulse penetrates and resets this focus. Note that the sinus impulse penetrated before the refractory stage of phase 4 (dotted area) of the ectopic cycle was due to begin, squeezing in through a narrow range of normal conduction after phase 3 (squared area).

In Fig. 16-2, again in the top panel, note the discharge of the parasystolic focus (P). However, because of a broader gap of normal conduction and because of an ectopic rhythm that is harmonious with the sinus rhythm, every third sinus impulse penetrates and resets the parasystolic focus to produce a ventricular ectopic beat every third beat, with the exact coupling intervals often thought to represent reentry or an afterpotential mechanism.

In summary, according to Rosenbaum and associates, the theory and clinical characteristics of parasystole can be reconciled as follows:

1. The parasystolic focus is comprised of a small group of slightly to moderately injured Purkinje fibers.
2. The rate of discharge of the parasystolic focus depends on the degree of enhanced automaticity in the Purkinje fibers or the injured fascicle.
3. Entrance block results from a combination of phase 3 block and phase 4 block, with a narrow or absent normal conduction period between them. One-way block is common in phase 3 and also occurs during phase 4 if accompanied by slight hypopolarization and a shift of the threshold potential toward zero.

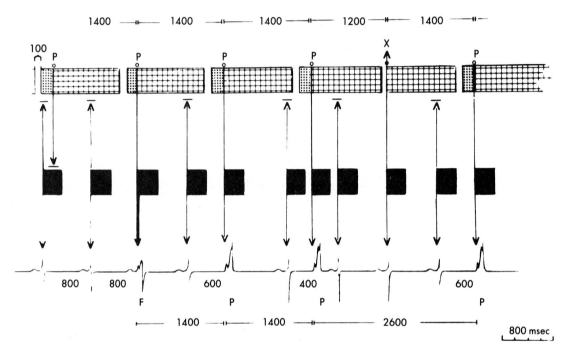

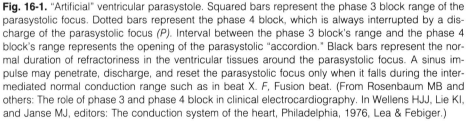

Fig. 16-1. "Artificial" ventricular parasystole. Squared bars represent the phase 3 block range of the parasystolic focus. Dotted bars represent the phase 4 block, which is always interrupted by a discharge of the parasystolic focus *(P)*. Interval between the phase 3 block's range and the phase 4 block's range represents the opening of the parasystolic "accordion." Black bars represent the normal duration of refractoriness in the ventricular tissues around the parasystolic focus. A sinus impulse may penetrate, discharge, and reset the parasystolic focus only when it falls during the intermediated normal conduction range such as in beat X. *F,* Fusion beat. (From Rosenbaum MB and others: The role of phase 3 and phase 4 block in clinical electrocardiography. In Wellens HJJ, Lie KI, and Janse MJ, editors: The conduction system of the heart, Philadelphia, 1976, Lea & Febiger.)

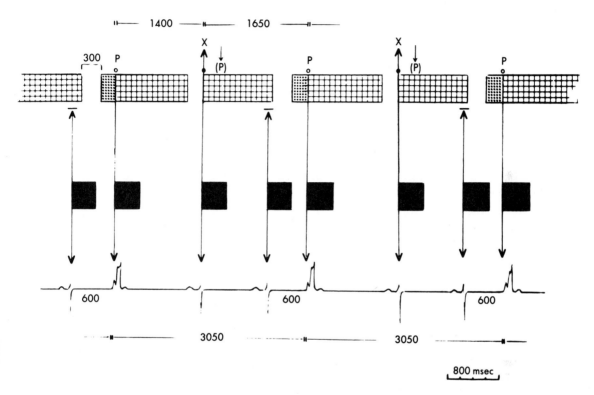

Fig. 16-2. Demonstration of how parasystole can give rise to a fixed coupling if the variables of the model are properly adjusted. *P,* Parasystolic focus; *X,* beat. (From Rosenbaum MB and others: The role of phase 3 and phase 4 block in clinical electrocardiography. In Wellens HJJ, Lie KI, and Janse MJ, editors: The conduction system of the heart, Philadelphia, 1976, Lea & Febiger.)

Exit block

In the presence of exit block no excitation of the heart from the parasystolic focus can arise. Exit block is therefore present when an expected parasystolic impulse is not propagated, even though the ventricles appear nonrefractory on the surface ECG. The rate of the parasystolic focus with exit block is usually faster than that of the dominant rhythm.[15] The concept of exit block has been experimentally demonstrated time and again.[36,38-43]

Entrance block keeps extraneous impulses from invading and resetting the ectopic focus, and exit block limits the number of impulses propagated from the regularly firing ectopic pacemaker. Parasystole cannot exist unless the focus is protected by entrance block, nor can it excite the heart unless exit block is at least transiently absent; persistent exit block results in concealed parasystole.

Exit block should not be confused with normal refractoriness in surrounding tissue. For example, if the ectopic focus discharges just before or during the QRS, there may be a fusion beat; if it is a little later, it cannot emerge because of normal refractoriness in surrounding tissue—but this is not exit block. On the other hand, if the parasystolic impulse fires when the ventricles are apparently nonrefractory and does not result in a propagated impulse, exit block exists.

Cranefield[44] proposes that the cause of exit block is concealed conduction, in that the zone of protection around the parasystolic focus can be incompletely penetrated from both sides (the sinus conducted impulse and the parasystolic one). Every time a sinus impulse enters this zone but fails to traverse it, refractoriness is the result; likewise, every time a parasystolic impulse enters and is blocked, the same occurs. Therefore the period during which it is possible for an impulse to emerge successfully from the zone surrounding the parasystolic focus may be shorter than appears on the surface ECG. According to Cranefield, exit block can be relieved by a local increase in catecholamines, a local improvement in perfusion, sinus slowing, or summation.

The patterns of exit block are generally of the type II variety, but type I may also occur[37] (Wenckebach conduction of the emerging impulse). First and third degree blocks would not be detected on the ECG.

Classical ventricular parasystole

Classical ventricular parasystole implies an automatic focus with absolute protection by virtue of entrance block; it is recognized because of the perfect regularity of the ectopic rhythm and the marked variation in the coupling intervals of the ectopic beats (no fixed coupling), with or without fusion. Absolute regularity, when associated with no fixed coupling, is an indication that the protected focus has not been reset by the dominant rhythm; when the interectopic intervals are multiples of a common denominator, absolute entrance block can be assumed.[37,38,45,46] This type of parasystole may or may not manifest exit block, and it may be intermittent. The rate of the parasystolic pacemaker and the degree of exit block can vary with cardiotropic drugs, electrolyte abnormalities, or autonomic impulses, making it difficult at times to determine the precise mechanism of a given arrhythmia.[15]

"No fixed coupling" is recognized by marked variations in the intervals between the ectopic beats and the preceding beats of the dominant rhythm. The term "coupling" is inappropriate in the setting of parasystole, although we shall continue to use it since there is no acceptable alternative. Coupling strictly refers to the interval between the dominant (usually sinus) beat and the coupled beat; and a coupled beat is one that is related to—dependent on—the preceding beat to which it owes its existence. As the quintessence of parasystole is *independence*, there is no coupling, constant or varying. The ectopic impulse propagates into the ventricular tissue when the ventricles are not refractory at the time of the ectopic discharge. One should realize, however (as is explained in the section, "Fixed coupling in parasystole"), that fixed coupling does not preclude a diagnosis of parasystole any more than variable coupling proves parasystole. Exact coupling has been reported in arrhythmias assumed to be parasystolic[47-49]; and variable coupling is seen in those arrhythmias assumed supported by reentry.[50]

Interectopic intervals as simple multiples of a common denominator. The interectopic intervals reflect the rate of the parasystolic focus, although the impulses themselves need not appear regularly. The times at which the parasystolic impulses activate the ventricles are not related to the sinus rhythm; rather, they are related to each other since the interval between any two parasystolic complexes depends on the firing rate of the ectopic focus and therefore equals that interval or is some multiple of it. A variance of $\pm$ 0.10 second or more is commonly allowed since the exit of the parasystolic impulse may occasionally be delayed because of refractoriness of the surrounding ventricular tissue as a result of the preceding sinus conducted impulse. In such a case the parasystolic impulse would be delayed in evoking a QRS complex because of local slow conduction.

Fusion beats. Fusion occurs between the dominant and the parasystolic impulses and is a mathematical certainty that is eventually seen if a long enough tracing is taken. Fusion beats are, however, not essential to the diagnosis. They occur when the fixed frequency of the parasystolic focus coincides with the activation of the ventricles from the sinus impulse.

Classical parasystole without exit block

Classical parasystole without exit block is most common when the rate of the parasystolic focus is slower than that of the sinus rhythm, allowing all parasystolic beats to fall within the nonrefractory period. With faster parasystolic rates, the diagnosis of parasystole is made when it can be shown that the sporadic appearance of the nonparasystolic rhythm does not reset the ectopic rhythm.

Classical parasystole without exit block may behave exactly like the simplest of all pacemakers, the "fixed-rate" one. The fixed-rate pacemaker fires regularly, regardless of the competitive sinus rhythm because it cannot be shut off by a competing rhythm, with the result that the paced beats show a varying relationship to the sinus beats but are always a constant interval (or a multiple of that constant interval) from each other. The varying relationship to the dominant rhythm attests to one of its two cardinal characteristics—that it is *independent*; and the common denominator of the interectopic intervals declares that it is *undisturbable*, its second cardinal characteristic. The only differences in the ECG between artificial (pacemaker) and natural parasystole are (1) the "blip" that precedes and initiates all paced beats and (2) the parasystolic focus that can be modulated (but not actually discharged) by electrotonic potentials transmitted across the region of block.

A fixed-rate artificial pacemaker is shown in Fig. 16-3 so that you can observe the firing of the parasystolic focus and plot the interectopic intervals. It is easily appreciated in this tracing that the fusion beats (**F**) result from the simultaneous propagation within the ventricles of an ectopic impulse (paced beat in this case) and a conducted sinus impulse.

Note the parasystolic behavior of the fixed-rate pacemaker:

1. It is protected in the sense that nothing can shut it off.
2. Whenever its impulse falls at a time when the ventricles are responsive, a QRS accompanies the pacemaker blip.
3. Whenever it falls at a time when the ventricles are refractory, the blip appears, but no ventricular complex results.
4. Thus the longer interectopic intervals are multiples of the shortest interectopic interval (e.g., in the second strip, the long interectopic interval, 350 msec, equals four times the shortest interval, 87 msec).
5. Whenever the artificial discharge coincides with sinus conduction into the ventricles, a fusion beat results (F).
6. Because parasystole represents an independent rhythm and is not beholden to the preceding beat, it will appear at varying intervals after the sinus beats (variable coupling).

These six points are all characteristic of parasystole.

Parasystole is first suspected in the clinical tracing if ectopic beats show varying coupling intervals such as in Fig. 16-4, an example of classical parasystole without exit block. The eye-catching feature is that the interval between the ectopic beat and the preceding sinus beat is never the same. It is a decided change from the exact coupling of an extrasystole to the sinus beat, which is thought caused by reentry or afterpotentials.

One then seeks to demonstrate that the ectopic rhythm cannot be interrupted. This is accomplished by showing that the interectopic intervals have a common denominator. The first three ectopic beats in Fig. 16-4 indicate the shortest manifest

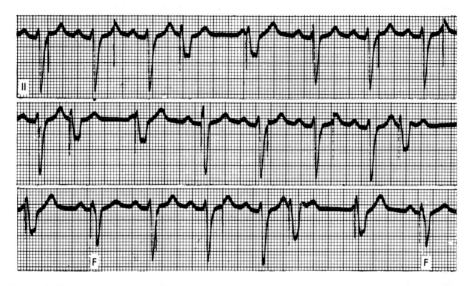

Fig. 16-3. Strips are continuous. Fixed-rate pacemaker for comparison with ventricular parasystole. The fusion *(F)* beats result from a collision within the ventricles of the paced beat (comparable to the parasystolic focus) and the sinus-conducted beat.

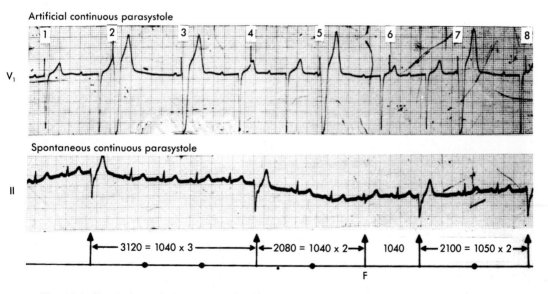

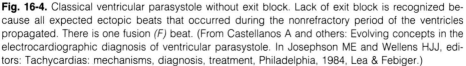

Fig. 16-4. Classical ventricular parasystole without exit block. Lack of exit block is recognized because all expected ectopic beats that occurred during the nonrefractory period of the ventricles propagated. There is one fusion *(F)* beat. (From Castellanos A and others: Evolving concepts in the electrocardiographic diagnosis of ventricular parasystole. In Josephson ME and Wellens HJJ, editors: Tachycardias: mechanisms, diagnosis, treatment, Philadelphia, 1984, Lea & Febiger.)

interectopic intervals. They are 145 and 146 hundredths of a second, respectively. All subsequent interectopic intervals are multiples of cycles between 143.5 and 156.5 hundredths of a second.

Fig. 16-5 illustrates the special pattern of fusion that occurs when, in the presence of bundle branch block (BBB), the ectopic focus is on the same side as the BBB. Note that the third beat in the bottom strip looks remarkably normal because the sinus impulse activated the unblocked left ventricle while the ectopic impulse was simultaneously activating the right side of the blocked branch to produce a normally narrow QRS.

In the presence of BBB, the parasystolic beats often arise on the side of the block and therefore have a shape characteristic of a block of the opposite bundle branch[6] (see Fig. 16-5). Some authorities claim that the pathology responsible for the BBB also provides the conditions necessary for parasystole, that is, slightly to moderately injured Purkinje fibers with consequent abnormal automaticity.[37,51,52]

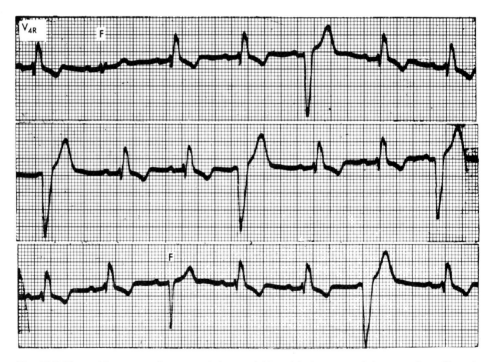

Fig. 16-5. Three strips are continuous and show a right ventricular parasystole competing with a sinus rhythm with RBBB.

This apparent relationship between BBB and parasystole might also explain the preponderance of ventricular parasystole over atrial and junctional parasystoles and the common link between parasystole and organic heart disease.[52]

Fig. 16-6 illustrates classical ventricular parasystole in the presence of atrial fibrillation. The diagnosis of fusion is made with less assurance in such a case since it is never known exactly when the next fibrillatory impulse will be conducted to the ventricles. However, in Fig. 16-6 it is reasonably certain that the third beat from the end of the second strip (**x**) is a fusion beat since, assuming parasystole, this is precisely where an ectopic beat would be expected. It is therefore reasonable to conclude that the beat in question is mainly conducted from the fibrillating atria but contains a small distorting contribution from the ventricular ectopic focus.

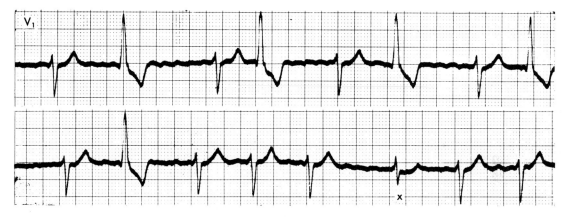

Fig. 16-6. Atrial fibrillation and parasystole.

Classical parasystole with exit block

The exit block in ventricular parasystole is usually of the type II variety.[37] It is recognized when an anticipated ectopic beat fails to appear, although the ventricles are nonrefractory, assuming the usual criteria for ventricular parasystole are also present. Fig. 16-7 is an example of classical ventricular parasystole with exit block. In the bottom strip, midway between the two complexes, an ectopic beat is expected to fuse with the sinus impulse, but it does not appear.

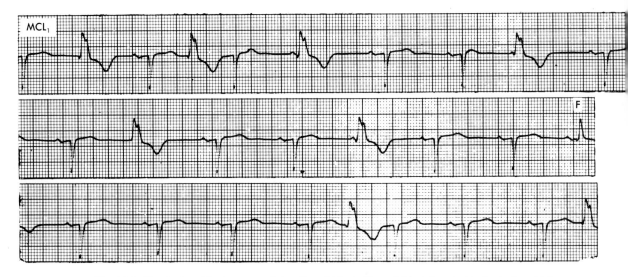

Fig. 16-7. Classical ventricular parasystole with exit block. The exit block is noted in the bottom tracing; midway between the first two complexes, a ventricular ectopic beat was due but did not occur, even though the ventricles were nonrefractory.

Concealed parasystole

Concealed parasystole is seen only during sinus slowing.[53,54] The explanation for the concealment of the parasystolic focus with faster rhythm is a refractory period in the area of protection (exit block) that is longer than that of the faster sinus rhythm. Thus the parasystolic focus maintains its fixed rate but does not exit into the surrounding myocardium until the underlying rhythm drops below a critical rate.

Modulated ventricular parasystole

Any pacemaker that is in contact with surrounding depressed myocardium that is exhibiting entrance, but not exit, block may experience modulation of its rhythm by the electrotonic effects in the surrounding tissue.[55] A series of studies initiated in Moe's laboratory[2-6,8,12] have demonstrated electrotonic modulation of a protected automatic focus. Considering the clinical and experimental observations of the past and the studies from Moe's group,[2-6,8,12,13] we now know that entrance block is caused by abnormal tissue and not by the normal refractoriness associated with rapid rhythms and that it may or may not be absolute. That is, the ectopic focus can be totally shielded from the influence of extraneous impulses, or it can be modulated when subthreshold electrotonic depolarizations are transmitted across the depressed barrier. Early studies demonstrating this electrotonic link were accomplished through computer model simulations and were later confirmed in a biological model. The electrotonic theory is based on the following premises:

1. The cycle length of a pacemaker can be altered by partial depolarization.
2. If the partial depolarization occurs early in phase 4 depolarization of the parasystolic focus, the next discharge is delayed.[53]
3. If the partial depolarization occurs later in phase 4, the next expected discharge from the parasystolic focus is early (captured by the invading impulse) because, with the membrane potential closer to threshold, an additional partial depolarization across the zone of protection causes it to fire prematurely.[2] The ectopic pacemaker may in fact be entrained by the dominant pacemaker. In such a case there would be fixed coupling to the dominant pacemaker over a wide range of frequencies.[8,55]
4. In spite of the entrance block, the parasystolic focus is not entirely independent of the electrical influences surrounding it.[56]
5. The parasystolic cycle may be modulated (prolonged or shortened) depending on (a) the amplitude of the electrotonic events, and (b) the relationship of the two cycle lengths (parasystolic and sinus) to each other.

Thus the premise that the interectopic intervals are simple multiples of a common denominator is clearly not an obligatory feature of a parasystolic rhythm.[41]

Intermittent parasystole

Intermittent parasystole may have absolute protection,[45,57-59] or the protection may be limited to the initial portions of the cycle (phase 3).[45,60-62]

ENTRANCE BLOCK DURING THE ENTIRE CYCLE. Intermittent parasystole with entrance block during the entire cycle has been described by Sherf and associates[57-59] and Pick and Langendorf[45] as characterized by long nonparasystolic intervals interspersed with a series of parasystolic beats. In almost all cases of intermittent parasystole the first beat of each series had fixed coupling.[15] The intermittent character of the parasystolic rhythm may be caused either by a cessation of automatic activity[52,53] or by a periodic loss of protection.[44] Sherf and associates[57,58] believe the fixed coupling of the first beat of the parasystolic period is caused by the sinus beat forcing the discharge through electrotonic interaction; and others believe it is caused by temporary loss of protection of the parasystolic focus, resulting in its being discharged and reset.[15,27,49]

ENTRANCE BLOCK ONLY DURING EARLY CYCLE. Intermittent parasystole with protection only during the early cycle has been described by many authors,[45,60-65] with most cases limiting the protection to the initial half of the cycle (phase 3 protection). In this case the fixed coupling interval at the outset of the parasystolic period is not essential to the diagnosis.[37]

Cranefield[44] has postulated that entrance block may be temporarily relieved because of summation (Fig. 16-8). Thus, if neighboring fibers in the depressed segment of tissue are activated simultaneously, evoking subthreshold action potentials, the two currents then summate, reach threshold, and evoke an action potential that can propagate. If this propagation occurs, the parasystolic focus is reset by the two invading impulses, causing intermittent parasystole. Electrotonic modulation of the parasystolic focus may also explain some cases of intermittent parasystole.[15]

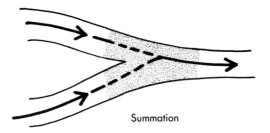

Summation

Fig. 16-8. Summation may occur when two currents from depressed areas join to form a current that can be propagated, although each current on its own could not be propagated.

Parasystolic accelerated idioventricular rhythm

With faster ventricular ectopic rates and no exit block, the number of ectopic beats may be more than the sinus rhythm and may indeed resemble an accelerated idioventricular rhythm (AIVR) or ventricular tachycardia.[45,46,57,66] In such a case there is no way to recognize the rhythm as parasystolic unless there are interruptions with nonparasystolic beats that do not reset the ectopic focus.[37] Fig. 16-9 shows a continuous parasystolic AIVR without exit block. The proof is seen in the bottom tracing when the nonparasystolic beats fail to reset the parasystolic focus.

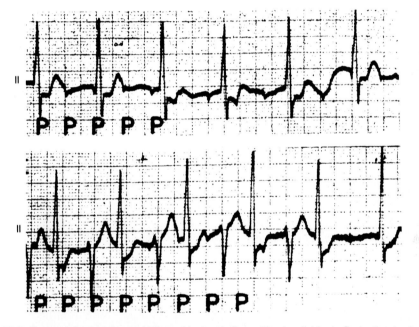

Fig. 16-9. Parasystolic accelerated idioventricular rhythm without exit block. Protection is demonstrated in the bottom strip by the appearance of nonparasystolic beats that failed to affect the ectopic cycle length. The resulting electrocardiographic pattern resembles that of bidirectional tachycardia. (From Castellanos A and others: Evolving concepts in the electrocardiographical diagnosis of ventricular parasystole. In Josephson ME and Wellens HJJ, editors: Tachycardias: mechanisms, diagnosis, treatment, Philadelphia, 1984, Lea & Febiger.)

Fixed coupling in parasystole

If, by chance, rates of the parasystolic focus and the sinus node are mathematically related, fixed coupling may be seen.[47] For example, if the sinus rate is 70 beats/min and the rate of the parasystolic focus is 35 beats/min, there is a fixed relationship (which is coincidental rather than real) between the sinus beat and the parasystolic one, and an ectopic beat will appear, following every other normal beat at a fixed interval.

Supernormality is also recognized as a mechanism for fixed coupling in parasystole.[39,67-69] Fixed coupling may result when the impulse from the parasystolic focus is subthreshold, and is effective only when it falls during the supernormal phase. An artificial example of fixed coupling caused by supernormality can be seen in Fig. 16-10. A subthreshold fixed-rate pacemaker is firing at a regular rate throughout the tracing. It is effective only when it falls during the supernormal phase of excitability.

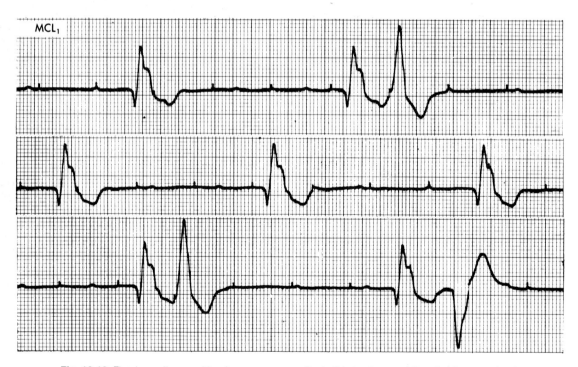

Fig. 16-10. Fixed coupling resulting from supernormality. In this tracing a subthreshold pacemaker is effective only when it fires during the supernormal period.

Reversed coupling and modulation of the ectopic pacemaker by the dominant pacemaker (electrotonic influences) have already been mentioned as possible causes of constant coupling in parasystole.[8,55]

Paired ectopic ventricular beats

Kuo and Surawicz[70] postulated that, when paired ventricular ectopic beats are seen in parasystole, the mechanism is that of reentry within the parasystolic focus or its vicinity. These authors noted that paired ventricular ectopic beats appear more frequently in patients with no fixed coupling (presumably parasystole) than in those with fixed coupling.

Atrial parasystole

Atrial or junctional parasystole is less common than ventricular parasystole and is more difficult to diagnose.[71-73] This difficulty arises because the anomalous ventricular complex is easier to identify and because an atrial and possibly a junctional parasystolic discharge will interrupt and reset the sinus rhythm, producing what is called "reversed coupling."[39] Since the sinus node is reset by the ectopic impulse, the interval between the atrial or junctional parasystolic beat and the sinus P wave will be the same each time (exact coupling). However, instead of the usual situation in which the ectopic beat is coupled to the preceding sinus beat, the reverse is true; the sinus beat is coupled to the ectopic beat.

Fig. 16-11 provides examples of atrial parasystole. In Fig. 16-11, *A*, the parasystolic P waves are very similar to the sinus P waves. Note that the coupling interval between the atrial parasystolic beat and the preceding sinus P wave varies but that the interval between it and the following sinus P wave is constant (reversed coupling). In this tracing the common denominator of the interectopic intervals is 57, making this a parasystolic tachycardia at a rate of 107 beats/min. In Fig. 16-11, *B*, you see fusion beats; the coupling interval becomes longer and longer until the two impulses fuse within the atria.

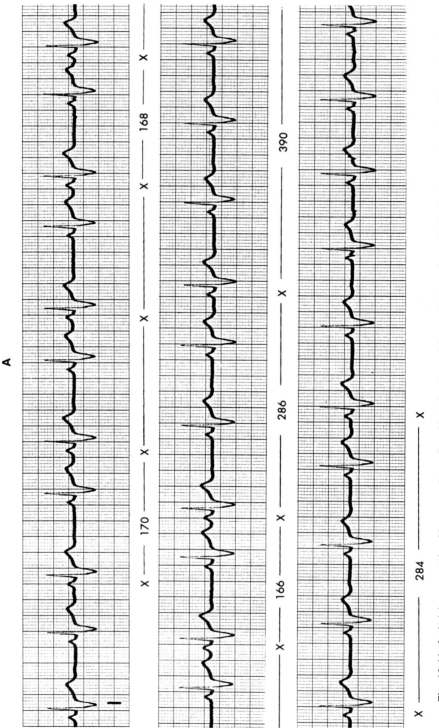
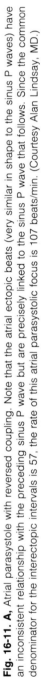

Fig. 16-11. A, Atrial parasystole with reversed coupling. Note that the atrial ectopic beats (very similar in shape to the sinus P waves) have an inconsistent relationship with the preceding sinus P wave but are precisely linked to the sinus P wave that follows. Since the common denominator for the interectopic intervals is 57, the rate of this atrial parasystolic focus is 107 beats/min. (Courtesy Alan Lindsay, MD.)

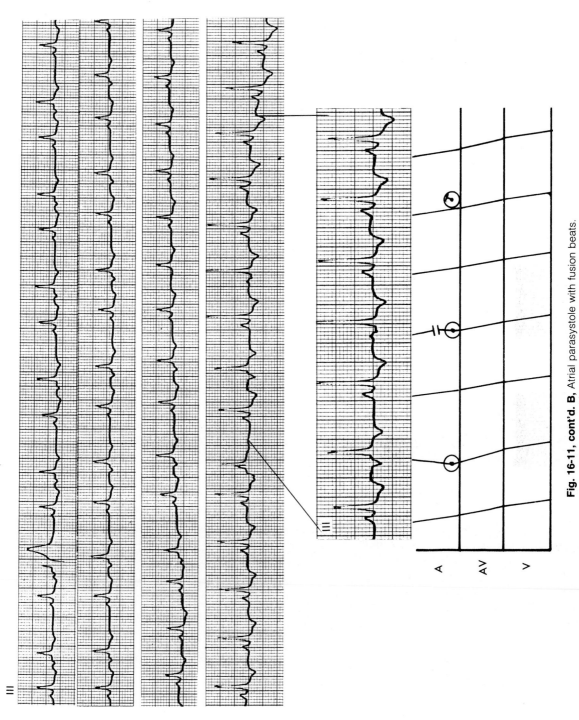

Fig. 16-11, cont'd. B, Atrial parasystole with fusion beats.

Clinical significance of parasystole

Ventricular parasystole is generally regarded as a benign rhythm.[37,74] Since parasystole is an independent, autonomous rhythm that cannot be interrupted, it follows that its impulses (like the blip of a fixed-rate pacemaker) must from time to time land on the T waves of the competitive sinus beats. Because of this inevitable R-on-T incidence, parasystole may be thought dangerous. It is, however, an empirical observation that a parasystolic beat rarely occurs on the T wave because the effective refractory period of nonparasystolic beats is usually equal to or slightly longer than the QT interval.[37] Moreover, there is no acceptable evidence that, if parasystolic (automatic) beats arrived in the vulnerable period, they would provoke ventricular tachycardia or ventricular fibrillation, even in the setting of acute myocardial infarction.[74-78]

The benign nature of ventricular parasystole may result because the parasystolic rhythm is usually not fast or sustained and it is easily suppressed by antiarrhythmic drugs.[75] For example, lidocaine slows the rate of the focus and walls it off by compounding the depression in the area of entrance block surrounding the focus.[77] In addition, ventricular parasystole also occurs in apparently healthy individuals.[74]

Summary

Parasystole is usually ventricular, but it may also be atrial or, less commonly, junctional or SA nodal. The ECG characteristics of parasystole are variable intervals between ectopic beats and the preceding normal beats and, in its classic form, interectopic intervals that have a common denominator (i.e., the focus is never reset, thanks to a zone of protection surrounding it [entrance block]). Microelectrode studies have further shown that entrance block is caused by one-way block in depressed tissue. Thus the protection associated with a parasystolic focus is an abnormal mechanism. This protection can be continuous or intermittent, with or without exit block, producing the classical form of parasystole in which the cycle length of the ectopic focus is not influenced at all by extraneous impulses. Parasystole may also be concealed and may demonstrate a classical form when it emerges. The parasystolic focus can be modulated by electrotonic subthreshold currents traversing the band of depressed tissue and producing the nonclassical form of parasystole. Although the parasystolic focus is never actually reset by the extraneous rhythm, its cycle length can be altered in that early beats cause a delay in parasystolic discharge and late beats cause an acceleration of the discharge. Exit block exists when an expected parasystolic impulse does not appear in spite of a nonrefractory ventricle.

REFERENCES

1. Jalife J, Michaels DC, and Langendorf R: Modulated parasystole originating in the sinoatrial node, Circulation 74:40, 1986.
2. Jalife J and Moe GK: Effect of electrotonic potentials on pacemaker activity of canine Purkinje fibers in relation to parasystole, Circ Res 39:801, 1976.
3. Moe GK and others: A mathematical model of parasystole and its application to clinical arrhythmias, Circulation 56:968, 1977.
4. Jalife J and Moe GK: A biological model of parasystole, Am J Cardiol 43:761, 1979.
5. Antzelevitch C, Jalife J, and Moe GK: Characteristics of reflection as a mechanism of reentrant arrhythmias and its relationship to parasystole, Circulation 61:182, 1980.
6. Jalife J and Antzelevitch C: Pacemaker annihilation: diagnostic and therapeutic implications, Am Heart J 100:128, 1980.
7. Ferrier GR and Rosenthal JE: Automaticity and entrance block induced by focal depolarization of mammalian ventricular tissue, Circ Res 47:238, 1980.
8. Jalife J, Antzelevitch C, and Moe GK: The case for modulated parasystole, PACE 5:811, 1982.
9. Cranefield PF: The conduction of the cardiac impulse, Kisco, NY, 1975, Futura Publishing Co, Inc.
10. Wit AL and Cranefield PF: Triggered activity in cardiac muscle fibers of the simian mitral valve, Circ Res 38:85, 1976.
11. Singer DH, Baumgarten GM, and Ten Eick, RE: Cellular electrophysiology of ventricular dysrhythmia: studies on diseased and ischemic heart, Prog Cardiovasc Dis 24:97, 1981.
12. Antzelevitch C and others: Parasystole, reentry, and tachycardia: a canine preparation of cardiac arrhythmias occurring across inexcitable segments of tissue, Circulation 68:1101, 1983.
13. Antzelevitch C, Jalife J, and Moe GK: Electrotonic modulation of pacemaker activity; further biological and mathematical observations on the behavior of modulated parasystole, Circulation 66:1225, 1982.
14. Lamanna VR, Antzelevitch C and Moe GK: Effects of lidocaine on conduction through depolarized canine false tendons and on a model of reflected reentry, J Pharmacol Exp Ther 221:353, 1982.
15. El-Sherif N: The ventricular premature complex: mechanisms and significance—an update. In Mandel WS, editor: Cardiac arrhythmias, their mechanisms, diagnosis and management, Philadelphia 1987, JB Lippincott Co.
16. Watanabe Y: Reassessment of parasystole, Am Heart J 81:451, 1971.
17. Scherf D and Bornemann C: Parasystole with a rapid ventricular center, Am Heart J 62:320, 1961.
18. Scherf D and others: Parasystole, Am J Cardiol 11:527, 1963.
19. Scherf A, Bornemann C, and Yildiz M: AV nodal parasystole, Am Heart J 60:179, 1960.
20. Eliakim M: Atrial parasystole, Am J Cardiol 16:457, 1965.
21. Cranefield PF, Wit AL, and Hoffman BR: Genesis of cardiac arrhythmias, Circulation 47:190, 1973.
22. Fleming GG: Triple rhythm of the heart due to ventricular extrasystoles, Q J Med 5:318, 1912.
23. Kaufmann R and Rothberger CJ: Beitrag zur Kenntnis der Entstelungsweise extrasystolischer Allorhythmien, Z Ges Esp Med 5:3490, 1917; 7:119, 1919; 9:103, 1919; 11:40, 1920; 13:1, 1922.
24. Katz LN and Pick A: Clinical electrocardiography. II. The arrhythmias, Philadelphia, 1956, Lea & Febiger.
25. Watanabe Y: Reassessment of parasystole, Am Heart J 81:451, 1971.
26. Steffens TG: Intermittent ventricular parasystole due to entrance block failure, Circulation 44:442, 1971.
27. Cohen H, Langendorf R, and Pick A: Intermittent parasystole—mechanism of protection, Circulation 48:761, 1973.
28. Vedoya R: Parasistolia, Buenos Aires, 1944, A Lopez.
29. Scherf D and Schott A: Extrasystoles and allied arrhythmias, London, 1953, William Heinemann.
30. Scherf D and Chick FB: Experimental parasystole, Am Heart J 42:212, 1951.
31. Schamroth L: Ventricular parasystole with slow manifest ectopic discharge, Br Heart J 24:731, 1962.
32. Singer DH, Lazzara R, and Hoffman BF: Interrelationships between automaticity and

conduction in Purkinje fibers, Circ Res 21:537, 1967.

33. Singer DH, Lazzara R, and Hoffman BF: Interrelationships between automaticity and conduction in Purkinje fibers, Circ Res 21:537, 1967.

34. Kao CY and Hoffman BF: Graded and decremental responses in heart muscle fibers, Am J Physiol 194:187, 1958.

35. Van Dam RT, Moore EN, and Hoffman BR: Initiation and conduction of impulses in partially depolarized cardiac fibers, Am J Physiol 204:1133, 1963.

36. Castellanos A and others: Evolving concepts in the electrocardiographic diagnosis of ventricular parasystole. In Josephson ME and Wellens HJJ, editors: Tachycardias: mechanisms, diagnosis, treatment, Philadelphia, 1984, Lea & Febiger.

37. Rosenbaum MB and others: The role of phase 3 and phase 4 block in clinical electrocardiography. In Wellens HJJ, Lie KI, and Janse MJ, editors: The conduction system of the heart, Philadelphia, 1976, Lea & Febiger.

38. Cranefield PF, Klein HO, and Hoffman BF: Conduction of the cardiac impulse. I. Delay, block, and one-way block in depressed Purkinje fibers, Circ Res 28:199, 1971.

39. Pick A: The electrophysiologic basis of parasystole and its variants. In Wellens HJJ and others: Exit block, Am J Cardiol 28:402, 1971.

40. Fisch C, Greenspan K, and Anderson GJ: Exit block, Am J Cardiol 28:402, 1971.

41. Greenspan K, Anderson GJ, and Fisch C: Electrophysiologic correlate of exit block, Am J Cardiol 28:197, 1971.

42. Hoffman BF: The genesis of cardiac arrhythmias, Prog Cardiovasc Dis 8:319, 1966.

43. Watanabe Y: Reassessment of parasystole, Am Heart J 81:451, 1971.

44. Cranefield PF: The conduction of the cardiac impulse, Mt Kisco, 1975, Futura Publishing Co, Inc.

45. Pick A and Langendorf R: Interpretation of complex arrhythmias, Philadelphia, 1979, Lea & Febiger.

46. Schamroth L: The disorders of cardiac rhythm, Oxford, 1980, Blackwell Scientific Publications, Ltd.

47. Langendorf R and Pick A: Parasystole with fixed coupling, Circulation 35:304, 1967.

48. Levy MN, Lee MH, and Zieike H: Feedback mechanism responsible for fixed coupling in parasystole, Circ Res 31:846, 1972.

49. Schamroth L and Marriott HJL: Intermittent ventricular parasystole with observations on its relationship to extrasystolic bigeminy, Am J Cardiol 7:799, 1961.

50. Mack I and Langendorf R: Factors influencing the time of appearance of premature systoles (including a demonstration of cases with ventricular premature systoles due to re-entry but exhibiting variable coupling), Circulation 1:910, 1950.

51. Pick A: Parasystole, Circulation 8:243, 1953.

52. Rosenbaum MB and others: Relationship between increased automaticity and depressed conduction in the main intraventricular conduction fascicles of the human and canine heart, Circulation 49:818, 1974.

53. Nau GJ and others: Concealed ventricular parasystole uncovered in the form of ventricular escapes of variable coupling, Circulation 64:199, 1981.

54. Castellanos A and Castillo CA: Concealed ventricular parasystole exposed by abrupt cessation of pacing, Chest 82:362, 1982.

55. Moe GK, Antzelevitch C, and Jalife J: Premature contractions: reentrant or parasystolic? In Harrison DC, editor: Cardiac arrhythmias, Boston, 1981, G.K. Hall.

56. Weidmann S: Effect of current flow in the membrane potential of cardiac muscle, J Physiol (London) 115:2277, 1951.

57. Scherf D and Schott A: Extrasystoles and allied arrhythmias, Chicago, 1973, Year Book Medical Publications, Inc.

58. Scherf D and Boyd LJ: Three unusual cases of parasystole, Am Heart J 39:650, 1950.

59. Scherf D and others: Intermittent parasystole, Cardiologia 30:16, 1957.

60. Cohen H, Langendorf R, and Pick A: Intermittent parasystole—mechanism of protection, Circulation 48:761, 1973.

61. Steffens T: Intermittent ventricular parasystole due to entrance block failure, Circulation 44:442, 1971.

62. Castellanos A and others: Electronic pacemaker models of parasystole, PACE 5:537, 1982.

63. Castellanos A and others: A search for modulation in intermittent ventricular parasystole, PACE 3:73, 1980.

64. Kinoshita S and Tanabe Y: Second degree entrance block in intermittent parasystole, Chest 67:236, 1975.

65. Kinoshita S: Mechanisms of ventricular parasystole, Circulation 58:715, 1978.

66. Marriott HJL and Menendez MM: AV dissociation revisited, Prog Cardiovasc Dis 8:522, 1966.

67. Soloff IA and Fewell JW: Supernormal phase of ventricular excitation in man: its bearing on the genesis of ventricular premature systoles and a note on atrioventricular conduction, Am Heart J 59:869, 1960.

68. Spear JF and Moore EN: The effect of changes in rate and rhythm on supernormal excitability in the isolated Purkinje system of the dog. A possible role in re-entrant arrhythmias, Circulation 50:1144, 1974.

69. Pick A and Langendorf R: Parasystole and its variants, Med Clin North Am 60:125, 1976.

70. Kuo CS and Surawicz B: Coexistence of ventricular parasystole and ventricular couplets: mechanism and clinical significance, Am J Cardiol 44:435, 1979.

71. Chung KY, Walsh TJ, and Massie E: Atrial parasystole, Am J Cardiol 14:255, 1964.

72. Chung EK: Diagnosis and clinical significance of parasystole. In Sandoe E, Flensted-Jensen E, and Olesen KH, editors: Symposium on cardiac arrhythmias, Elsinore, 1970, Astra.

73. Eliakim M: Atrial parasystole. Effect of carotid sinus stimulation, Valsalva maneuver, and exercise, Am J Cardiol 16:457, 1965.

74. El-Sherif N: The ventricular premature complex: mechanism and significance. In Mandel WS, editor: Cardiac arrhythmias, their mechanisms, diagnosis and management, Philadelphia 1987, JB Lippincott Co.

75. Salazar J and McKendrick CS: Ventricular parasystole in acute myocardial infarction, Br Heart J 32:377, 1978.

76. Luceri RM and others: Ventricular parasystole in inferior myocardial infarction, Clin Res 30:830A, 1982 (abstract).

77. Lazzara R: Accelerated ventricular rhythms in acute myocardial infarction and the differential effects of lidocaine, Circulation 56:III66, 1977 (abstract).

78. Kotler MN and others: Prognostic significance of ventricular ectopic beats with respect to sudden death in the late post-infarction period, Circulation 47:959, 1973.

CHAPTER 17

Concealed conduction

As long as the cardiac impulse is traveling in the specialized conduction system, it writes nothing in the surface tracing because of the small amount of tissue involved. However, if an impulse travels a limited distance within the system, even though it leaves no trace of its own on the record, it can interfere with the formation or propagation of another impulse. When this interference can be recognized in the tracing because of an unexpected conduction delay or postponement of an impulse, it is known as *concealed conduction.* Therefore concealed conduction can be defined as the propagation of an impulse within the specialized conduction system of the heart, which can be recognized only from its effect on the subsequent beat or cycle.

Historical background

The first indirect electrocardiographical evidence of concealed AV conduction came in 1925 when Lewis and Master[1] demonstrated in the canine heart the effect of blocked impulses on subsequent conduction. During the same period Ashman[2] was performing similar experiments on the turtle heart. Twenty years before this time Erlanger[3] had noted concealed conduction in his studies on complete heart block and had postulated with Engelmann that delayed conduction was caused by incomplete penetration of the junctional tissues, causing partial refractoriness.

In 1927 Kaufmann and Rothberger[4] were the first to apply clinically the concept of concealed conduction. They proposed that the alternation of ventricular cycle length seen in a case of atrial flutter with 2:1 ventricular response was secondary to concealed deeper penetration into the AV junction by every other blocked flutter wave (diagrammatically illustrated in Fig. 17-1).

The term concealed conduction was not introduced until 1948, when Langendorf[5] succinctly defined it in the title of his published paper: "Concealed A-V Con-

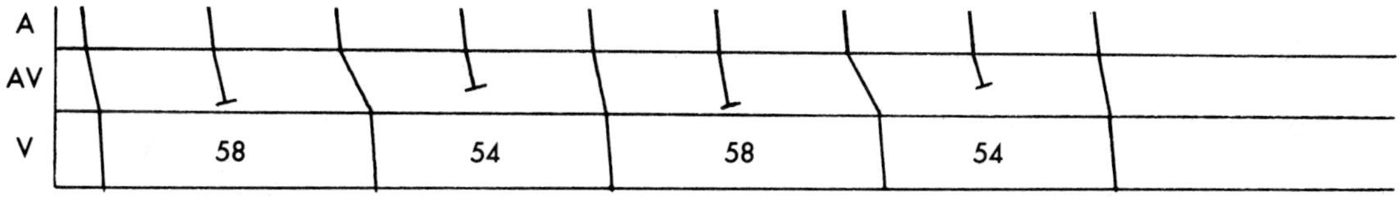

Fig. 17-1. Diagram of atrial flutter with 2:1 AV conduction and alternation of the ventricular cycle length secondary to concealed deeper penetration of alternate blocked impulses (the first clinical invocation of concealed conduction). (From Kaufmann R and Rothberger CJ: Z Ges Exp Med 57:600, 1927.)

duction: the Effect of Blocked Impulses on the Formation and Conduction of Subsequent Impulses."

In 1950 Soderstrom[6] and, later, Moe, Abildskov, and Mendez[7] showed that the irregular ventricular response in atrial fibrillation was a function of concealed conduction.

The mechanism of concealed conduction was outlined in detail in 1956 by Katz and Pick[8] and was demonstrated experimentally as a possibility in any part of the conduction system in 1961 by Hoffman, Cranefield, and Stuckey.[9] Finally, in 1969, direct evidence of concealed AV conduction was obtained in His bundle recordings performed by Lau and co-workers.[10]

An understanding of this mechanism has proved to be most useful in interpreting arrhythmias that would otherwise be unexplainable in the surface ECG.

Concealed conduction in atrial fibrillation

The most common display of concealed conduction is seen in atrial fibrillation.[11] In this arrhythmia literally hundreds of impulses per minute are available for conduction to the ventricles. If hundreds of impulses are crowded into the space of 1 minute, it stands to reason that there can be little measurable variation in their spacing. The AV node would then be expected to conduct whenever it became nonrefractory, which would be at regular intervals. This, however, is not what happens. The ventricular response to atrial fibrillation is chaotically irregular because numerous impulses are competing for pathways in the AV junction. Some penetrate incompletely, leaving the AV junction refractory yet not producing a QRS complex (concealed conduction); others are blocked; and a few get through, resulting in (1) haphazard activation of the ventricles and (2) reduction in the number of impulses that pass the AV barrier. In fact, the more rapid is the bombardment of the AV node by vagrant impulses from the fibrillating atria, the more the concealed conduction and the slower the ventricular response.

Fig. 17-2, *A*, is a regular supraventricular tachycardia at a rate of 148 beats/min. In Fig. 17-2, *B*, atrial fibrillation has developed in the same patient, with the ventricular rate reduced to less than 100 beats/min. In this patient it is evident that the AV junction is able to conduct 148 beats/min *(A);* yet when atrial fibrillation ensues, the AV junction can conduct only 100 beats/min because of concealed conduction.

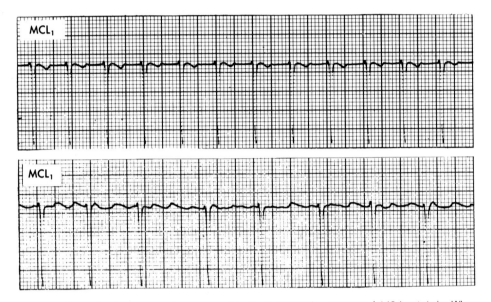

Fig. 17-2. Top strip shows a regular supraventricular tachycardic at a rate of 148 beats/min. When atrial fibrillation develops (bottom strip), AV conduction to the ventricles is reduced to less than 100 beats/min.

Interpolated ventricular extrasystoles with concealed retrograde conduction

Ventricular extrasystoles often conduct retrogradely all the way to the atria. In fact, Kistin and Landowne[12] showed that this happened nearly half the time. It is therefore likely that a majority of ectopic ventricular impulses are conducted at least as far as the AV junction. This conduction is evident only if it has an effect on the next cycle; and this effect is most likely if the next beat is due soon such as the beat after an *interpolated* ventricular premature beat (VPB) sandwiched between two consecutive sinus beats. If the VPB penetrates retrogradely into the fast pathway of the AV junction, the next sinus beat travels down the nonrefractory slow pathway. Thus the PR interval of the sinus beat following the VPB is prolonged.

Fig. 17-3 graphically illustrates such a case. In fact, the PR interval after the VPB is so long that it creates the impression of supraventricular prematurity in the following beat. When the ventricular rhythm is irregular, the atrial rhythm often seems irregular also. The laddergram indicates the regularity of the sinus rhythm and the concealed retrograde conduction from the VPB.

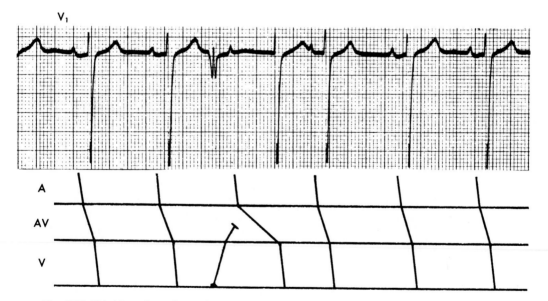

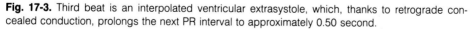

Fig. 17-3. Third beat is an interpolated ventricular extrasystole, which, thanks to retrograde concealed conduction, prolongs the next PR interval to approximately 0.50 second.

In Fig. 17-4 there are three interpolated VPBs, all of which are followed by concealed retrograde conduction up the fast pathway. Note in the laddergram that the sinus P waves are right on time, a fact not immediately perceived in the tracing. The PR prolongation after each VPB varies, depending on how soon the P wave follows the VPB. The closer it is, the longer the PR interval (a shorter RP results in a longer PR); and the later the P is, the shorter the PR.

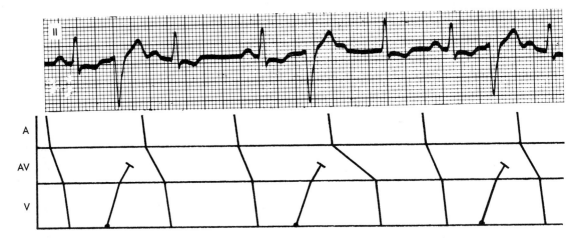

Fig. 17-4. The second, fifth, and eighth beats are interpolated ventricular extrasystoles that prolong the ensuing PR intervals by concealed retrograde conduction.

Fig. 17-5 shows the progressive effect of interpolated ventricular bigeminy on the PR interval, producing a Wenckebach-like effect. Three of the P waves in this tracing are detectable only because of the way they distort the T waves, especially since this distortion is at a time when a sinus P wave is expected (see laddergram). The first VPB is interpolated, and its retrograde concealed conduction lengthens the following PR interval. Since the sinus rhythm is regular and the VPBs are precisely coupled, the next sinus P wave falls earlier on the downslope of the ectopic T—resulting in an even longer PR interval. This sequence continues, with the sinus P waves falling progressively closer to the preceding ectopic beat. Thus the fifth P wave of the series ends such a short RP interval that it is not conducted. The first three VPBs are interpolated; the fourth is not, and the Wenckebach-like cycle begins again.

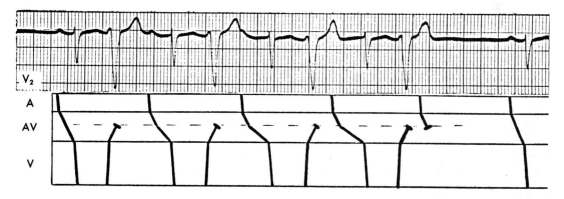

Fig. 17-5. Interpolated ventricular bigeminy produces a Wenckebach-like effect because of retrograde concealed conduction. The first ventricular premature beat (VPB) lengthens the next PR, which automatically "pushes" the next couplet (sinus beat + VPB) to the right, bringing the ectopic beat nearer to the next P wave (shorter RP). Thus the next retrograde conduction is closer to the next descending impulse, and the PR is prolonged still further. This sequence is repeated until finally, after the fourth extrasystole, the descending impulse fails to get through.

Fig. 17-6 is another example of the same mechanism. In this case, however, because of the slower sinus rate, the P waves are quite evident, and the PR lengthening is easily appreciated. The sequence consists of two VPBs that are interpolated and a third that is not. The third VPB is followed by a ventricular escape beat.

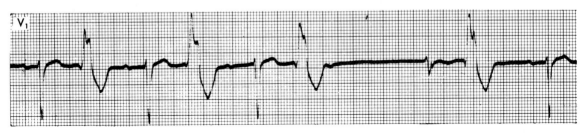

Fig. 17-6. Another example of ventricular bigeminy with concealed retrograde conduction producing progressive lengthening of the PR interval until the fourth sinus impulse fails to get through. After the "dropped" beat, the cycle ends with a ventricular escape beat.

Concealed junctional extrasystoles

Concealed junctional extrasystoles discharge the AV junction while both anterograde and retrograde conduction is blocked. Such an event is totally silent on the surface ECG; and yet its diagnosis may be extremely important in the management of the patient, for concealed junctional beats can imitate type I (Wenckebach) and type II AV block[5,13-15] and are themselves thought to indicate significant junctional disease.[16]

Wenckebach periodicity may be imitated in the presence of concealed junctional bigeminy since the PR may progressively lengthen until a beat is dropped.[5] This sequence is diagrammatically illustrated in Fig. 17-7.

Type II AV block may be imitated if a single concealed junctional extrasystole suddenly prevents conduction of a sinus impulse (Fig. 17-8) or if concealed penetration involves the proximal His-Purkinje system as well.[17,18] Since the development of type II AV block is a widely accepted indication for a permanent implanted pacemaker, one has a serious responsibility to rule out concealed junctional extrasystoles.

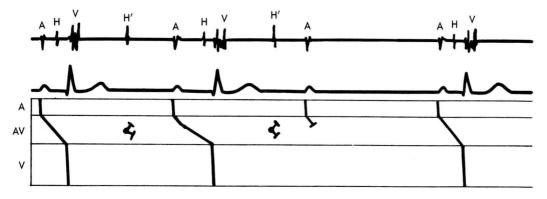

Fig. 17-7. Diagrammatic representation of how concealed junctional extrasystoles can imitate Wenckebach conduction. The His bundle recording, ECG, and laddergram are shown depicting concealed junctional bigeminy mimicking the Wenckebach phenomenon. Note that the first functional extrasystole lengthens the following AH and PR intervals; the next extrasystole then prevents conduction altogether and simulates the dropped beat of a Wenckebach period. Key to His bundle records: *A,* atrial activation; *H,* His bundle activation; *V,* ventricular activation; *H',* junctional extrasystole.

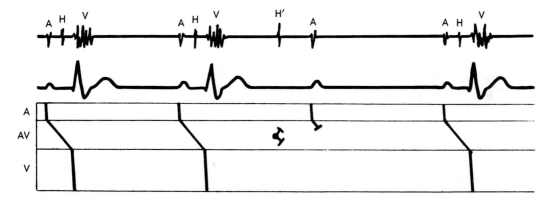

Fig. 17-8. Diagrammatic representation of how concealed junctional extrasystoles can mimic type II AV block. Without prior lengthening of the PR interval, the junctional extrasystole prevents conduction of the next sinus impulse. Key to abbreviations as in Fig. 17-7.

ECG CLUES TO CONCEALED JUNCTIONAL EXTRASYSTOLES. Although concealed junctional extrasystoles can be documented only with the aid of His bundle electrograms, which may indeed be necessary if there is a question of pacing the patient, they can be strongly suspected from the following clues[19]:

1. Abrupt, unexplained lengthening of the PR interval
2. The presence of apparent types I and II AV block in the same tracing
3. Apparent type II block in the presence of a normal QRS
4. The presence of manifest junctional extrasystoles elsewhere in the tracing

In the top tracing of Fig. 17-9 there is an abrupt and unexplained lengthening of the PR interval. This lengthening is certainly not caused by the Wenckebach phenomenon since the next sinus impulse is conducted with a shorter PR interval and there are no nonconducted beats. In the bottom tracing there is the same, abrupt, unexplained lengthening of the PR interval followed by two normally conducted beats and then what looks like an interpolated VPB with concealed retrograde conduction to the atria, manifested by the long PR interval. Herein lies the clue to the abrupt unexplained PR prolongations. The laddergram illustrates their explanation: if instead of a VPB the bizarre beat is a junctional extrasystole with aberration, the otherwise unexplained lengthening of the first three PR intervals becomes understandable—they are caused by the effect of concealed junctional extrasystoles.

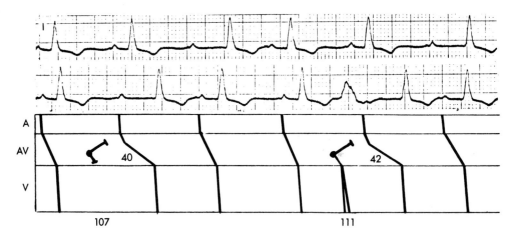

Fig. 17-9. Strips are not continuous. In the top strip the two longer PR intervals and ventricular cycles are caused by concealed junctional extrasystoles (as diagrammed under the beginning of the bottom strip). Further along in the bottom strip there is a junctional extrasystole conducted to the ventricles with left bundle branch block (LBBB) aberration, producing the same effect on the next PR interval. (Courtesy Dr. Leo Schamroth, Johannesburg.)

Concealed conduction affecting impulse formation

In the bottom tracing of Fig. 17-10 there is a sudden unexpected interruption of an accelerated junctional rhythm. The junctional rate averages 64 beats/min and is dissociated from the slightly slower sinus rhythm. In the top tracing the junctional rhythm is interrupted when a sinus impulse (P wave in the T of the third junctional beat) is conducted to the ventricles (ventricular capture); then after two normal sinus beats the accelerated junctional rhythm takes over again. Toward the end of the bottom tracing the same thing almost occurs a second time, but the sinus impulse fails to reach the ventricles. It does, however, discharge the AV pacemaker and interrupt the junctional rhythm. Thus concealed conduction is recognized because an expected beat fails to appear.

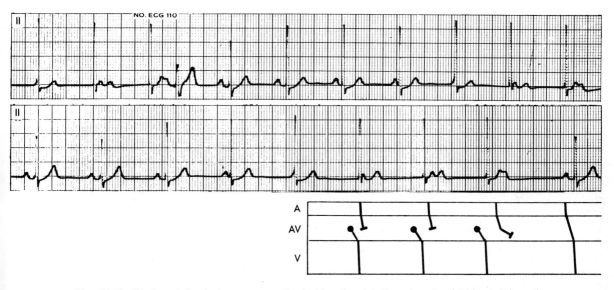

Fig. 17-10. AV dissociation between an accelerated junctional rhythm at a rate of 74 beats/min and a slightly slower sinus rhythm. In the top strip the fourth beat is a ventricular capture conducted with aberration. At the end of the bottom strip there is another attempted capture, but the sinus impulse fails to reach the ventricle. It does, however, reach and discharge the junctional pacemaker (see laddergram).

In Fig. 17-11 another junctional rhythm has a sudden unexpected interruption. Each junctional beat is followed by a retrograde P' wave, and the RP' interval lengthens with each beat. It is only when the RP' interval has lengthened critically that the junctional rhythm is abruptly interrupted. The readiest explanation is illustrated in the laddergram. Delayed retrograde conduction has permitted reentry with a resulting abortive reciprocal beat. The retrograde impulse with the longest RP' interval turns down toward the ventricles but fails to reach its destination. It does, however, succeed in discharging and thus resetting the junctional focus, leaving in its tracks an unexpected pause.

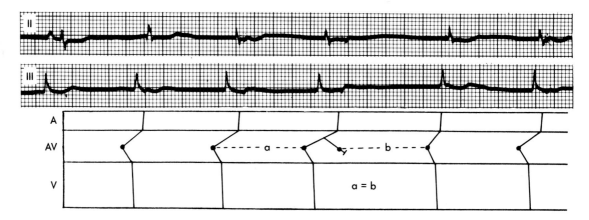

Fig. 17-11. In lead II the first beat is a sinus beat. Then a mildly accelerated junctional rhythm takes over at a rate of 62 beats/min with retrograde conduction to the atria. The RP lengthens progressively (potential retrograde Wenckebach), and after the fourth beat a longer ventricular cycle develops. The same sequence is repeated twice in lead III, for which the mechanism is diagrammed. A critical degree of retrograde conduction delay enables the retrograde impulse to reenter a downward path and discharge and reset the junctional pacemaker, although it fails to reach the ventricles.

Fig. 17-12 illustrates yet another form of concealed retrograde conduction. In this tracing there is a junctional escape rhythm of 36 beats/min resulting from an underlying sinus bradycardia and arrhythmia. Three VPBs can be seen in the two strips. In the top strip these VPBs do not disturb the basic junctional cycle length, which varies between 161 and 166. However, the VPB in the second strip postpones the junctional beat. We can infer from this that the ventricular ectopic impulse has traveled retrogradely into the AV junction, discharged the junctional pacemaker, and reset its rhythm.

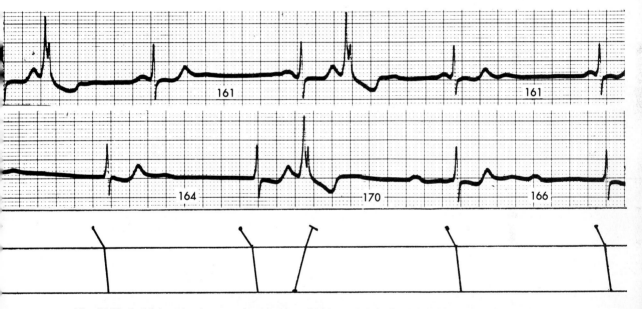

Fig. 17-12. An idiojunctional pacemaker at a rate of 36 beats/min is dissociated from an irregular but even slower sinus rhythm. The two ventricular premature beats (VPBs) in the top strip do not interfere with the regularity of the junctional firing, but the one in the bottom strip does. The mechanism is diagrammed below the second strip. This VPB, through concealed retrograde conduction to the AV junction, resets the idiojunctional pacemaker.

Fig. 17-13 is an interesting example of how consecutive atrial premature beats (APBs) can suggest some degree of AV block. Note in the top tracing that there is an APB in the second and fourth T waves. On each occasion it is immediately followed by a second one, which is late enough in the cycle to conduct normally to the ventricles; yet it is not conducted, suggesting AV block, and the pause ends with a junctional escape beat. Compare this to the bottom tracing from the same patient, in which on two occasions a single APB with the same coupling interval as in the top tracing is conducted. One would think that if some APBs premature enough to land on the T wave can be conducted, certainly the second of each pair of APBs in the top strip, which land well beyond the T wave, could be easily conducted. The explanation for this failure of conduction is that the first of each pair of APBs in the top strip has penetrated the AV junction and left it refractory so that the second of the pair is blocked.

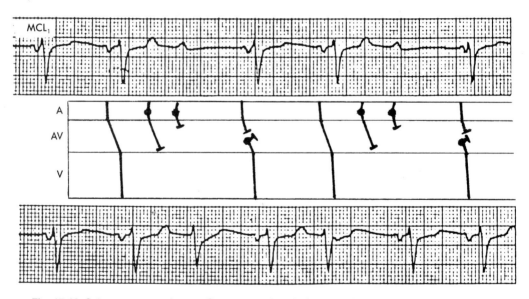

Fig. 17-13. Strips are not continuous. On two occasions in the top strip there are pairs of atrial premature beats (APBs), neither of which is conducted. The first is not conducted because of refractoriness resulting from the preceding sinus conducted beat. The second is not conducted because of incomplete penetration of the junction by the preceding APB.

In Fig. 17-14 the same mechanism explains the failure of the second of a pair of APBs to be conducted when the first of the pair is conducted with right bundle branch block (RBBB) aberration at the end of the tracing. The underlying rhythm is sinus with nonconducted atrial bigeminy. For a more exhaustive listing of complex manifestations of concealed conduction see Chan and Pick.[19]

V₁

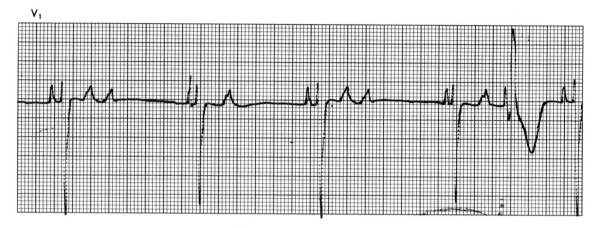

Fig. 17-14. Bigeminal nonconducted atrial premature beats (APBs). After the first and third ventricular complexes there are two APBs in a row; the second of them is not conducted, probably because of incomplete penetration into the AV junction by the preceding APB. At the end of the strip an APB is conducted with right bundle branch block (RBBB) aberration. There is an artifact in the second sinus P wave.

Summary

Conduction of the impulse through the heart is reflected on the surface ECG when the atrial or ventricular myocardium is activated. When the impulse is traveling within the SA node and perinodal fibers or within the AV node or His-Purkinje system, the amount of electrical current generated is too small to be seen on the surface ECG and is therefore "concealed." These currents can, however, be recorded, using invasive technics such as SA nodal and His bundle electrograms. The existence of concealed conduction can be determined by its effects on the beats that follow it. For example, after a P wave it is known that the impulse has travelled through the AV node and the His-Purkinje system because a QRS appears. If the QRS does not appear, it would be known that this normal concealed conduction failed somewhere along that pathway. During atrial fibrillation concealed conduction into the His-Purkinje system from the fibrillating atria is responsible for the irregular ventricular response in that not all impulses reach the ventricular myocardium but do leave the conduction system refractory. Concealed conduction retrogradely into the fast pathway of the AV node is often observed after an interpolated ventricular extrasystole, causing a long PR interval because the next sinus beat finds only the slow intranodal pathway available. Junctional extrasystoles that are blocked in both directions are concealed and affect the sinus impulse that follows.

REFERENCES

1. Lewis T and Master AM: Observations upon conduction in the mammalian heart. A-V conduction, Heart 12:209, 1925.
2. Ashman K: Conductivity in compressed cardiac muscle; supernormal phase in conductivity in compressed auricular muscle in the turtle heart, Am J Physiol 74:140, 1925.
3. Erlanger J: On the physiology of heart block in mammals, with especial reference to the causation of Stokes-Adams disease, J Exp Med 7:676, 1905.
4. Kaufmann R and Rothberger CJ: Der-Uebergang von Kammerallorhythmien in Kammer-Arrhythmie in klinischen Fällen von Vorhofflattern, Alternans der Reisleitung, Z Ges Exp Med 57:600, 1927.
5. Langendorf R: Concealed A-V conduction: the effect of blocked impulses on the formation and conduction of subsequent impulses, Am Heart J 35:542, 1948.
6. Sodorstrom N: What is the reason for the ventricular arrhythmia in cases of atrial fibrillation? Am Heart J 40:212, 1970.
7. Moe GK, Abildskov JA, and Mendez C: An experimental study of concealed conduction, Am Heart J 67:338, 1964.
8. Katz LN and Pick A: Clinical electrocardiography. I. Arrhythmias, Philadelphia, 1956, Lea & Febiger.
9. Hoffman BF, Cranefield PF, and Stuckey JH: Concealed conduction, Circ Res 9:194, 1961.
10. Lau SH and others: A study of atrioventricular conduction in atrial fibrillation and flutter in man using His bundle recordings, Circulation 40:69, 1965.
11. Langendorf R and others: Ventricular response in atrial fibrillation: role of concealed conduction in the AV junction, Circulation 32:69, 1965.
12. Kistin AD and Landowne M: Retrograde conduction from premature ventricular contractions, a common occurrence in the human heart, Circulation 3:738, 1951.
13. Langendorf R and Mehlman JS: Blocked (nonconducted) A-V nodal premature systoles imitating first and second degree heart block, Am Heart J 34:500, 1947.

14. Rosen KM, Rahimtoola SH, and Gunnar RM: Pseudo A-V block secondary to premature nonpropagated His bundle depolarization. Documentation by His bundle electrocardiography, Circulation 42:367, 1970.

15. Pick A: Mechanisms of cardiac arrhythmias: from hypothesis to physiologic fact, Am Heart J 86:249, 1973.

16. Narula OS: His bundle electrocardiography and clinical electrophysiology, Philadelphia, 1975, FA Davis Co.

17. Cohen AC, Langendorf R, and Pick A: Intermittent parasystole; mechanism of protection, Circulation 48:761, 1973.

18. Castellanos A and others: Pseudo AV block produced by concealed extrasystoles arising below the bifurcation of the His bundle, Br Heart J 36:457, 1974.

19. Chan AQ and Pick A: Reentrant arrhythmias and concealed conduction, Am Heart J 97:644, 1979.

CHAPTER 18

Supernormality

Supernormal excitability was first described in 1912 for nerves[1] and in 1938 for heart muscle.[2] With the advent of the microelectrode, supernormal excitability was first demonstrated in 1953 in isolated Purkinje fibers from sheep and calves.[3] Since that time intracellular stimulation methods have demonstrated supernormal excitability in the bundle branch–Purkinje system[4] and in Bachmann's bundle[5] but not in the AV node,[6] bundle of His,[4] or working myocardium.[5]

The supernormal period

The supernormal period occurs at the end of phase 3. It is that period during which a stimulus of less than the normally required intensity can initiate a propagatable action potential.

Supernormal excitability is diagnosed when the myocardium responds to a stimulus that is ineffective when applied earlier or later in the cycle. During the supernormal period the cell has recovered enough to respond to a stimulus; and since the membrane potential is still reduced, it requires only a little additional depolarization to bring the fiber to threshold. Thus a smaller stimulus than is normally required elicits an action potential during the supernormal phase of excitability.

The shaded areas in Fig. 18-1 illustrate the supernormal period and its relationship to the total refractory period. There is a point within this time that the current requirement for excitation is at its minimum. This point is indicated by an **X** within the shaded areas. Spear and Moore[7] have found that the duration of the supernormal phase remains the same in spite of changes in the action potential duration. Thus as the action potential shortens, the supernormal period occupies more of it.

Fig. 18-2 is an example of supernormal excitability. In this tracing a failing pacemaker is ineffective except when the pacing stimulus lands between the nadir and the end of the T wave.

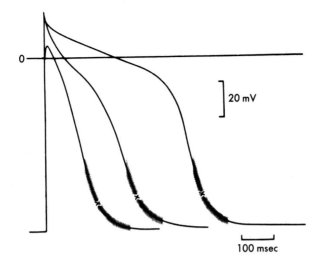

Fig. 18-1. Relationship between supernormal period and total refractory period. (X indicates moment of maximal supernormality.) Above are shown superimposed action potentials. The longest duration action potential was evoked at a basic cycle length of 800 msec. The shorter action potentials were successively evoked premature beats at cycle lengths of 460 and 251 msec. Shaded areas delineate the boundaries of the period of supernormal excitability. The X's within the shaded area indicate the point of minimal current requirements. (From Spear JF and Moore EN: Circulation 50:1174, 1974. By permission of the American Heart Association, Inc.)

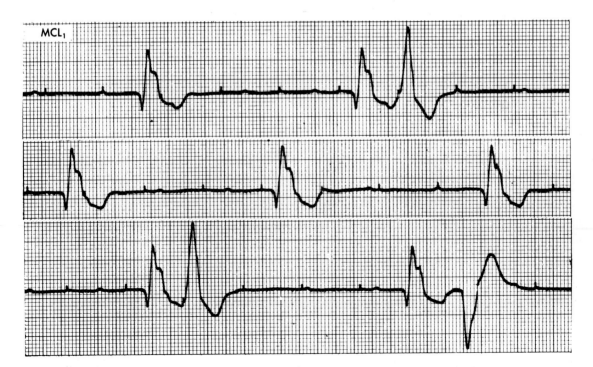

Fig. 18-2. Strips are continuous. Complete AV block with very slow left idioventricular rhythm. The implanted pacemaker is ineffective except on two occasions when the stimulus lands in the "supernormal" phase of excitability—toward the end of the T wave.

Supernormal conduction

Supernormal conduction is not better than normal, only better than expected. Conduction is better earlier in the cycle than later and occurs when block is expected.

Spear and Moore[7] have demonstrated the relationship between supernormal excitability and supernormal conduction. The mechanism is as follows: a conduction wave relies for its propagation on local currents flowing across the membranes just in front of the propagating action potential. If the downstream cells can be brought to threshold faster because of reduced current requirement for excitation during late repolarization, then conduction velocity is improved over that expected at a later time in diastole when current requirements to reach threshold are greater.

Supernormal conduction can be seen in Fig. 18-3. Most of the sinus impulses are conducted with right bundle branch block (RBBB). However, there are two early beats that are conducted normally, suggesting supernormal conduction in the right bundle branch (RBB). This is also an example of critical rate RBBB since the sinus impulses following the atrial premature beat (APB) end a longer cycle (overdrive suppression) and are conducted normally.

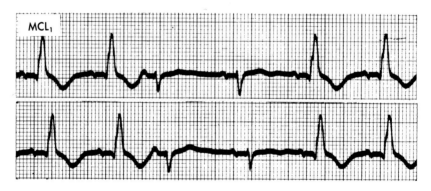

Fig. 18-3. Strips are not continuous. Supernormal conduction in the right bundle branch (RBB). The third beats in the two tracings are atrial premature beats (APBs) with normal conduction in the face of an underlying right bundle branch block (RBBB) with much longer cycles.

Concealed supernormal conduction

In Fig. 18-4 there are two instances of manifest supernormal conduction (fifth beat in each tracing) and two instances of concealed supernormal conduction (after the first beat in each tracing). Supernormal conduction is evident just beyond the middle of each strip. The sinus P waves deforming the ST segment in the top strip and the T wave in the bottom represent impulses that are conducted, whereas later sinus impulses, with an expected better chance of conduction, are blocked.

Concealed supernormal conduction is not quite so easy to recognize. Apart from the two instances of capture caused by manifest supernormal conduction, notice the irregularity of the junctional escape rhythm in the face of a significant degree of AV block. The following principle often facilitates a diagnosis: when an independent rhythm (in this case junctional) manifests two cycle lengths, subtract the shorter from the longer, *starting from the end of the long cycle.* At that point look for possible clues that may explain what has lengthened this cycle beyond the shorter ones. Applying this principle to the tracing at hand, note that just preceding the spot to which you have measured in the longer cycle, there is a sinus P wave. Clearly this sinus P wave is causally related to the lengthened cycle and implies penetration of that sinus impulse into the AV junction, thus discharging and resetting the junctional pacemaker. The postponement of the next expected junctional beat earmarks this as concealed conduction.

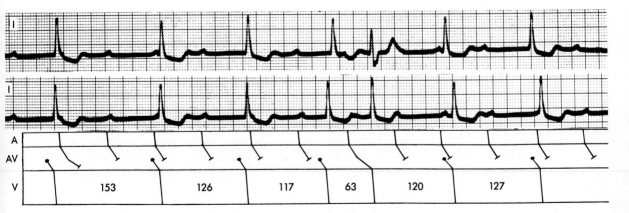

Fig. 18-4. Strips show a significant degree of AV block with a junctional escape rhythm at a rate of 48 beats/min. The first cycle in each strip is longer than the other cycles because the atrial impulse immediately following the first QRS is conducted into the AV junction and resets the junctional pacemaker (see laddergram). The fifth beat in each strip is conducted from the somewhat later atrial impulses, deforming the ST segment or T wave of the preceding beat. Since these atrial impulses are much earlier in the cycle than many that are not conducted at all, they may be considered examples of supernormal conduction; and since the impulses after the first QRS do not reach the ventricles and their conduction is only inferred, they are examples of concealed supernormal conduction.

Mimics of supernormal conduction

When conduction is better earlier than later, supernormality is certainly a possibility. However, other mechanisms should also be considered, some of which are listed below.[8-10] Keep in mind that you may not always be able to prove your point conclusively.

1. Concealed junctional extrasystoles
2. Phase 4 (paradoxical critical rate)
3. Reentry with ventricular echo
4. The gap phenomenon

CONCEALED JUNCTIONAL EXTRASYSTOLES. In Fig. 18-5 the underlying sinus rhythm is regular at 68 beats/min. Note that each time there is a shorter RP interval, it is complemented by a shorter PR interval, suggesting supernormal conduction of these alternate beats. A much more likely explanation, postulated by Langendorf[11] in 1948, is that the longer PRs are the result of concealed junctional extrasystoles, as illustrated in the laddergram.

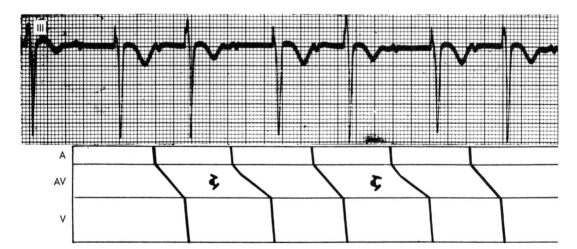

Fig. 18-5. Concealed junctional extrasystoles mimicking supernormal conduction.

PHASE 4 (PARADOXICAL CRITICAL RATE).[12-15] Enhanced phase 4 depolarization within the bundle branch system may result in bundle branch block (BBB) (phase 4 block, see Chapter 11). In such a case the maximal diastolic potential immediately follows repolarization, from which point the membrane potential is steadily reduced. Thus an action potential initiated early in the cycle (immediately after repolarization) would have a steeper and higher phase 0 and consequently better conduction than would an action potential initiated later in the cycle.

In Fig. 18-6 the underlying rhythm is a sinus bradycardia at 50 beats/min with a faster junctional escape rate of 56 beats/min producing AV dissociation. If the fibers of the RBB have enhanced automaticity, late-arriving impulses resulting from the bradycardia find a reduced membrane potential, and conduction is blocked. Since diastolic depolarization begins immediately after repolarization, the membrane potential is maximum early in the cycle; in fact, the earlier the better. Note that all the beats except two early ones are conducted with RBBB. When ventricular capture occurs (fifth beat), there is much less evidence of BBB, suggesting that conduction occurred either before the membrane potential could be reduced or because the impulse arrived during the phase of supernormal excitability in the RBB.

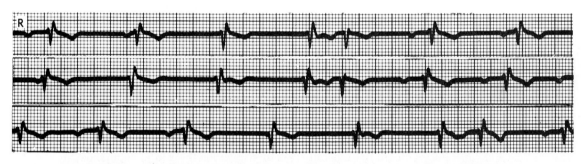

Fig. 18-6. Strips are continuous. A junctional rhythm with right bundle branch block (RBBB) aberration is dissociated from a slightly slower sinus rhythm. The three early beats are ventricular captures; and the first two are conducted with much less evidence of RBBB, suggesting conduction during the "supernormal" phase of the RBB or conduction before reduction of the membrane potential.

CONCEALED REENTRY. Fig. 18-7 is another example of simulated supernormal conduction. A shorter PR interval (fourth beat) unexpectedly interrupts what starts as a Wenckebach sequence. Since the P wave of this impulse is close to the preceding T wave, one might suspect supernormal conduction. A more likely explanation is that, after the lengthened PR interval of the third beat, there is reentry with retrograde conduction (see laddergram). The descent of the next atrial impulse thwarts this attempt at an atrial echo. However, further (anterograde) reentry produces a ventricular echo as the impulse returns to the ventricles, making it appear that the atrial impulse was conducted during a period of supernormality.

THE GAP PHENOMENON. The gap phenomenon was originally described by Moe, Mendez, and Han[16] in 1965 as a zone in which premature atrial stimuli encountered AV block, whereas if the stimulus were earlier or later, AV conduction was accomplished. Since that time as many as six types of gaps have been described for anterograde conduction.[17]

The more commonly encountered gaps, thought functional in nature, are dependent on a difference in refractoriness between the cells at two different levels in the AV conduction system so that a premature atrial beat is blocked in the His-Purkinje system but not in the AV node. This is because the shortest time between two atrial impulses needed for the AV node to conduct (functional refractory period) is less than the effective refractory period of the His-Purkinje system.

Fig. 18-8 diagrammatically illustrates the mechanism of the gap phenomenon. In Fig. 18-8, *A,* a premature atrial beat is not conducted to the ventricles because the impulse traverses the AV node rapidly enough to arrive while the His-Purkinje system is still in its effective refractory period. In Fig. 18-8, *B,* with a shorter coupling interval the impulse travels more slowly through the AV node, which is in its relative refractory period. By the time this impulse traverses the AV node, the His-Purkinje system has completed its effective refractory period, and conduction is possible. Ventricular activation results.

Fig. 18-9 diagrammatically illustrates another level for the gap phenomenon, in which the effective refractory period of the His-Purkinje system exceeds both the functional and the effective refractory period of the AV node, meaning that the His-Purkinje system and not the AV node is the site of conduction delay. In Fig. 18-9, *A,* a premature atrial beat is blocked within the His-Purkinje system. In Fig. 18-9, *B,* at a shorter coupling interval, a premature atrial beat is delayed in the proximal His-Purkinje system, probably in the bundle branches,[15] giving the distal portion time to recover. Ventricular activation results.

From these two examples you can see that the gap phenomenon depends on conduction delay in fibers activated during their relative refractory period when conduction velocity is slower than it would have been if activation had occurred later in the cycle. Other types of gap phenomenon are described in which the required conduction delay is in the bundle of His,[18] the proximal AV node,[17] or the atria.[18]

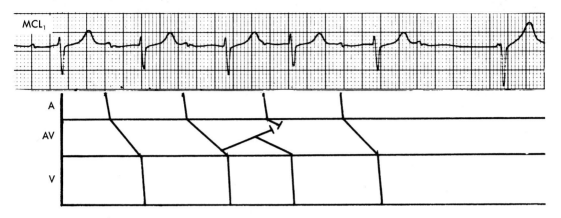

Fig. 18-7. Concealed reentry as a mimic of supernormal conduction.

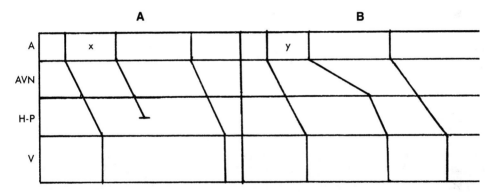

Fig. 18-8. Diagrammatic representation of the mechanism of the gap phenomenon. **A,** The initial block is in the His-Purkinje system. **B,** The required conduction delay is in the AV node.

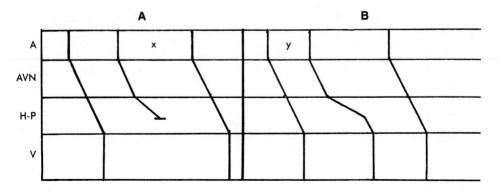

Fig. 18-9. Diagrammatic representation of the mechanism of another type of gap phenomenon. **A,** The initial block is low in the His-Purkinje system. **B,** The required conduction delay is in the bundle branches.

The gap phenomenon has also been described in a retrograde direction[19]; and, in fact, it is thought to occur more frequently during retrograde than during antero-grade conduction. The site of retrograde block is the AV node or upper reaches of the His-Purkinje system, whereas the gap-produced retrograde delay in conduction is lower in the His-Purkinje system.

Summary

During the supernormal period, located at the end of phase 3 of the action potential, a stimulus that could not elicit a propagated action potential before that time or after it can do so. That is, a stimulus of less-than-normal intensity can result in a propagated action potential if it occurs during the supernormal period. There are two factors responsible for this phenomenon: (1) the availability of fast sodium channels, and (2) the proximity of the membrane potential to threshold potential. The same mechanism is responsible for supernormal conduction. That is, faster conduction results if the downstream cells can be brought to threshold potential more easily because the stimulus arrives during that point in the repolarization process when enough fast sodium channels are available for a propagated action potential.

REFERENCES

1. Adrian ED and Lucas K: On the summation of propagated disturbances in nerve and muscle, J Physiol 44:68, 1912.
2. Cranefield PE, Hoffman BE, and Siebens AA: Anodal excitation of cardiac muscle, Am J Physiol 190:383, 1957.
3. Weidmann S: Effects of calcium ions and local anesthetics on electrical properties of Purkinje fibers, J Physiol 129:568, 1955.
4. Spear JF and Moore EN: The effect of changes in rate and rhythm on supernormal excitability in the isolated Purkinje system of the dog. A possible role in re-entrant arrhythmias, Circulation 50:1144, 1974.
5. Childers RW, Merideth J, and Moe GJ: Supernormality in Bachmann's bundle: an in vivo and in vitro study, Circ Res 22:363, 1968.
6. Puech P and others: Supernormal conduction in the intact heart. In Narula OS, editor: Cardiac arrhythmias: electrophysiology, diagnosis, and management, Baltimore, 1979, The Williams & Wilkins Co.
7. Spear JF and Moore EN: Supernormal excitability and conduction. In Wellens HJJ, Lie KI, and Janse MJ, editors: The conduction system of the heart: structure, function and clinical implications, Philadelphia, 1976, Lea & Febiger.
8. Moe GK and others: An appraisal of "supernormal" A-V conduction, Circulation 38:5, 1968.
9. Damato AN and others: Observations on the mechanism of one type of so-called supernormal A-V conduction, Am Heart J 82:725, 1971.
10. Gallagher JJ and others: Alternative mechanisms of apparent supernormal atrioventricular conduction, Am J Cardiol 31:362, 1973.
11. Langendorf R: Concealed A-V conduction: the effect of blocked impulses on the formation and conduction of subsequent impulses, Am Heart J 35:542, 1948.
12. Singer DH, Lazzara R, and Hoffman BF: Interrelationships between automaticity and conduction in Purkinje fibers, Circ Res 21:537, 1967.
13. Rosenbaum MB, and others: The mechanisms of intermittent bundle branch block: relationship to prolonged recovery, hypopolarization, and spontaneous diastolic depolarization, Chest 63:666, 1973.
14. Pick A and Fishman AP: Observations in heart block. Supernormality of A-V and intra-

ventricular conduction and ventricular parasystole under the influence of epinephrine, Acta Cardiol 5:270, 1950.

15. Hoffman BF: Physiology of A-V transmission, Circulation 24:506, 1961.

16. Moe GK, Mendez C, and Han J: Aberrant A-V impulse propagation in the dog heart. A study of functional bundle branch block, Circ Res 16:261, 1965.

17. Damato AN and others: Gap phenomena: antegrade and retrograde. In Wellens HJJ, Lie KI, and Janse MJ, editors: The conduction system of the heart: structure, function, and clinical implications, Philadelphia, 1976, Lea & Febiger.

18. Wu D and others: Nature of gap phenomenon in man, Circ Res 34:682, 1974.

19. Akhtar M and others: The gap phenomenon during retrograde conduction in man, Circulation 49:811, 1974.

CHAPTER 19

Laddergrams

Laddergrams are simple line drawings in tiers that represent different levels of the heart (SA node, atria, AV junction, and ventricles). The lines from tier to tier reflect the conduction sequence within the heart and are best drawn with a slant to represent the progress of the impulse. The lines are precisely aligned with the corresponding ECG events (P waves and QRS complexes) so that AV conduction, in particular, can be accurately extrapolated. The number of tiers used depends on what is being illustrated. Three will serve most purposes: one for atrial activation (A), one for AV conduction (AV), and the third for ventricular activation (V) such as in Fig. 19-1. Other tiers may be added when necessary. For example, if you wish to illustrate type I or II SA block, a narrow tier is added to the atrial tier for SA nodal activation; if you want, you can even use another tier between the ones for SA nodal and atrial activation to illustrate conduction through the perinodal fibers. If necessary, several divisions may be made of the AV tier (node, His bundle, and Purkinje fibers), and an extra tier may be tacked on below the ventricular tier to permit illustration of ventricular ectopic activity and microreentry mechanisms. In short, *the laddergram can be tailored to fit your need.*

Fig. 19-1 shows the simplest of laddergrams, using the three basic tiers. A gentle slope is used to indicate the passage of time as the impulse spreads through the atrium (complex a); this sloping line should begin in the atrial tier at a spot directly under the beginning of the P wave. Some authorities do not slant the atrial line at all but draw it straight down from the onset of the P wave, especially when it is apparent that the SA node is pacing the heart (complex b). Others make a dot at the top of the atrial tier to indicate the point of origin of the impulse (complex c). Sometimes, as a visual aid when the mechanism is more complicated, an arrowhead is used (complex d) to indicate the direction of impulse spread. It does not really matter which method you use, as long as it illustrates what you want.

When constructing a laddergram, first mark what you can see and then draw what is inferred. For example, using a straightedge, draw the atrial lines right under the beginning of the P waves so that the sinus rhythm is accurately reflected in the laddergram. Then draw in ventricular activity. If you have determined that the ventricular complexes are the result of conduction from the atria, indicate this by beginning the slope at the top of the ventricular tier right under the beginning of the QRS complex and ending at the bottom of the V tier at a point corresponding to the end of the QRS complex. Then join the two lines to reflect what is inferred, that is, AV conduction.

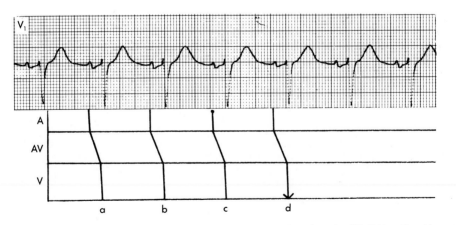

Fig. 19-1. Four methods *(a-d)* used to illustrate the same complex. *A,* atria; *AV,* AV junction; *V,* ventricles.

Illustrating supraventricular ectopic mechanisms

ATRIAL PREMATURE BEATS. In Fig. 19-2 a laddergram illustrates atrial premature beats (APBs). The leading point is placed midway down the atrial tier to indicate an ectopic focus.

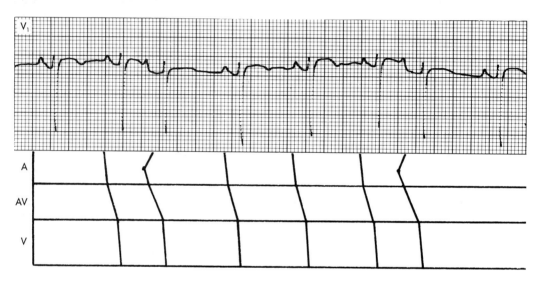

Fig. 19-2. Atrial premature beats.

NONCONDUCTED APBs. In Fig. 19-3, *A*, there is one nonconducted APB. Block is represented as being in the AV junction, although the impulse may never have penetrated the node at all. The level of the block cannot be known without His bundle electrograms; but since the point of this particular laddergram is to illustrate a nonconducted APB, the block may be indicated anywhere after the atrial tier and before the ventricular tier. If, however, you wish to illustrate that the block is in the AV node as opposed to the His-Purkinje system, the laddergram may look like Fig. 19-3, *B*, with the divisions of the AV conduction system delineated. The beat following the pause is a junctional escape (note the shorter PR interval).

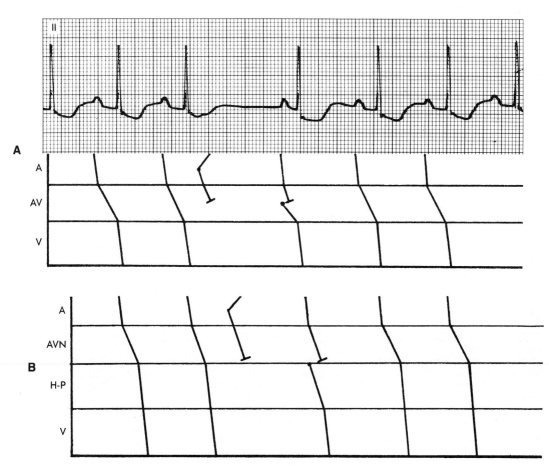

Fig. 19-3. *A*, Atria; *AVN*, AV node; *H-P*, His-Purkinje system; *V*, ventricles.

AV NODAL REENTRY. Laddergrams are particularly helpful in illustrating AV nodal reentry (AVNR). Reflecting lines are drawn in the AV tier, as seen in Figs. 19-4 and 19-5. The lines proceeding anterogradely conduct to the ventricles and meet the V tier directly under the onset of the QRS. The lines proceeding retrogradely show conduction to the A tier. The P′ wave is not seen in AVNR tachycardia, or it may distort the end of the QRS. It is drawn on the laddergram whether it is seen or not. If the mechanism involves an accessory pathway, the P′ wave occurs between the QRS complexes.

When constructing this laddergram, first draw in all the P′ waves. Remember that in AVNR the P′ waves are simultaneous with the QRSs. Then draw in the ventricular complexes, slanting them slightly anterogradely to indicate a supraventricular mechanism. Now you are ready to illustrate the AVNR mechanism. Draw a

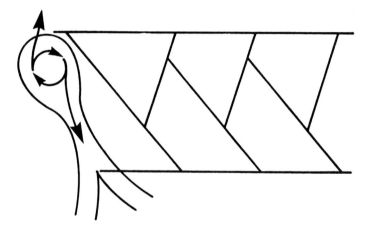

Fig. 19-4. A laddergram and diagrammatic illustration of the AV nodal reentry mechanism. Note that atrial and ventricular activations are simultaneous.

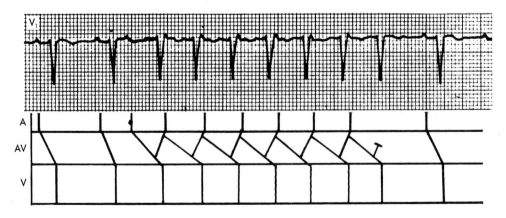

Fig. 19-5. AV nodal reentry.

straight line from the end of the APB to the top of the V tier where the first QRS of the tachycardia begins. A short distance up this line, illustrate retrograde conduction by drawing a line from this point to the beginning of the first retrograde line in the A tier. The next anterograde line will begin a short distance down the retrograde line in the AV tier and end at the top of the V tier where the next QRS begins; thus you continue until the tachycardia terminates.

ATRIAL FLUTTER. Fig. 19-6 shows atrial flutter at a rate of 306 beats/min. The normal response of the AV node to a rapidly firing atrial ectopic focus is Wenckebach conduction, which is reflected in this tracing by the group beating (pairs) and the alternating relationship of the F′ wave to the following QRS. When drawing the laddergram for atrial tachycardia or flutter, it is important to remember that the P′ immediately preceding the QRS is not necessarily the one to have conducted. Besoain-Santander, Pick, and Langendorf[1] long ago pointed out that the AV conduction time in atrial flutter is considerably prolonged, owing to the effect of concealed conduction of the numerous atrial impulses. They calculated that the usual "FR" interval during 2:1 conduction probably measured 0.26 to 0.46 second. (The FR interval in atrial flutter is measured in the inferior leads from the nadir of the negative component of the flutter wave to the beginning of the QRS.)

ATRIAL FLUTTER WITH WENCKEBACH CONDUCTION. In Fig. 19-6 there is a Wenckebach sequence of 3:2. Note the paired ventricular complexes and the alternating FR relationship. In constructing the laddergram, proceed as above by first drawing in the atrial impulses, then the ventricular ones, and finally AV conduction. Remember that the FR interval in atrial flutter will usually be greater than 0.26 second. In this case the shortest one is 0.30 second.

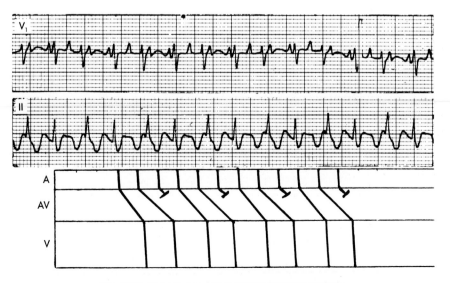

Fig. 19-6. Atrial flutter with 3:2 Wenckebach periods.

ATRIAL FLUTTER WITH EXIT BLOCK OUT OF THE FLUTTER FOCUS. To graph the tracing in Fig. 19-7, you need an additional tier because pairing of the flutter waves themselves must be accounted for (in V_1 the flutter wave is a positive peak). When beats are grouped in pairs, one should always think of 3:2 Wenckebach conduction. Although in atrial flutter it is undecided whether the mechanism is intra-atrial reentry or enhanced automaticity, either mechanism could exhibit an exit block out of the flutter focus.

To construct such a laddergram, draw an extra tier above the atrial tier to accommodate the ectopic focus. Then draw the atrial waves in the A tier and measure the length of the Wenckebach period (the distance between the two F waves beginning the short cycle); in this case it is 0.56 second. Since a 3:2 Wenckebach conduction is assumed, 0.56 second is divided by 3 (0.19 sec). Now plot the discharge of the ectopic focus at 0.19-second intervals, beginning at a spot in the F tier immediately preceding the Wenckebach period (just before the F wave ending the long cycle). The first two ectopic discharges are conducted with lengthening conduction time, and the third is blocked, creating the atrial bigeminy. Now the ventricular beats can be drawn in the V tier, and AV conduction can be established, revealing in addition a 5:4 AV Wenckebach conduction.

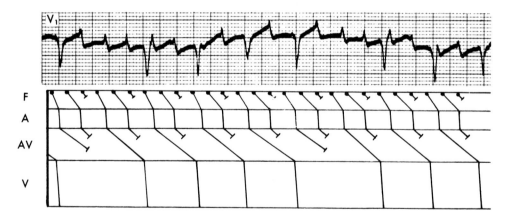

Fig. 19-7. Atrial flutter with 3:2 Wenckebach conduction out of the flutter focus *(F)*; in the AV junction there is 2:1 conduction at a higher level and 5:4 Wenckebach conduction at a lower level.

Illustrating SA block

SA conduction problems are illustrated by drawing an extra tier at the top of the laddergram. This segment represents the SA node and the perinodal fibers, silent zones on the surface ECG.

SA WENCKEBACH CONDUCTION. Fig. 19-8 has all the classical signs of Wenckebach conduction: group beating, shortening RR intervals, and pauses less than twice the shortest cycle (see Chapter 13). However, since the PR intervals are short and all are equal, the Wenckebach period must be higher in the conduction system between the sinus node and the atrial musculature.

In constructing this laddergram you may wish to illustrate only SA conduction, as we have, since there is no AV or ventricular problem. After drawing a tier for sinus and atrial activity, fill in what you can see—the P waves. The events in the SA node and perinodal fibers are concealed and must be extrapolated from the pattern of their activity, the PP intervals. Now measure the distance between the P waves ending the long cycles and divide that number by 4, which represents the number of P waves seen plus the one assumed to be lost (240 ÷ 4 = 60). This number (0.60 sec) represents the sinus cycle. Begin shortly before the P wave ending the pause and walk out the sinus cycle at the top of the SA tier. Now you can indicate conduction between sinus firing and atrial activation and clearly show a Wenckebach sequence.

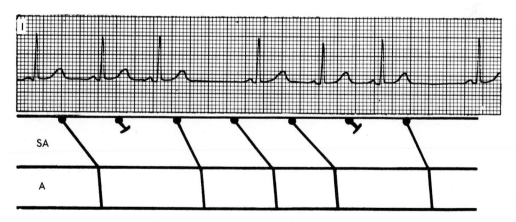

Fig. 19-8. 4:3 sinus Wenckebach conduction.

SA WENCKEBACH CONDUCTION WITH JUNCTIONAL ESCAPE. Fig. 19-9 is another SA Wenckebach. This time the pauses are interrupted by junctional escape beats, so the AV and V tiers are used in addition to the SA and A segments.

You could begin this laddergram without spotting the mechanism; constructing the laddergram, however, is an excellent way to arrive through a logical fashion at the mechanism. First draw the P waves into the A tier. In so doing, you will note the group of four, suggesting 5:4 Wenckebach conduction. There is noticeable shortening of the PP interval between the first and the second cycle, and the longest PP intervals are less than twice the shortest; therefore this must indeed be 5:4 sinus Wenckebach conduction. The ventricular complexes are now drawn into the laddergram. All of them are of supraventricular origin, so begin your line at the top of the V tier directly under the beginning of the QRS and slant it anterogradely.

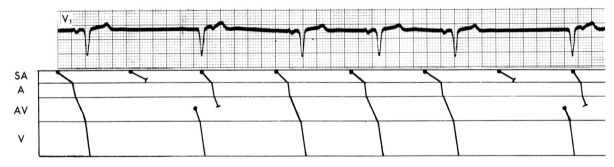

Fig. 19-9. 5:4 sinus Wenckebach conduction with junctional escape beats.

The two junctional escape beats are illustrated by placing dots in the AV tier just ahead of the junctional complexes and connecting the dots to the ventricular complex in the V tier. Now calculate the whole Wenckebach period as before by measuring the distance between the P waves ending the pauses. Count the number of P waves between pauses, add one for the missing P wave, and divide this number (5) into the total Wenckebach cycle ($525 \div 5 = 105$). The sinus cycle is 105, which is walked out in the SA tier beginning just before a P wave ending the longest atrial cycle (located immediately after the junctional escape beat). Now connect these dots with the lines in the A tier, and the illustration of 5:4 SA Wenckebach conduction with junctional escape beats is complete.

Fig. 19-10 is another SA Wenckebach conduction. Why not cover our laddergram and try plotting this one on your own?

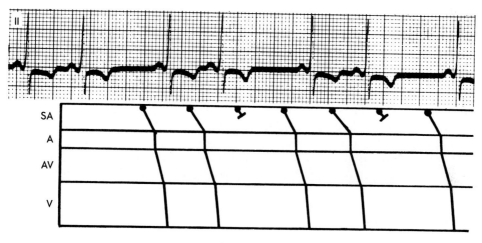

Fig. 19-10

Illustrating junctional ectopic mechanisms

The junctional ectopic focus is represented within the AV tier by a dot or by simply making that point the leading edge of conduction. However, the time of the junctional discharge is not known from the surface ECG. The location of the retrograde P′ with respect to the QRS is not even helpful because whether or not and where the retrograde P′ wave appears are determined by the speed of retrograde conduction as compared to anterograde conduction (Fig. 19-11). The RP′ interval is not a measure of retrograde conduction per se but represents the difference between anterograde and retrograde conduction (Fig. 19-12).

JUNCTIONAL RHYTHM WITH RECIPROCAL BEATS. Figs. 19-13 and 19-14 are examples of a junctional rhythm with progressively lengthening retrograde conduction culminating in reciprocal beats. In both cases retrograde conduction is slower than anterograde conduction.

To construct the laddergram, first draw in the P waves, showing their retrograde pathway by starting the slant up and forward from the bottom of the A tier. Then draw in the ventricular lines, reflecting their supraventricular origin by slanting them from the top of the V tier down. Now pick a reasonable spot in the AV tier preceding the ventricular lines to indicate the junctional discharge. The exact location of this position in the AV tier is not important since this information is not known without a His bundle electrogram; but keep the distance between the junctional impulse and its propagation through the ventricles consistent. Now you can establish anterograde and retrograde conduction. Note that retrograde conduction is lengthening until there is sufficient delay to permit the impulse to find a responsive downward pathway and return to the ventricles.

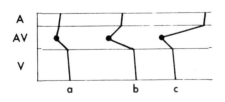

Fig. 19-11. Relationship of atrial to ventricular activation depends on the rate of conduction in each direction. In *a* retrograde atrial conduction is faster than anterograde ventricular conduction; in *b* anterograde conduction is faster still. In *c* the opposite is true.

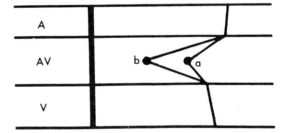

Fig. 19-12. RP interval of junctional beats remains unchanged provided the difference between retrograde and anterograde conduction remains the same.

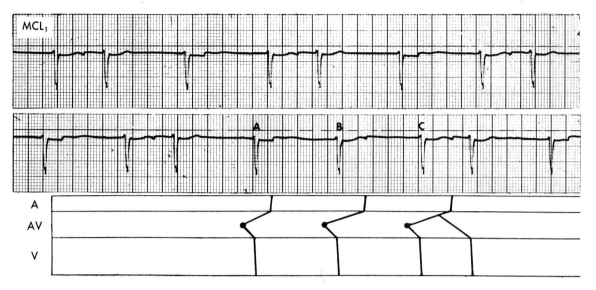

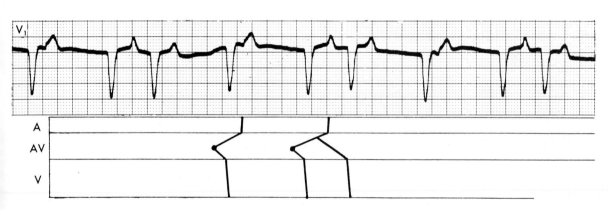

Fig. 19-13. Junctional rhythm with reciprocal beats.

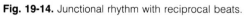

Fig. 19-14. Junctional rhythm with reciprocal beats.

JUNCTIONAL ESCAPE. Fig. 19-15 illustrates a sinus bradycardia that results in a junctional escape rhythm. First mark off the sinus impulses and then the retrograde P′ waves, noting that the first negative P′ is not as deep as the ones that follow. This is obviously a fusion beat since the sinus impulse was expected at that same time. Fusion is illustrated by the two lines opposing each other in the same tier. Now mark the ventricular complexes and establish AV conduction. Note that the PR interval of the third complex is shorter by 0.04 second than the preceding ones and therefore is not conducted to the ventricles. The third beat and those following it are junctional. This is illustrated by placing the dot in the AV tier just preceding the ventricular lines. Now anterograde and retrograde conduction from the junctional focus is drawn, as is the sinus conducted beat.

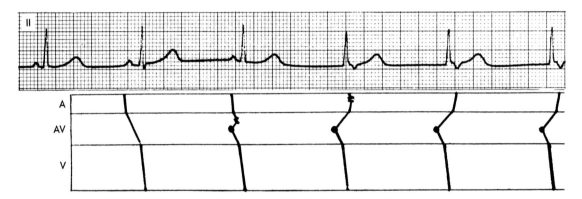

Fig. 19-15. Sinus bradycardia resulting in a junctional escape rhythm. There is one atrial fusion beat.

ACCELERATED IDIOJUNCTIONAL RHYTHM WITH WENCKEBACH EXIT BLOCK.

One of the manifestations of digitalis toxicity in atrial fibrillation is an accelerated idiojunctional rhythm with Wenckebach block (out of or below the junctional pacemaker). Fig. 19-16 is such a case, and the laddergram is useful in illustrating this mechanism. In lead V_2 there is group beating and shortening RR intervals, two of the indications of Wenckebach block. Paired beats are noted in lead V_4, and the absolute regularity of the independent junctional pacemaker is seen in V_3.

In constructing this laddergram for V_4, begin by drawing in the ventricular lines; the atrial tier can be left empty in atrial fibrillation. Since pairs usually reflect 3:2 Wenckebach conduction, you will divide by three once you determine the length of the full Wenckebach period (the distance between two Rs ending the long cycle). This length is 184, and the distance between junctional impulses is 63. Begin to plot these intervals at the center of the AV tier just preceding the first beat of one of the Wenckebach cycles (the QRS ending the pause) and then establish AV conduction. Conduction time lengthens, the third junctional impulse is finally blocked, and the sequence begins again (3:2 Wenckebach conduction).

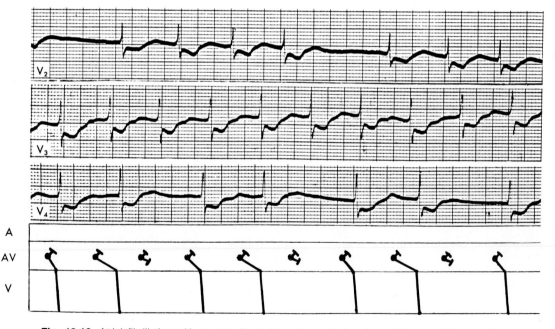

Fig. 19-16. Atrial fibrillation with an accelerated junctional rhythm (rate, 98 beats/min) and 3:2 Wenckebach conduction below or exit block from the junctional pacemaker.

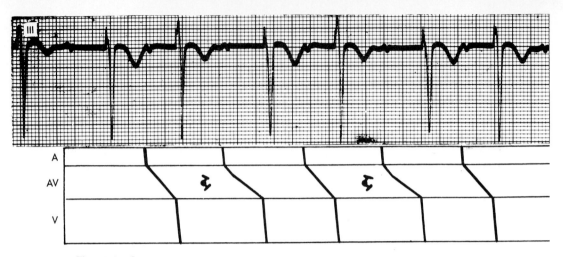

Fig. 19-17. Concealed junctional extrasystoles produce alternating PR and RR intervals.

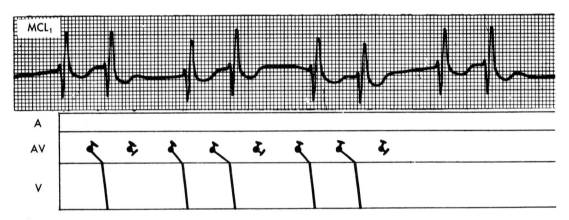

Fig. 19-18. Junctional tachycardia with 3:2 Wenckebach conduction below or exit block from the junctional pacemaker and RBBB.

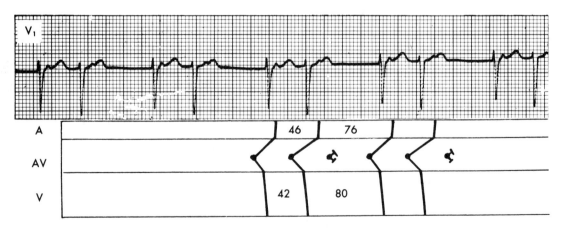

Fig. 19-19. Junctional tachycardia with simultaneous bidirectional (anterograde and retrograde) 3:2 Wenckebach conduction producing bigeminal grouping.

CONCEALED JUNCTIONAL BEATS. Useful applications of the laddergram are the illustration of both the concealed junctional extrasystoles and the blocked beat of the junctional tachycardia with Wenckebach exit block. Figs. 19-17 to 19-19 are examples of how nicely these mechanisms can be illustrated with the laddergram. The concealed junctional beat is drawn as a dot with both retrograde and antero-grade block.

Illustrating ventricular ectopic beats

A ventricular ectopic beat is reflected in the laddergram by drawing the line begin-ning at the bottom of the V tier at a spot directly under the beginning of the ectopic QRS. Then draw the line forward and upward to indicate clearly the ventricular origin of the impulse (Fig. 19-20). We have extended the retrograde conduction into the AV tier because one half of all ventricular ectopies have retrograde conduc-tion into the atria and we are assuming some retrograde AV nodal penetration.

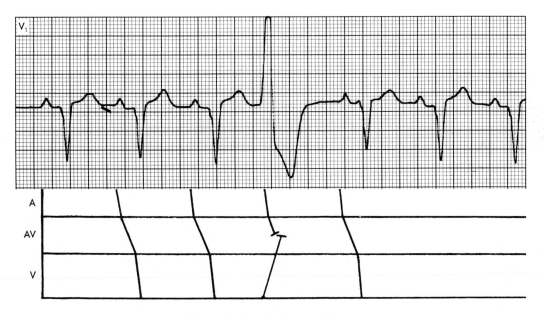

Fig. 19-20. Ventricular ectopic beat.

VENTRICULAR FUSION. Ventricular fusion complexes are illustrated in the laddergram by showing two lines meeting within the V tier; one line begins at the bottom of the V tier (ventricular ectopic beat) and the other enters the V tier from the AV tier (a supraventricular impulse). You can usually tell by the PR interval and the shape of the complex how much of the line in the V tier should be ventricular in origin and how much should be supraventricular (Fig. 19-21).

In Fig. 19-22 four fusion beats are indicated (1 to 4) in which the PR intervals progressively lengthen. It is evident that the QRS complexes become more and

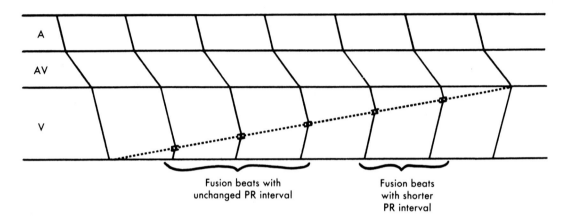

Fusion beats with
unchanged PR interval

Fusion beats
with shorter
PR interval

Fig. 19-21. Laddergram illustrating progressively "higher" levels of fusion within the ventricles. The first beat represents a pure sinus beat; the last beat, a pure ventricular ectopic beat. Note that at first the PR interval remains the same as that of the sinus beat (as long as the sinus impulse invades the ventricles before, or no later than, the ectopic center fires); but when the ectopic center fires before the sinus impulse arrives, the PR becomes shorter than that of the sinus beat.

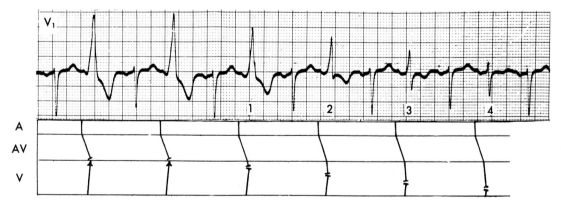

Fig. 19-22. Ventricular fusion.

more normal in contour as the supraventricular impulse captures more and more of the ventricular myocardium.

In Fig. 19-23 there is an atrial fusion beat because of an underlying atrial parasystole (longer strip in 16-11, *B*). Fusion is always illustrated on the laddergram by two opposing lines in the same tier. You can use your imagination to illustrate the atrial parasystolic focus; we have chosen to represent it by a dot within a circle in the atrial (A) tier. Note that the parasystolic focus fired once without capturing the atria because of refractoriness caused by the previous sinus beat.

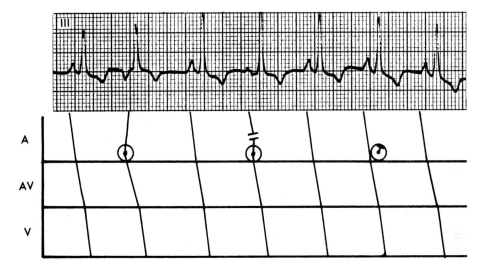

Fig. 19-23. Atrial fusion because of atrial parasystole. For a longer tracing see Fig. 16-11, *B*. (Courtesy Alan Lindsay, MD, Salt Lake City.)

VENTRICULAR MICROREENTRY. If you wish to illustrate the mechanism for ectopic impulse formation within the ventricles, an extra ectopic (E) tier can be added at the bottom of the V tier. In Fig. 19-24 two possible microreentry mechanisms are illustrated in the E tier.

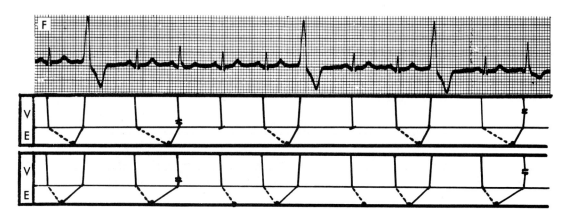

Fig. 19-24. If reentry is the mechanism for these ventricular extrasystoles, the laddergrams depict two possible explanations for the lengthening coupling intervals: Wenckebach-like conduction occurring in the afferent limb (upper diagram) and in the efferent limb (lower diagram) of the reentry circuit.

Now it is your turn

We have outlined the principles necessary for constructing laddergrams. Now try your hand at drawing the rather intricate diagrams needed to illustrate the mechanisms of Figs. 19-26 to 19-28. After your best attempt, turn the page and see if you have illustrated the mechanisms correctly (completed figures on pp. 360 and 361). Fig. 19-25 reviews the three mechanisms for reciprocal beating.

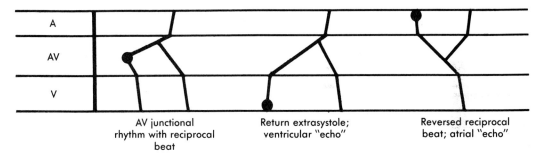

AV junctional
rhythm with reciprocal
beat

Return extrasystole;
ventricular "echo"

Reversed reciprocal
beat; atrial "echo"

Fig. 19-25. Three forms of reciprocal beating ("echo" beats).

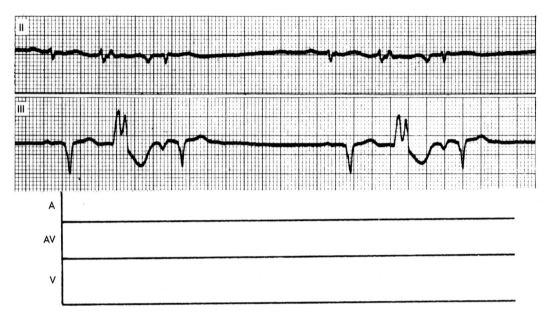

Fig. 19-26

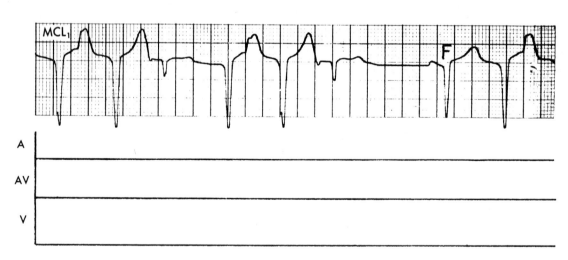

Fig. 19-27

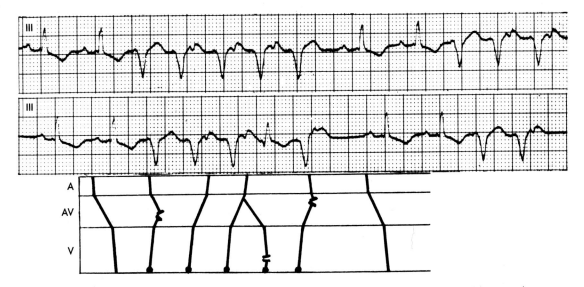

Fig. 19-28. Ventricular tachycardia with retrograde conduction to the atria, a reciprocal beat, and ventricular fusion.

REFERENCE

1. Besoain-Santander M, Pick A, and Langendorf, R: A-V conduction in auricular flutter, Circulation 2:604, 1950.

CHAPTER 20

An approach to arrhythmias

Many disturbances of rhythm and conduction are recognizable at first glance. For example, usually one can immediately spot atrial flutter with 4:1 conduction, atrial fibrillation with rapid ventricular response, or sinus rhythm with right bundle branch block (RBBB). There are, however, a significant number of dysrhythmias that defy immediate recognition, and it is for them that we require a systematic attack. The following five-point approach evolved after analyzing the reasons for mistakes made in diagnosing arrhythmias, and it is therefore designed to avoid the common errors of omission and commission. Before outlining this systematic approach, it is worth making some observations about the principles of monitoring.

Principles of monitoring

USE A LEAD CONTAINING MAXIMAL INFORMATION. V_1, or an approximation thereof, clearly supplies the most information. Even though all the information gleaned from leads is not immediately useful, why let available data go down the drain? An example of valuable information collected from monitoring in MCL_1 is found in the study of Gozensky and Thorne,[1] who monitored with this lead from the outset of the establishment of the coronary care unit in their hospital. They noted the taller left "rabbit ear" configuration in left ventricular ectopy, which was later confirmed by invasive studies[2] and today is widely used as an aid in the differential diagnosis between aberration and ectopy.

An example of lost information that might have been helpful is the fact that we do not yet really know whether there is any prognostic difference between left and right ventricular extrasystoles. If in the early years of the coronary care unit V_1 had been used as the monitoring lead, distinction between left and right ventricular premature beats would have been possible from the outset, and this information might well be in hand today. However, a counterfeit lead II was used for many years—a lead in which left bundle branch block (LBBB), RBBB, and left and right ventricular ectopics *can* look identical (Fig. 20-1). For this reason if for no other, lead II is one of the least satisfactory leads for constant monitoring. What is the virtue of a monitoring lead that can look similar in these four conditions?

ENSURE A MECHANICALLY CONVENIENT MONITORING SYSTEM. For most systems a maximum of three wires and electrodes is appropriate, and they should be strategically placed so as not to interfere with physical examination of the heart or with the application of emergency countershock.

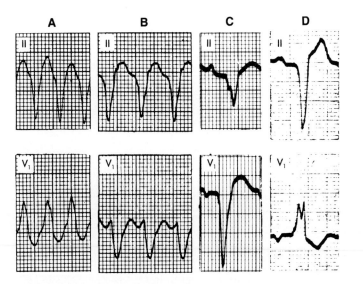

Fig. 20-1. Leads II and V_1. **A,** Left ventricular tachycardia. **B,** Right ventricular tachycardia. **C,** LBBB. **D,** RBBB. Note that lead II has a QS configuration in all four conditions and that V_1 contains far greater morphological contrast.

ONE LEAD IS NOT ENOUGH. In most situations it is obvious that a single monitoring lead is all that is convenient and practicable. However, it is important to appreciate the limitations of a single lead and to know when to obtain additional leads and which leads to obtain.

In Fig. 20-2 note that in V_1 and V_2 the pattern of the ventricular tachycardia is very similar to the conducted RBBB pattern—so much so that most observers would be content to call the tachycardia "supraventricular." However, another lead (aVF in this case) reveals the obvious and striking differences in the two patterns.

Another reason a single lead may be inadequate is that it may fail to reveal inconspicuous items in the tracing such as P waves or pacemaker spikes. Fig. 20-3 illustrates the invisibility of a pacemaker spike.

More than one lead is helpful when the distinction between ectopy and aberration is uncertain in a right chest lead. In Fig. 20-4 the pattern of the tachycardia in MCL_1 could be either left ventricular or supraventricular with RBBB aberration. A look at MCL_6 indicates with reasonable certainty that the origin of the tachycardia is supraventricular (Chapter 12).

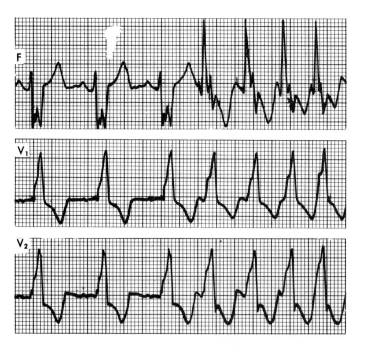

Fig. 20-2. First three beats are sinus beats conducted with RBBB; the next four beats are ventricular tachycardia produced by artificially stimulating the left ventricle. Note the great similarity of the QRS complexes in V_1 and V_2 during both rhythms and the marked dissimilarity in aVF.

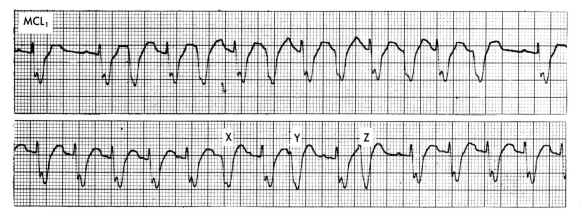

Fig. 20-3. Strips are not continuous. Beats X, Y, and Z are paced beats, as are the alternate ventricular complexes in the top strip, beginning with the third beat; but the pacemaker blips are not visible in this monitoring lead, causing one to suspect spontaneous ventricular ectopy. An additional deception is that this is a demand pacemaker in which the demand mode is not functioning so that it is behaving like a fixed-rate model, imitating ventricular parasystole. The underlying rhythm is sinus tachycardia, sometimes with 1:1 conduction (beginning and end of second strip) and sometimes with 2:1 conduction (beginning and end of top strip).

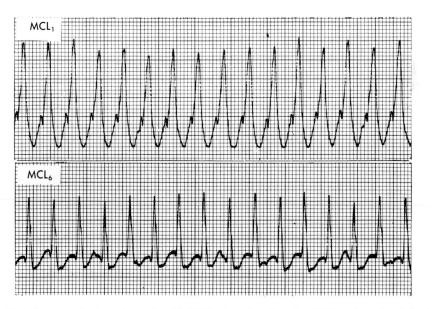

Fig. 20-4. Supraventricular tachycardia with RBBB aberration. From lead MCL₁ alone, the distinction cannot be made between left ventricular tachycardia and supraventricular tachycardia with RBBB aberration. However, the qRs pattern in MCL₆ immediately identifies it as supraventricular.

KNOW WHEN TO USE WHICH OTHER LEADS. A monitoring lead that satisfactorily fulfills most of the requirements is the modified CL_1 (MCL_1), introduced in 1968.[3] The positive electrode is placed at the C_1 (V_1) position, the negative electrode at the left shoulder, and the ground (which may be placed anywhere) usually at the right shoulder. This pattern leaves a clear platform for emergency cardioversion and an unencumbered precordium for physical examination. In addition, since it closely imitates V_1, this lead affords several diagnostic advantages:

1. One can immediately distinguish between left ventricular ectopy (QRS mostly positive) and right ventricular ectopy (QRS mostly negative) in most instances.
2. RBBB and LBBB can be recognized with ease.
3. P waves are sometimes best or only seen in a right chest lead.
4. Most important of all, a right chest lead gives the best opportunity for the differential diagnosis between VT and aberration (Chapter 12).

The only disadvantages of lead MCL_1 are that it fails to recognize shifts of axis and is therefore useless for spotting the development of hemiblock and that the polarity of the P wave is not as informative as it is in lead II. However, these disadvantages are minor in comparison with the advantages, especially in view of the fact that many times in a right chest lead an ectopic P wave can easily be differentiated from a sinus P wave because of its shape. When it is diphasic, the sinus P wave is usually $+-$(⋀); the ectopic or retrograde P wave, when diphasic, is usually $-+$ (⋀). This is illustrated in Fig. 20-5.

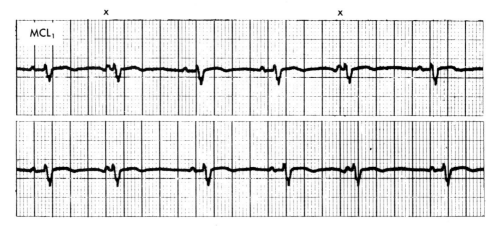

Fig. 20-5. The second and fifth beats in each strip are atrial premature beats. Note the $-+$ polarity of the ectopic P waves (X).

When MCL_1 fails to provide the answer, try a left chest lead by placing the positive electrode at the C_6 (V_6) position to obtain an MCL_6, a reasonable imitation of V_6. If you want to simulate lead III (M_3) for the purpose of recording the polarity of the retrograde P′, place the positive electrode low on the left flank below the diaphragm (leaving the negative electrode at the left shoulder). Fig. 20-6 illustrates an AV circus movement tachycardia in both MCL_1 and M_3. Note that the retrograde P′ is separate from the QRS.

A left chest lead (V_6 or MCL_6) is not reliable for distinguishing between left and right ventricular ectopy since the QRS in both may be either positive or negative.

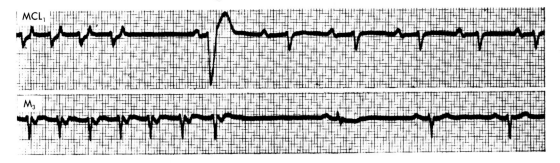

Fig. 20-6. Each lead shows the end of a run of AV circus movement tachycardia with the retrograde P wave just following the QRS complex. In the second half of each strip, sinus rhythm resumes. Note that the retrograde and sinus P waves are both predominantly positive in MCL_1, whereas in M_3 the retrograde P waves show the more familiar inversion so characteristic of retroconduction in an inferior lead. On each occasion, after the tachycardia ceases, the returning beat is an escape beat.

For examples of the sort of information that can be derived from a right chest lead that is not usually available in lead II, look at Fig. 20-7. In Fig. 20-7, *A*, the rSR′ pattern of the sinus beats is typical of RBBB; the qR pattern with early peak in the first extrasystole is typical of ectopy of left ventricular origin; and the rS pattern of the second extrasystole is typical of a right ventricular origin. In Fig. 20-7, *B*, the atrial fibrillation is interrupted by a burst of bizarre beats that are certain to evoke the "lidocaine reflex"; but the telltale shape (rSR′) of the first of these wide beats tell us that it is a run of aberrantly conducted beats rather than a run of ventricular tachycardia.

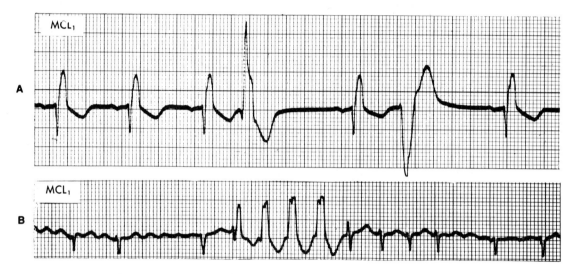

Fig. 20-7. A, Patterns of RBBB (sinus beats), left ventricular ectopy (fourth beat), and right ventricular ectopy (sixth beat) are readily recognized. **B,** Short run of aberrantly conducted beats during atrial fibrillation. The aberration is recognized by the characteristic triphasic (rSR′) contour of the first anomalous beat.

A systematic approach

Failing a diagnosis that is obvious, a systematic five-point approach is in order:
1. Know the causes
2. Milk the QRS
3. Cherchez le P
4. Who is married to whom
5. Pinpoint the primary disturbance

KNOW THE CAUSES. Knowing the possible causes is the first step in any medical diagnosis. It is part of the equipment that you carry with you—prepared at a moment's notice to use when faced with an unidentified arrhythmia.

The eight basic arrhythmias are early beats, unexpected pauses, tachycardias, bradycardias, bigeminal rhythms, group beating, total irregularity, and regular nonsinus rhythms at normal rates. Their most common causes, except for tachycardias, are outlined and illustrated below.

Causes of early beats (Fig. 20-8)

Extrasystoles *(A to C)*
Parasystole *(D)*
Capture beats *(E)*
Reciprocal beats *(F)*
Better conduction interrupting poorer conduction *(G)*
Supernormal conduction during AV block *(H)*
Rhythm resumption after inapparent bigeminy *(I)*

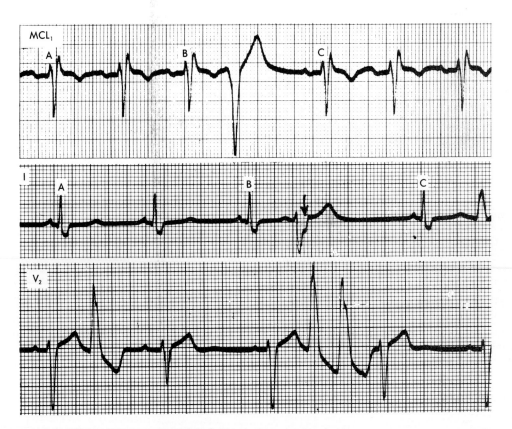

Fig. 20-8. A, Ventricular premature beats.

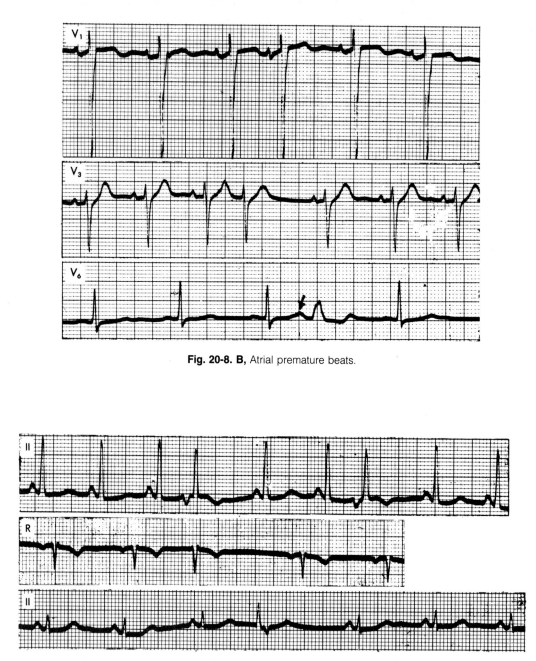

Fig. 20-8. B, Atrial premature beats.

Fig. 20-8. C, Junctional premature beats.

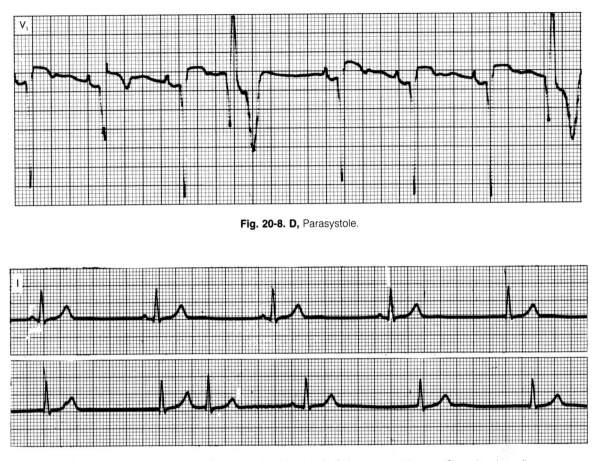

Fig. 20-8. D, Parasystole.

Fig. 20-8. E, Capture beat (bottom strip, third beat). Strips are continuous. Sinus bradycardia causes AV dissociation. The junction is escaping at a rate of approximately 43 beats/min. One of the sinus beats in the bottom strip is conducted (capture).

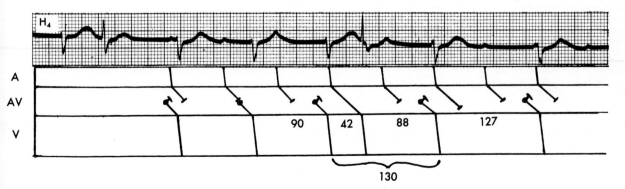

Fig. 20-8. F, Supernormal conduction during AV block. The junctional rhythm is interrupted twice by aberrantly conducted beats, both presumably caused by supernormal conduction since later impulses fail to be conducted to the ventricles.

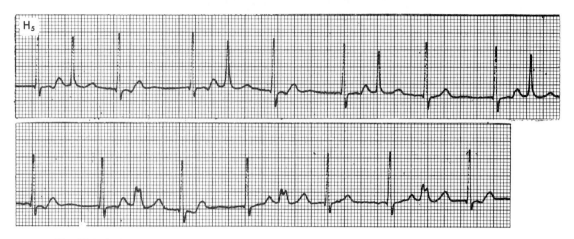

Fig. 20-8. G, Reciprocal beats. Continuous strips from a Holter monitoring lead. Throughout the tracing the beats are grouped in threes. The first of each trio is a junctional beat, which is followed by retrograde conduction to the atria and a reciprocal beat showing varying degrees of LBBB aberration. The third beat in each trio is probably a second reciprocal beat, with the preceding retrograde conduction failing to reach the atria.

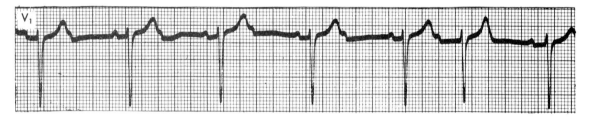

Fig. 20-8. H, Better conduction interrupting poorer conduction. The sixth beat is early because it is the second beat of a 3:2 Wenckebach period interrupting 2:1 conduction. At a faster atrial rate the early beat might develop aberration and be difficult to distinguish from a ventricular premature beat (VPB).

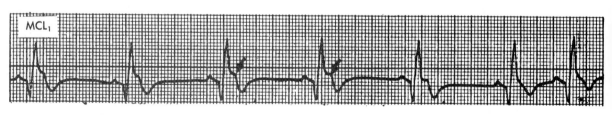

Fig. 20-8. I, Sinus rhythm with nonconducted atrial bigeminy. The atrial extrasystoles deform the shoulder of the ST segment *(arrows).* In the penultimate beat the deformity disappears, and two consecutive sinus beats result in a shorter cycle.

Causes of pauses (Fig. 20-9)
Nonconducted atrial extrasystoles *(A)*
Second degree AV block *(B and C)*
Second degree SA block *(D and E)*
"Sick sinus" variants *(F)*
Concealed conduction *(G)*
Concealed junctional extrasystoles *(H)*
Pacemaker pauses *(I)*

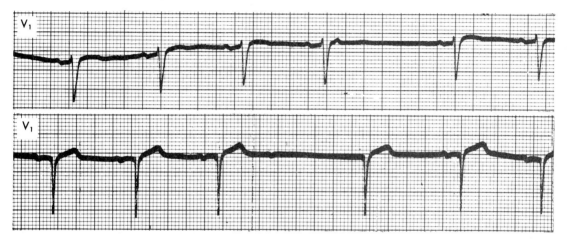

Fig. 20-9. A, Nonconducted atrial extrasystoles.

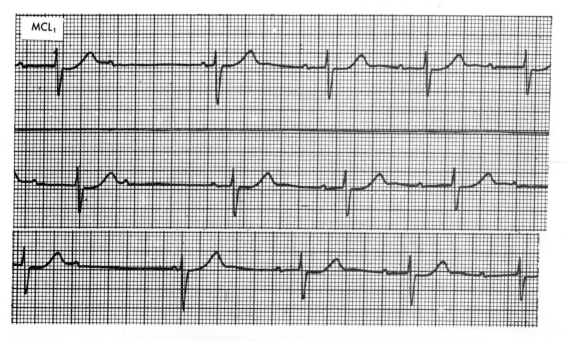

Fig. 20-9. B, Type I second degree AV block.

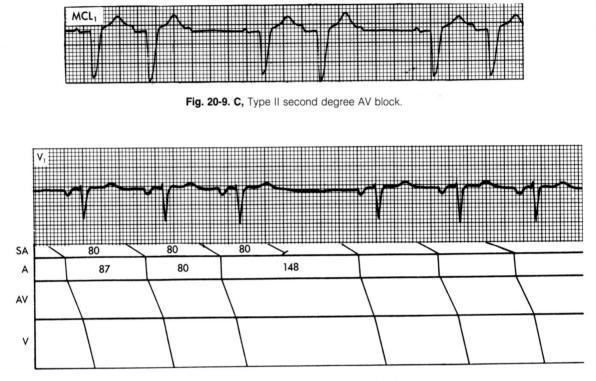

Fig. 20-9. C, Type II second degree AV block.

Fig. 20-9. D, Type I second degree SA block.

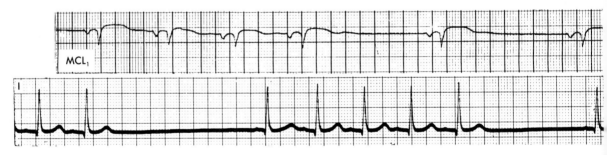

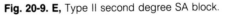

Fig. 20-9. E, Type II second degree SA block.

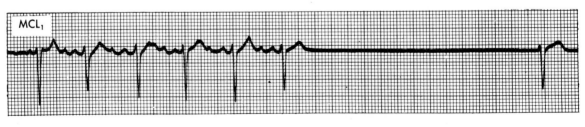

Fig. 20-9. F, Sick sinus (tachycardia-bradycardia) syndrome.

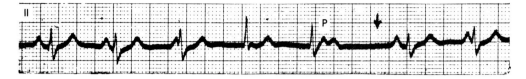

Fig. 20-9. G, Concealed conduction. The missing beat *(arrow)* results from incomplete penetration into the AV junction by a sinus impulse, postponing the next beat of an accelerated idiojunctional rhythm (rate, 86 beats/min).

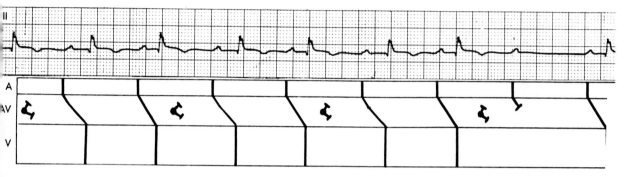

Fig. 20-9. H, Concealed junctional extrasystoles every third beat, causing lengthening of the subsequent PR and preventing AV conduction altogether toward the end of the strip *(laddergram).*

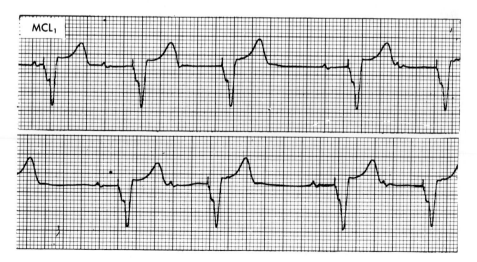

Fig. 20-9. I, Pacemaker pauses. The pauses in this tracing result from the pacemaker's sensing the T wave.

Causes of bradycardia (Fig. 20-10)

Sinus bradycardia *(A)*

SA block *(B)*

Nonconducted atrial bigeminy *(C)*

AV block *(D)*

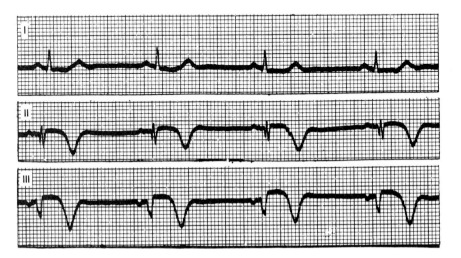

Fig. 20-10. **A,** Sinus bradycardia.

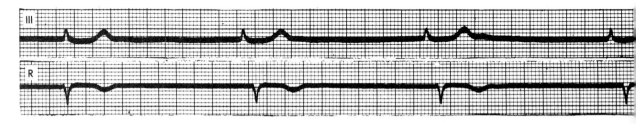

Fig. 20-10. B, Sick sinus. No atrial activity is visible, and the idiojunctional escape rate is 29 beats/min. Absence of the P waves could be caused by generator failure, exit block, atrial paralysis, or an inadequate sinus impulse.

Basic pattern

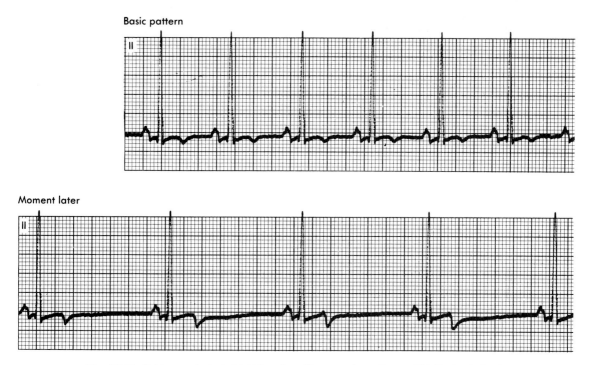

Moment later

Fig. 20-10. C, Nonconducted atrial bigeminy. (Courtesy Janet Bacon, RN, Portland, Ore.)

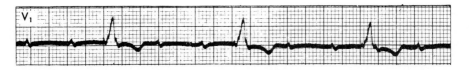

Fig. 20-10. D, AV block. Sinus rhythm (rate, 126 beats/min) with 3:1 block, producing a ventricular rate of 42 beats/min.

Causes of bigeminy (skeleton classification) (Fig. 20-11)

Extrasystoles *(A)*

Parasystole *(B)*

3:2 conduction *(C to F)*

Reciprocal beating *(G)*

Fortuitous pairing in atrial fibrillation *(H)*

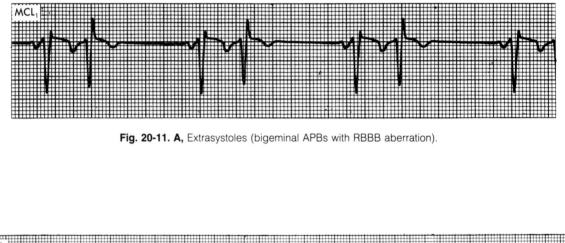

Fig. 20-11. A, Extrasystoles (bigeminal APBs with RBBB aberration).

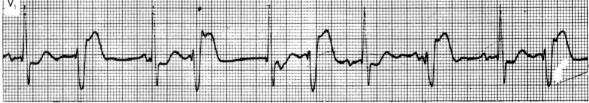

Fig. 20-11. B, Parasystole producing bigeminy with varying "coupling." Note that although the relationship of the ventricular ectopic beats to the preceding supraventricular beats varies markedly, the interval between consecutive ectopic beats is constant.

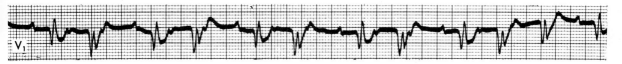

Fig. 20-11. C, 3:2 conduction of Wenckebach type during sinus tachycardia (rate, 132 beats/min), leaving the ventricular complexes in pairs except for one threesome. The beats ending the shorter cycles are conducted aberrantly compared with the first beat of each pair.

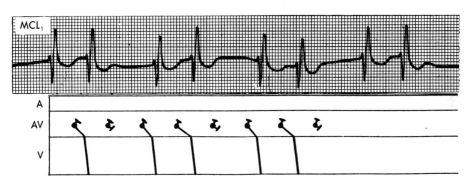

Fig. 20-11. D, 3:2 conduction. Junctional tachycardia with no sign of atrial activity; 3:2 Wenckebach conduction below the junctional pacemaker, leaving the ventricular complexes paired.

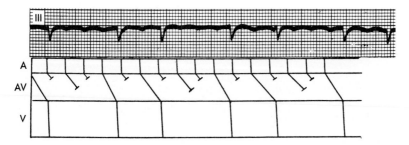

Fig. 20-11. E, 3:2 conduction. Atrial flutter with alternating 2:1 and 4:1 conduction, resulting in paired ventricular complexes; there is 2:1 "filtering" at a higher level in the AV junction combined at a lower level with 3:2 Wenckebach conduction of the alternate beats that pass the filter.

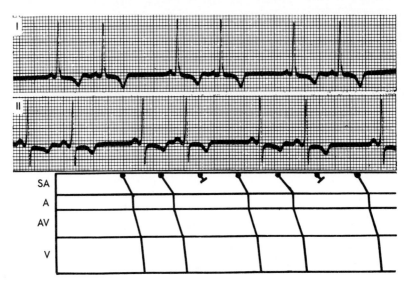

Fig. 20-11. F, 3:2 sinus Wenckebach conduction results in pairing of sinus beats.

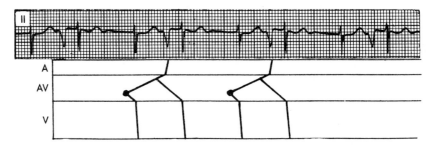

Fig. 20-11. G, Reciprocal beating during a junctional rhythm with delayed retrograde conduction produces bigeminy.

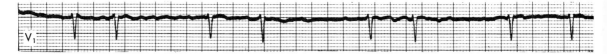

Fig. 20-11. H, Fortuitous pairing in atrial fibrillation. Occasionally, presumably by chance or by some nuance of concealed conduction, the beats in atrial fibrillation are conducted after alternately longer and shorter cycles.

Common causes of group beating (Fig. 20-12)

Supraventricular tachycardia with Wenckebach periods *(A)*

Atrial flutter with 2:1 "filtering" at upper level in the junction and Wenckebach periodicity below *(B)*

Sinus rhythm with two or more consecutive extrasystoles *(C)*

Recurrent bursts of tachycardia, ventricular or supraventricular *(D)*

Every third beat an interpolated ventricular extrasystole

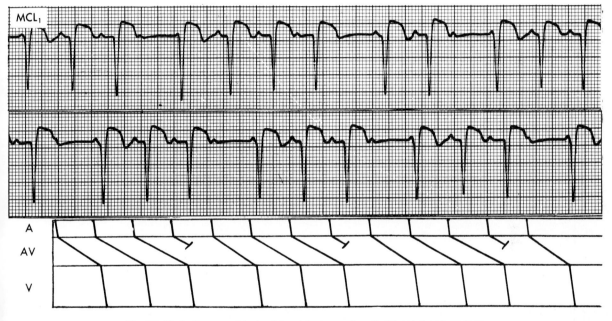

Fig. 20-12. A, Supraventricular (sinus) tachycardia with Wenckebach periods.

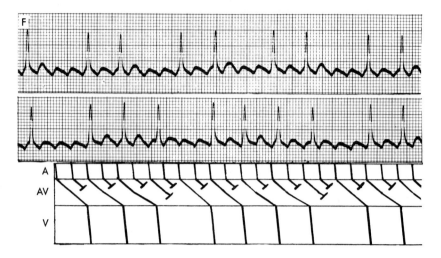

Fig. 20-12. B, Atrial flutter with 2:1 "filtering" at upper level in the junction and Wenckebach periodicity below (see laddergram).

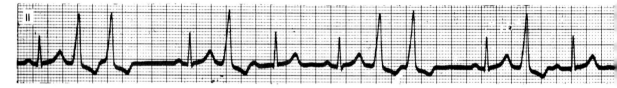

Fig. 20-12. C, Sinus rhythm with two consecutive extrasystoles. The first and third trios consist of a sinus beat followed by a pair of ventricular extrasystoles; the second and fourth consist of a ventricular extrasystole interpolated between two sinus beats.

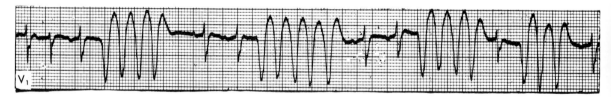

Fig. 20-12. D, Recurrent bursts of ventricular tachycardia.

Common causes of chaotic irregularity
Atrial fibrillation
Atrial flutter with varying AV conduction
Chaotic (multifocal) atrial tachycardia
Shifting (wandering) pacemaker with atrial extrasystoles
Sinus rhythm with multifocal extrasystoles
Mixed ventricular rhythms

MILK THE QRS. In arrhythmia detection, give priority to ventricular behavior. In general, it matters little what the atria are doing so long as the ventricles are behaving themselves.

When measuring the QRS duration, be sure to check at least two leads because initial or terminal forces may be isoelectric in a particular lead, causing the QRS to appear narrow in that lead only (Fig. 20-13).

If the QRS is of normal duration, you know that the rhythm is supraventricular; but if it is wide and bizarre, you have to decide whether it is supraventricular with ventricular aberration or ectopic ventricular. Your knowledge of the ECG in the distinction between aberrancy and ectopy will enable you to get the most out of the QRS milking process (Chapter 12).

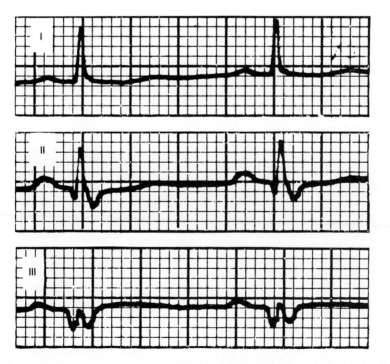

Fig. 20-13. From lead I, no one would think that this patient has intraventricular block with a QRS interval of 0.11 second, as seen in leads II and III. By Einthoven's equation, since the terminal 0.06 second of the QRS in lead II and that in lead III are almost identical negative deflections, this part of the QRS in lead I is isoelectric.

CHERCHEZ LE P. If the shape of the QRS does not help you make a diagnosis, turn to the P wave for help. In the past the P wave, as the key to arrhythmias, has certainly been overemphasized. However, there are times when it holds the diagnostic clue and must be accorded the starring role.

In one's search for P waves, there are several clues and caveats to bear in mind.

The S$_5$ lead. This lead was introduced by French cardiologists in 1952. It is obtained by placing the positive electrode at the fifth right interspace close to the sternum (just below the C$_1$ position) and the negative electrode on the manubrium of the sternum. This placement will sometimes greatly magnify the P wave, rendering it readily visible when it may have been virtually indiscernible in other leads. Fig. 20-14 illustrates this amplifying effect and makes the diagnosis of atrial tachycardia with 2:1 block immediately apparent. If it succeeds, this technique is certainly preferable to invasive ones (atrial wire or esophageal electrode).

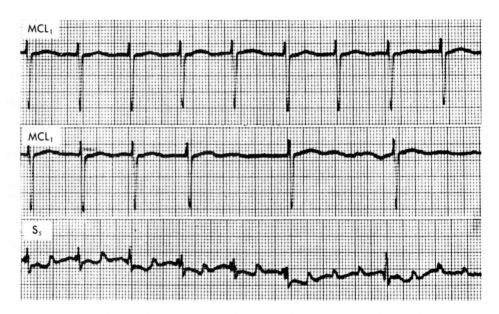

Fig. 20-14. S$_5$ lead. Top strip of MCL$_1$ shows barely perceptible P' waves of an atrial tachycardia. Second strip shows the effect of carotid sinus stimulation: the ventricular rate halves because of increased AV block, and additional P' waves become barely visible through the artifact. In contrast, the strip of lead S$_5$ has prominent P waves.

The Bix rule. Whenever P waves of a supraventricular tachycardia are exactly halfway between the ventricular complexes, you should always suspect that additional P waves are hiding within the QRS complex—a point emphasized by the late Harold Bix of Vienna and Baltimore. In the top strip of Fig. 20-15 the P' wave is midway between the QRS complexes. Moments later the conduction pattern alters (middle strip) and exposes the lurking P' waves. It is clearly important to know if there are twice as many atrial impulses as are apparent because, if there are, there is the ever present danger, especially if the atrial rate should slow somewhat, that the ventricular rate may double or almost double. It is better to be forewarned and take steps to prevent such potentially disastrous acceleration.

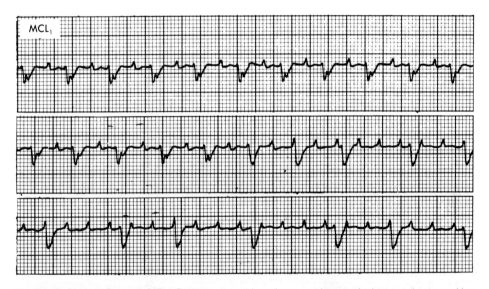

Fig. 20-15. Bix rule *(top strip)*. The P waves are midway between the ventricular complexes, making one suspect a hidden P' wave.

The haystack principle. If you were searching for a needle in a haystack, you would obviously prefer a small to a large haystack. Therefore, whenever you cannot find an elusive P wave or pacemaker spike, give the lead with the least disturbance of the baseline (the smallest ventricular complexes) a chance to help you. There are some leads that no one would think of looking at to solve an arrhythmia (aVR, for example). The patient whose tracing you see in Fig. 20-16 died because no one thought to apply the haystack principle and look in aVR. He had a runaway pacemaker at a discharge rate of 440 beats/min with a halved ventricular response of 220 beats/min. Lead aVR was the lead with the smallest ventricular complex, and it was the only lead in which the pacemaker "blips" were plainly visible (arrows). The patient went into shock and died because none of the attempted therapeutic measures affected the tachycardia, when all that was necessary was to disconnect the wayward pulse generator.

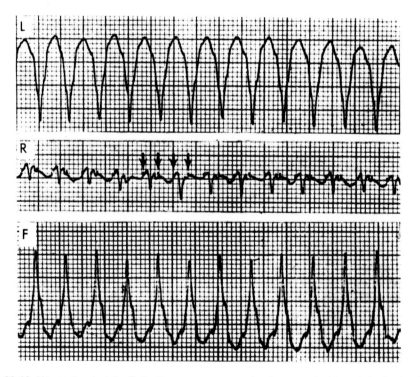

Fig. 20-16. Haystack principle. Patient's runaway pacemaker is recognizable only in the lead with the least disturbance of the baseline, in this case aVR.

Mind your Ps. "Mind yours Ps" means to be wary of things that look like P waves and particularly applies to P-like waves that are adjacent to the QRS complex—they may be part of the QRS complex. This is a trap for the unwary sufferer from the "P-preoccupation syndrome," to whom anything that looks like a P wave is a P wave. For example, the strips of V_1 and V_2 in Fig. 20-17 would be diagnosed by many as a supraventricular tachycardia for the wrong reasons. In V_1 the QRS seems not to be very wide and appears to be preceded by a small P wave. In V_2 an apparently narrow QRS is followed by what appears to be a retrograde P wave. In fact, the P-like waves in both these leads are part of the QRS complex. If the QRS duration is measured in V_3, it is found to be 0.14 second. To attain a QRS of that duration in V_1 and V_2, one needs to include the P-like waves in the measurement.

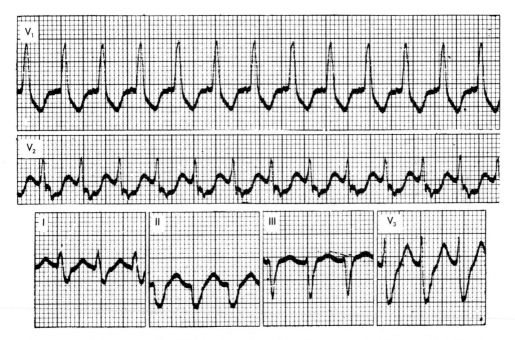

Fig. 20-17. Mind your "Ps." The QRS duration in leads I and V_3 measures 0.14 second. Therefore the P-like waves in the other leads must be part of the QRS.

Find a break. It is at a break in rhythm that you are most likely to spot the solution. For example, look at Fig. 20-18. At the beginning of the strip where the rhythm is regular at a rate of 200 beats/min, it is impossible to know whether the tachycardia is ectopic atrial, ectopic junctional, or reciprocating in the AV junction. A fourth possibility is that the little peak is part of the QRS and not a P wave at all. Further along the strip there is a pause in the rhythm. The commonest cause of a pause is a nonconducted atrial extrasystole; and, sure enough, there at the arrow is the culprit—in this situation a diagnostic ally. As a result of the pause, the P wave can be seen in front of the next QRS; therefore the mechanism is atrial tachycardia.

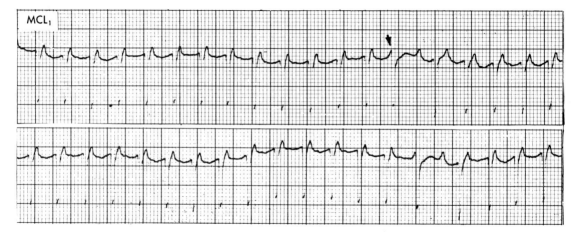

Fig. 20-18. Focus on the break in rhythm *(arrow),* and it gives you the answer: the P′ wave precedes the QRS rather than follows it.

WHO IS MARRIED TO WHOM? Establishing relationships is often the crucial step in arriving at a firm diagnosis. This principle is illustrated in Fig. 20-19, in which a junctional rhythm is dissociated from sinus bradycardia. On three occasions there are bizarre early beats of a qR configuration that is nondiagnostic. The fact that they are seen *only* when a P wave is emerging beyond the preceding QRS tells us that they are "married to" the preceding P waves and establishes them as conducted (capture) beats with RBBB aberration rather than ventricular extrasystoles.

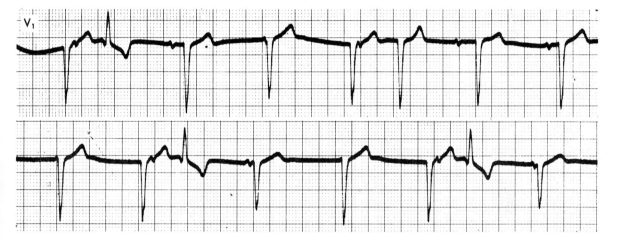

Fig. 20-19. Who is married to whom? Strips are continuous. Early beats are consistently preceded by a sinus P wave just emerging beyond the QRS and are therefore conducted (capture) beats. The underlying rhythm is sinus bradycardia producing AV dissociation.

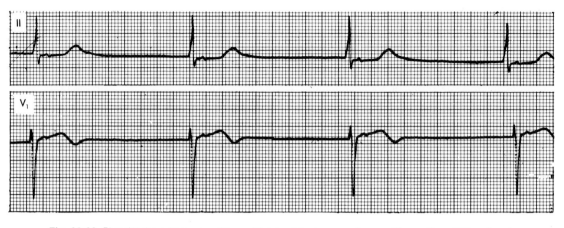

Fig. 20-20. Pinpoint the primary condition, which is sick sinus syndrome with resulting AV junctional escape (rate, 31 beats/min) with retrograde conduction.

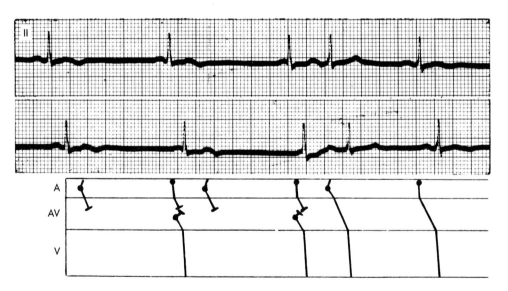

Fig. 20-21. Strips are continuous. Sinus rhythm with atrial bigeminy; most of the APBs are not conducted, with resulting junctional escape.

PINPOINT THE PRIMARY DISTURBANCE. One must never be content to let the diagnosis rest with a phenomenon such as AV dissociation, escape, or aberration, which are always secondary to some primary disturbance.

In Fig. 20-20 there is a junctional rhythm with retrograde conduction at a rate of 31 beats/min. Show this strip to most observers and ask for a *diagnosis*. Almost certainly the answer will be "junctional rhythm." But this is not a diagnosis. No junctional rhythm could possibly hold sway in the presence of a normal sinus node. The diagnosis—the primary disturbance—is a sick SA node; and junctional rhythm is a secondary escape mechanism.

Fig. 20-21 presents a chance to review several of the points under "A systematic approach," p. 368. This tracing was sent thousands of miles with the note: "This patient needed a pacemaker for this funny sort of block—what is it?"

After observing the presence of bradycardia and of two premature supraventricular beats, probably the first thing that you notice is AV dissociation and the different shapes of the Ts. The P′ wave is a common reason for such distortion, and the diagnosis "falls into your lap": conducted and nonconducted bigeminal atrial premature beats (APBs) with junctional escape beats.

Failing this approach, the diagnosis could have been reached by any of the following methods:

1. Review the causes of bradycardia. Nonconducted atrial bigeminy is third on the list and elicits from you a careful examination of the T waves, in which you find the nonconducted APBs.
2. If you were motivated by the injunction to "find the break," you would concentrate on the early beats since they represent the "break" in the otherwise regular rhythm. Attention would then be directed to the T waves and the hidden Ps.
3. If you had recited the causes of early supraventricular beats, you would have thought first of atrial extrasystoles.

REFERENCES

1. Thorne D and Gozensky C: Rabbit ears: an aid in distinguishing ventricular ectopy from aberration, Heart Lung 3:634, 1974.
2. Wellens HJJ and others: The value of the electrocardiogram in the differential diagnosis of a tachycardia with a widened QRS complex, Am J Med 64:27, 1978.
3. Marriott HJL and Fogg E: Constant monitoring for cardiac dysrhythmias and blocks, Mod Concepts Cardiovasc Dis 39:103, 1970.

Glossary

A wave (HBE) Represents atrial activation.

aberrant ventricular conduction The *temporary* abnormal intraventricular conduction of supraventricular impulses; also called "ventricular aberration" or "aberrancy."

abnormal automaticity A type of altered automaticity occurring in cells that do not normally possess that property; occurs in severely depressed myocardial cells.

absolute refractory period The period during which the cell will not respond to a second stimulus of even greater strength or duration than was necessary to discharge it in its nonrefractory state.

accelerated idiojunctional rhythm An ectopic junctional rhythm at a rate exceeding the normal firing rate of the junction without retrograde conduction to the atria.

accelerated idioventricular rhythm A rhythm of ectopic ventricular origin, faster than the normal rate of the His-Purkinje system but slower than 100 beats/min without retrograde conduction to the atria.

accelerated junctional rhythm An ectopic junctional rhythm at a rate exceeding the normal firing rate of junctional tissue and with or without retrograde atrial conduction.

accessory pathway An extra muscular tract between atrium and ventricle.

action potential A very precise rapid sequence of changes in the electrical potential across the cell membrane, consisting of 5 phases, 0 to 4, and representing the electrical cardiac cycle; phases 0 to 3 comprise electrical systole, and phase 4, electrical diastole

    depressed fast response action potential The action potential produced when not all of the fast sodium channels are available to depolarize the fiber.

    fast response action potential The action potential produced when all of the fast sodium channels are available for depolarization, resulting in rapid upstroke velocity and maximal amplitude for phase 0 and consequent optimal conduction velocity.

    slow response action potential The action potential produced when only slow channels are available to depolarize the fiber.

afterdepolarization A depolarization caused by a transient inward sodium current; if such a depolarization reaches threshold potential, propagated action potentials may occur; the resultant beats represent "triggered activity."

    delayed afterdepolarization A transient inward sodium current that occurs after phase 3 has been completed; if threshold potential is achieved, triggered activity may result.

    early afterdepolarization A transient depolarization during phase 3 of the action potential; if threshold potential for the slow channels is achieved, triggered activity may result.

AH interval (HBE) Represents AV nodal conduction time, measured from the A wave on the HBE to the earliest onset of the His bundle potential.

altered automaticity Automatic activity resulting from either a loss of fast sodium channels such as would occur in depressed tissue (abnormal automaticity) or a steepening of phase 4 depolarization in pacemaker cells (enhanced normal automaticity).

allorhythmia A repetitive arrhythmic sequence.

AN region Area in which the atrial fibers merge with AV nodal tissue.

anterograde conduction Forward conduction (i.e., from atria or from AV junction to the ventricles).

APB Atrial premature beat.

atrial fibrillation Erratic electrical activity of the atria; said to be "controlled" when the ventricular rate has been decreased by drugs.

atrial flutter An atrial ectopic tachycardia with rates that can range from 230 to 380 beats/min; type I and II are distinguished from each other by their rates and because type I is more easily cardioverted. In type I the atrial rate is 290 to 310 beats/min but can range from 230 to 350 beats/min; in type II the atrial rate is 360 to 380 beats/min but can range from 340 to 430 beats/min.

atrial tachycardia A rapid heart rate of 100 to 250 beats/min, with the ectopic focus in the atria; may be paroxysmal and easy to treat or incessant and difficult to treat. The focus for incessant atrial tachycardia is usually located in the atrial septum.

    chaotic atrial tachycardia An atrial ectopic tachycardia resulting from multifocal activity; often associated with chronic lung disease.

automatic Capable of spontaneous activity arising without external cause.

automaticity The capability of a cell to depolarize spontaneously, reach threshold potential, and initiate an action potential.

    altered automaticity The steepening of normal phase 4 depolarization in pacemaker cells or the abnormal automaticity of cells (with reduced membrane potentials) not ordinarily possessing that property.

AV dissociation The independent beating of atria and ventricles.

AV junctional tachycardia An ectopic junctional rhythm at a rate exceeding 100 beats/min.

AVNR AV nodal reentry.

AV nodal reentry The arrhythmogenic mechanism in which two parallel pathways are established within the AV node, with one pathway (usually the slower one) conducting anterogradely to the ventricles and the other retrogradely to the atria.

AV reciprocating tachycardia A rapid rhythm caused by AV nodal reentry or AV reentry using an accessory pathway.

AV tract A muscular pathway between atrium and ventricle with one end inserted into conductive tissue.

bidirectional tachycardia Tachycardia in which the wide QRS complexes alternate in polarity in the observed lead.

bigeminy Any rhythm in which the beats are spaced in pairs.

bradycardia-tachycardia syndrome Any arrhythmia characterized by alternating slow and fast heart rates.

bypass tract A muscular tract between the atrium and the ventricle that excludes the AV node.

cardiac action potential The very precise rapid sequence of changes in the electrical potential across the cell membrane.

chaotic atrial tachycardia Atrial tachycardia with P' waves that are irregular in time and variable in shape; multifocal atrial tachycardia.

circus movement tachycardia Any reentry tachycardia; generally reserved for the AV reentry using an accessory pathway and the AV node.

CMT Circus movement tachycardia.

complete (third degree) AV block Exists when the opportunity for AV conduction is optimal and none occurs.

concealed accessory pathway An accessory pathway that conducts only in a retrograde direction, often producing a "concealed WPW syndrome."

concealed bigeminy Although the mechanism producing the bigeminal rhythm continues in effect, it is not always manifested on the ECG; recognized by finding only odd numbers of P waves between manifest extrasystoles.

concealed conduction The propagation and block of an impulse, usually within the specialized conduction system, that can be recognized only from its effect on the subsequent beat or cycle.

concealed junctional extrasystole A junctional impulse arising in and discharging the AV junction but failing to reach either atria or ventricles.

concealed reentry The reentrance and block of an impulse in a depressed pathway, leaving the pathway refractory to the passage of a subsequent impulse.

concealed supernormal conduction Supernormal conduction that is recognized only by its effect on subsequent conduction or impulse formation.

concealed Wolff-Parkinson-White (WPW) syndrome The condition in which an accessory pathway is present but is capable of only retrograde conduction; the ECG is normal, and the patient is prone to paroxysmal supraventricular tachycardia.

concentration gradient The gradient that exists across a membrane that separates a high concentration of a particular ion from a low concentration of the same ion.

connection A muscular pathway between atrium and ventricle apart from the conductive system.

coupling interval The interval between the dominant (usually sinus) beat and the coupled extrasystole.

decremental conduction Conduction that slows progressively because the effectiveness of the propagating impulse progressively decreases.

delta wave Slurring of the initial part of the QRS because of preexcitation.

depolarization The reduction of a membrane potential to a less negative value.

   rapid depolarization Phase 0 depolarization.

   slow diastolic depolarization (same as phase 4 depolarization) The reduction of the membrane potential during electrical diastole because of a slow influx of sodium into the cell; it is the normal property of pacemaker cells but may be abnormal if accelerated.

depressed fast response action potential The action potential produced when only some of the fast sodium channels are used to depolarize the fiber, resulting in decreased velocity and amplitude of phase 0 and consequent reduction in conduction velocity.

diastole (electrical) Phase 4 of the action potential.

diastole (mechanical) The relaxation of the heart's chambers.

diastolic potential The transmembrane potential of the cell during electrical diastole.

double tachycardia The simultaneous operation of two rapidly firing but independent foci, one controlling the atria and one the ventricles.

dV/dt The rate of change of voltage with respect to time; its units are in volts/second.

echo beat A reciprocal beat, that is, one that results from the return of an impulse to a chamber to reactivate it; may be either atrial or ventricular.

electrical potential gradient The gradient that exists when an electrical voltage difference exists across a membrane.

end-diastolic VPB A ventricular premature ectopic beat falling after the P wave (at the end of diastole); may or may not result in a fusion beat.

enhanced normal automaticity Automatic activity caused by steepening of phase 4 depolarization in pacemaker cells; occurs with excess catecholamines; easily suppressed with overdrive pacing.

entrance block A zone of depressed conduction surrounding a pacemaker focus, protecting it from discharge by an extraneous impulse but not necessarily from electrotonic influences.

excitability The property by which a cardiac cell can give rise to an action potential when driven by an adequate stimulus.

exit block The pathological failure of an expected impulse to emerge from its focus of origin and propagate.

fast response action potential The action potential produced when all of the fast sodium channels are available for depolarization, resulting in rapid upstroke velocity, maximal amplitude for phase 0, and consequent optimal conduction velocity.

fast sodium channels The membrane channels that open in response to voltage to allow sodium to enter the cell during phase 0 of the action potential.

flutter-fibrillation A supraventricular tachyarrhythmia with features of both atrial flutter and fibrillation.

functional refractory period The shortest interval at which a tissue is capable of conducting consecutive impulses; measured by the time intervening between the arrival of an initial impulse and the earliest subsequent conductible (premature) impulse at the distal end of the conducting tissue in question.

fusion The complex (ventricular or atrial) that results when two impulses collide within the same pair of chambers (ventricles or atria).

gap phenomenon A zone in which a premature stimulus encounters block, whereas an earlier or later stimulus is conducted.

gating mechanism The increasing duration of the action potential from the AV node to a point in the distal Purkinje system, beyond which point it again decreases.

H deflection (HBE) Represents His bundle activation.

H region The bundle of His from its AV nodal connection to its branching portion.

His bundle AV bundle; the cablelike fibers that are continuous from the AV node to the bundle branches.

His bundle electrogram (HBE) A direct recording of the electrical activity in the bundle of His.

His-Purkinje system The conduction system from the bundle of His to the distal Purkinje fibers inclusive.

HV interval (HBE) The conduction time through the His-Purkinje system, measured from the earliest onset of the His potential to the onset of ventricular activation as recorded on either the intracardiac bipolar His bundle lead or any of the multiple surface ECG leads.

idiojunctional rhythm A rhythm emanating from the AV junction but without retrograde conduction to the atria.

inhibition The effect of a weaker impulse, unable to conduct through a depressed segment, leaving that segment refractory so that a subsequent stronger impulse is also blocked.

interpolated ventricular premature beat (VPB) A ventricular extrasystole sandwiched between two consecutive beats of the dominant—usually sinus—rhythm.

isorhythmic AV dissociation AV dissociation during which the atria and the ventricles beat at approximately the same rate, preventing AV or VA conduction.

junction (AV) An area composed of the AV node and the nonbranching portion of the bundle of His.

junctional tachycardia A heart rate greater than 100 beats/min emanating from the AV junction; often related to digitalis toxicity and caused by triggered activity; may also be caused by altered automaticity.

Kent bundle Histologically specialized tissue anteriorly adjacent to the fibrous ring of the tricuspid valve; the term is often misassigned to the other AV connections responsible for Wolff-Parkinson-White syndrome.

longitudinal dissociation The insulation of parallel pathways from each other, usually in the AV junction.

Lown-Ganong-Levine syndrome A form of preexcitation characterized by a short PR interval and a normal QRS; associated with a tendency to supraventricular tachycardia.

macroreentry Reentry involving a large circuit (for example, both bundle branches).

Mahaim fibers Paraspecific conductive tracts running between AV node or His bundle and the muscle of the ventricular septum.

maximal diastolic membrane potential The greatest degree of negative transmembrane potential achieved by the cell during diastole.

maximal diastolic potential The most negative level of transmembrane potential achieved by the cell.

membrane conductance The degree of permeability of the membrane to particular ions.

membrane responsiveness The relationship between the membrane potential at the time of stimulation and the maximal rate of depolarization of the action potential.

microreentry Reentry involving a small circuit (for example, within Purkinje fibers).

multifocal Arising from more than two foci.

multiform Of varied shape; variform.

N region The body of the AV node.

NH (nodal-His) region Area in which the AV node merges with the bundle of His.

nonpacemaker cell A cell without the property of automaticity.

one-way conduction The passage of a current in only one direction through a fiber or fibers.

overdrive suppression The inhibitory effect of a faster pacemaker on a slower pacemaker; seen in healthy His-Purkinje cells but decreases with a decrease in membrane potential and loss of fast sodium channels.

overshoot In cellular electrophysiology, that part of phase 0 of the action potential that is greater than 0 mV.

PA interval (HBE) A measurement of intra-atrial conduction time, measured from the onset of the P wave on the standard ECG or from the atrial deflection of the high right atrial electrogram to the A wave on the HBE.

pacemaker cells Cells exhibiting the property of normal automaticity (e.g., cells of the sinus node, ventricular conduction system, and portions of the AV valves).

pacemaker current The time-dependent increase in inward sodium current that is peculiar to pacemaker cells; when threshold potential is reached, rapid depolarization occurs.

parasystole An independent ectopic rhythm that cannot be discharged by impulses of the dominant rhythm but which can be modulated by electrotonic influences; an abnormality of both automaticity and impulse conduction (entrance block).

paroxysmal supraventricular tachycardia (PSVT) An ectopic rhythm usually supported by an AV nodal reentry mechanism, circus movement using an accessory pathway and the AV node, or SA nodal reentry; may be initiated by an atrial premature beat, junctional premature beat, or ventricular premature beat with retrograde conduction.

perinodal fibers Atrial fibers surrounding the SA node.

phase 0 The rapid upstroke of the action potential that occurs after a cell reaches threshold potential; the result of the opening of fast sodium channels.

phase 1 The initial rapid repolarization phase of the action potential that results from an exodus of potassium from the cell.

phase 2 The plateau of the action potential that is particularly long in cardiac cells as a result of the influx of calcium and sodium ions through the slow channels.

phase 3 The terminal rapid repolarization phase of the action potential that begins with the closing of the slow channels; it is completed by an exodus of potassium from the cell and the activity of the sodium pump.

phase 3 aberration Ventricular aberration resulting from the arrival of the impulse in the ventricular fascicle during phase 3 of its action potential.

phase 4 Electrical diastole, the interval between action potentials; the resting phase of the electrical cardiac cycle; it is steadily maintained in nonpacemaker cells, but in pacemaker cells the membrane potential is slowly reduced until threshold potential is reached spontaneously (or it is driven there by an outside stimulus).

phase 4 aberration Ventricular aberration resulting from the arrival of the impulse in a spontaneously depolarizing ventricular fascicle late in diastole.

phase 4 depolarization The slow reduction of the membrane potential during electrical diastole; it is normal in pacemaker cells, although it may be abnormal if accelerated.

preexcitation Activation of part of the ventricular myocardium earlier than would be expected if the activating impulses traveled only down the normal routes.

pumps In cellular electrophysiology, the mechanism of active transport of ions across the cell membrane.

Purkinje fibers The terminal ramifications of the ventricular conduction system.

reciprocal beat The beat, atrial or ventricular, that results when the same impulse activates the same pair of chambers for the second time; also called echo beat.

reentry Reactivation of a tissue for the second or subsequent time by the same impulse.

reflection A form of reentry in which, after encountering delay in one fiber, the impulse enters a parallel fiber and returns retrogradely toward its source.

refractoriness The inability of a fiber to respond to a second stimulus after it has responded to a prior stimulus.

refractory period In cellular physiology, the time from phase 0 to the end of phase 3 of the action potential; divided into effective and relative periods.

   effective refractory period The time from phase 0 to approximately −60 mV during phase 3 of the action potential; that time during which it is impossible for the myocardium to respond to even a strong stimuli with a propagated action potential.

relative refractory period The time from approximately −60 mV during phase 3 of the action potential to its end; that time during which a depressed response to a strong stimulus is possible.

repolarization The process by which the cell is restored to its resting potential; occurs from phase 1 to the end of phase 3 of the action potential.

resting membrane potential The transmembrane voltage that exists when the heart muscle is at rest.

retrograde Wenckebach conduction Progressively lengthening conduction from the ventricles or AV junction to the atria that continues until an impulse fails to reach the atria.

"rule of bigeminy" The tendency of a lengthened ventricular cycle to precipitate a ventricular premature beat.

SA conduction time Conduction time from the sinus node to the atrial musculature, measured from the SA deflection in the SA nodal electrogram to the beginning of the P wave in the bipolar records or to the beginning of the high right atrial electrogram in the unipolar record.

SA electrogram A direct recording of the electrical activity of the SA node.

sarcolemma The membrane of a muscle cell.

short-PR–normal-QRS syndrome Describes itself; when associated with supraventricular tachycardia, sometimes called "Lown-Ganong-Levine syndrome."

sick sinus Sinus node dysfunction characterized by marked sinus bradycardia, SA block, sinus arrest, prolonged SA pauses, or the bradycardia–tachycardia syndrome.

sick sinus syndrome Sinus node dysfunction complicated by cerebral dysfunction secondary either to failure of escape mechanisms or to a tachycardia.

slow response action potential The action potential produced when none of the fast sodium channels are available for depolarization and the fiber is depolarized only through slower sodium-calcium channels to produce an action potential with a slow upstroke velocity, low amplitude, and consequent slow conduction.

sodium-potassium ATPase The enzyme that hydrolyzes adenosine triphosphate and thus provides the energy necessary for the active sodium-potassium exchange across the sarcolemma.

sodium pump A cellular mechanism that actively transports sodium out of the cell in exchange for potassium.

SSS Sick sinus syndrome.

summation The merging of weaker impulses to form a stronger wave front.

supernormal conduction Conduction that occurs when block is expected.

supernormal excitability The ability of the myocardium to respond to a stimulus that is ineffective when applied earlier or later in the cycle.

supernormal period A period at the end of phase 3 during which activation can be initiated with a lesser stimulus than is required at maximal repolarization.

third degree (complete) AV block A block that exists when the opportunity for conduction is optimal and none occurs.

threshold potential The transmembrane potential that must be achieved before an action potential can be initiated.

torsade de pointes (twisting of the points) A type of polymorphous but organized ventricular tachycardia that occurs against a background of long QT intervals and extrasystoles preceded by long coupling intervals; usually drug related.

torsades de pointes Refers to more than one episode.

triggered activity Rhythmic activity that results when a series of afterdepolarizations reach threshold potential.

triggered impulse An impulse that results when an afterdepolarization reaches threshold potential.

type A preexcitation Preexcitation in which the R wave is dominant in V_1, V_2, and/or V_E.

type B preexcitation Preexcitation in which the S or Q wave is dominant in V_1, V_2, and/or V_E.

unidirectional block Pathological failure of conduction in one direction while conduction is possible in the other direction.

V deflection (HBE) Represents ventricular activation.

VPB Ventricular premature beat.

WPW Wolff-Parkinson-White syndrome.

Index

A

Aberrant conduction
 atrial, 210-213
 ventricular, 197-217; *see also* Ventricular
  conduction, aberrant
Accelerated idiojunctional rhythm
 digitalis toxicity and, 74-75
  atrial fibrillation and, 78
 Wenckebach exit block and, 351-352
Accelerated idioventricular rhythm
 digitalis toxicity and, 80
 drug-induced, 184, 185
 fusion and, 276, 278-279
 parasystolic, 303
 reciprocal beat and, 134
 ventricular fusion and, 273
Accessory pathway in Wolff-Parkinson-White
  syndrome, 154-157
Action potential, 30, 31
 cardiac disease and, 179
 comparison with other potentials, 33
 electrocardiogram and, 42
 fast response, 87
 nodes and, 40
 slow response, 87, 88
Afterdepolarization, 56
 digitalis toxicity and, 60
 triggered activity and, 52-55
Age in QRS tachycardia, 220
AH interval, 15
AIVR; *see* Accelerated idioventricular rhythm
Altered automaticity, 45-52, 56
 early afterdepolarization and, 55
 parasystole and, 288-311; *see also*
  Parasystole
Alternating aberrancy, 214-215
Amiodarone
 digoxin and, 61
 torsades de pointes and, 187

Anesthetic
 drug-induced arrhythmia and, 175-176, 189
 fast sodium channel blockade and,
  176-177
Anoxia, 88
Anterograde conduction, 123
Antiarrhythmic drug
 automaticity and, 48
 proarrhythmic action of, 174-191
  abnormal conduction and, 180
  cardiac disease and, 178
  fast sodium channel blockade and,
   176-177
  membrane channel and, 175-176
  prolonged refractory period and, 182-183
  supraventricular arrhythmia and, 183
  ventricular tachyarrhythmia and, 183-189
Antidepressant, tricyclic, 184
Antidromic circus movement tachycardia
 QRS tachycardia and, 241
 Wolff-Parkinson-White syndrome and,
  163
APB; *see* Atrial premature beat
Artificial ventricular parasystole, 292
Ashman's phenomenon, 210-211
Asystole, ventricular, 258, 259
ATPase pump, 53
Atria; *see also* Atrial *entries*
 atrioventricular node reentry, 124
 second-in-a-row anomaly and, 209
Atrial beat
 ectopic, 206
 premature, 366, 370
  aberration and, 193
  atrioventricular node reentry and, 122
  concealed conduction and, 324-325
  laddergram and, 340
  nonconducted, 341
  sinoatrial node reentry and, 108

Atrial bigeminy
  alternating aberrancy and, 215
  nonconducted, 377
    sinus rhythm and, 372
Atrial conduction, aberrant, 210-213
Atrial extrasystole
  nonconducted, 373
  sinus node and, 107
  ventricular fusion and, 272, 273
Atrial fibrillation
  aberrancy in, 210-211
  accessory pathway and, 241
  atrioventricular node reentry and, 128
  concealed conduction in, 313-314
  digitalis toxicity and, 78
  sick sinus syndrome and, 114
  Wolff-Parkinson-White syndrome and,
    164-167
Atrial flutter
  aberrancy in, 213
  bigeminy and, 379
  laddergram and, 343
    exit block and, 344
  Wenckebach period and, 382
Atrial fusion, 268, 286-287
  laddergram and, 355
Atrial impulse, 248
Atrial pacemaker, wandering, 106-107
Atrial parasystole, 305-307
  atrial fusion and, 355
Atrial premature beat, 366, 370
  aberration and, 193
  atrioventricular node reentry and, 122
  concealed conduction and, 324-325
  laddergram and, 340, 341
  nonconducted, 341
  sinoatrial node reentry and, 108
Atrial tachycardia
  aberrancy in, 212-213
  digitalis toxicity and, 62
  sick sinus syndrome and, 114
Atrioventricular block, 247-267
  2 to 1, 254-255
  anatomy versus behavior and, 250
  bradycardia and, 377
  complete, 256, 258
  digitalis toxicity and, 65
  enhanced normal automaticity and, 49, 52
  high-grade, 256
  nonconducted beats and, 247-248
  phase 3 and 4, 200
  PR interval and, 247
  reclassification of, 260-266
  second degree, 374, 375

Atrioventricular block—cont'd
  supernormal conduction and, 331, 371
  type I and type II, 248-249
  ventricular asystole and, 258
  Wenckebach periodicity and, 252-253
  Wolff-Parkinson-White syndrome and, 162
Atrioventricular circus movement tachycardia,
    367
Atrioventricular dissociation, 224
Atrioventricular junction, 131
Atrioventricular node
  atrial fibrillation and, 313-314
  development of, 6-7
  origin of, 2
  reentry and, 102, 120-140
    dual pathways and, 120
    laddergram and, 342-343
    mechanism of, 122-124
    reciprocal beats and, 129-138
    supraventricular tachycardia and, 129
    tachycardia and, 125-126
    uncommon forms of, 126-128
  Wenckebach period and, 78
  Wolff-Parkinson-White syndrome and, 159
Atrioventricular ring, 1
Automaticity
  altered, 45-52, 56
    early afterdepolarization and, 55
    parasystole and, 288-311; see also
        Parasystole
  enhanced normal, 46, 48, 52, 56
    overdrive suppression and, 49, 52
  sinus node and, 106
Autonomic nervous system, 107
AV node; see Atrioventricular node
AVNR; see Atrioventricular node, reentry and

B

B-T ring; see Bulbotruncal ring
B-V ring; see Bulboventricular ring
Beat
  atrial premature; see Atrial premature beat
  capture, 371
    QRS tachycardia and, 224
  concealed junctional, 353
  early, causes of, 369-372
  ectopic
    atrial, 206
    bigeminy and, 275
    fusion and, 270
    laddergram and, 353
    paired, 305
    reciprocal beat and, 133
    slow response action potential and, 87

Beat—cont'd
  fusion, 268-287; *see also* Fusion
  junctional escape, 346-347
  nonconducted
    atrial premature, 341; *see also* Atrial
      premature beat
    atrioventricular block and, 247-248
  parasystole and; *see* Parasystole
  premature; *see* Premature beat
  reciprocal, 372
    atrioventricular node reentry and, 129-138
    bigeminy and, 380
    junctional rhythm and, 348, 349
    second-in-a-row anomaly, 208-209
    triggered, 60
  ventricular escape, 282
Bedside diagnosis of ventricular tachycardia, 226
Behavior in atrioventricular block, 250
Beta stimulation, 54
Bidirectional ventricular tachycardia, 70-71
Bigeminy
  atrial
    alternating aberrancy and, 215
    nonconducted, 372, 377
  causes of, 378-380
  concealed, 101
  ventricular
    digitalis toxicity and, 72
    ventricular fusion and, 272, 275
Bix rule, 385
  atrioventricular node reentry and, 126
Block
  atrial tachycardia and, 62
  atrioventricular, 247-267; *see also*
    Atrioventricular block
  bundle branch; *see* Bundle branch block
  entrance, 289-293, 302
  exit
    parasystole and, 294-295, 300
    Wenckebach, 78, 351-352
  left bundle branch; *see* Left bundle branch
    block
  right bundle branch; *see* Right bundle branch
    block
  sinoatrial, 110-113
    laddergram and, 345-347
  unidirectional, 88
Block/acceleration dissociation, 264
Blockade, fast sodium channel, 176-177
Blood supply, 107
Body temperature, 107
Bradycardia
  causes of, 376-378
  sick sinus syndrome and, 113

Bradycardia—cont'd
  sinus, 376
    digitalis toxicity and, 77, 81
Bradycardia-dependent bundle branch block,
    198
Bulbotruncal ring, 1
Bulboventricular ring, 1
Bundle branch
  development of, 8-10
  reentry within, 102
Bundle branch block
  atrioventricular block and, 255
  classical ventricular parasystole and, 298,
    298-299
  left; *see* Left bundle branch block
  phase 4 depolarization and, 333
  rate-dependent, 200
  right; *see* Right bundle branch block
  supraventricular tachycardia and, 242, 243
  ventricular fusion and, 270
Bundle of His
  branching portion of, 8-10
  electrogram of, 12-18
  reentry within, 102

C

Calcium
  delayed after depolarizaton and, 53, 54
  digitalis toxicity and, 60
Capture beat, 371
  QRS tachycardia and, 224
Cardiac tube, 1
Cell
  His-Purkinje, 48
  pacemaker, 47
Cellular electrophysiology, 19-44
  action potential and, 30, 31
    comparison with other action potentials, 33
    electrocardiogram and, 42
    nodes and, 40
  automaticity and
    excitability versus, 41
    normal, 37
  current flow in heart and, 20
  electrical cardiac cycle and, 24-30
  gating mechanism and, 34
  history of, 19
  membrane channels and, 24-25
  membrane potential and conduction velocity,
    35-37
  normal, 21-24
  overdrive suppression and, 38, 39
  refractory period and, 32-33
  supernormal period and, 35

Channel, membrane, 175-176
Circus movement, interrupted, 128
Circus movement tachycardia
  antidromic
    QRS tachycardia and, 241
    Wolff-Parkinson-White syndrome and,
      163-164
  atrioventricular, 367
  atrioventricular node reentry and, 129
  orthodromic, 154, 157, 159, 161-162
  persistent, 162
Classical ventricular parasystole, 294-300
CMT; see Circus movement tachycardia
Complete atrioventricular block, 256, 258, 259
Concealed bigeminy, 101
Concealed conduction, 312-327, 375
  atrial fibrillation and, 313-314
  historical background of, 312-313
  impulse formation and, 321-325
  interpolated ventricular extrasystoles and,
    315-318
  junctional extrasystoles and, 318-320
  supernormal, 331
Concealed junctional beat, 353
Concealed junctional extrasystole, 375
  supernormal conduction and, 332
Concealed parasystole, 301
Concealed reentry, 100
  supernormal conduction and, 334, 335
Concordant precordial pattern, 224
Conduction
  aberrant atrial, 210-213
  aberrant ventricular, 192-217; see also
    Ventricular conduction, aberrant
  abnormal; see also Automaticity, altered
    antiarrhythmic drug and, 180-181
    cardiac disease and, 178-179
  accessory pathway and, 241, 254-257
  atrioventricular node reentry and, 120, 121,
    126
    anterograde and retrograde, 123
  concealed, 312-317, 375
    atrial fibrillation and, 313-314
    historical background of, 312-313
    impulse formation and, 321-325
    interpolated ventricular extrasystoles and,
      315-318
    junctional extrasystoles and, 318-320
    supernormal, 331
  delayed, 85, 96
    Wenckebach-like, 98
  development of, 1-11
  infarction and, 99
  Mahaim fibers and, 68

Conduction—cont'd
  one-way block of, 89
  reciprocal beat and, 133
  retrograde
    atrioventricular node reentry and, 123
    concealed, 315-318
    reciprocal, 133
  supernormal, 328-337, 330
    atrioventricular block and, 371
  Wenckebach; see Wenckebach entries
Conduction velocity
  aberrant ventricular conduction and, 193
  drug-induced arrhythmia and, 178
  Purkinje fibers and, 94
  sinus node and, 107
Coronary occlusion, 88; see also Myocardial
    infarction
Coupling, fixed
  classical ventricular parasystole and, 295
  parasystole and, 293, 304-305
Critical rate bundle branch block, 200

D

Deflection
  His bundle electrogram and, 15
  right bundle branch block and, 207
Delayed afterdepolarization
  digitalis toxicity and, 60
  triggered activity and, 52-55
Delayed conduction
  reentry and, 85, 96
  Wenckebach-like, 98
Delta wave, 154-157
Dependence, 176-177
Depolarization
  altered automaticity and, 45, 46
  parasystole and, 290
  slow response and, 87-88
  supernormal conduction and, 333
Depressed fast response, 87
Digitalis; see also Digitalis toxicity
  atrial flutter and, 213
  atrioventricular node reentry and, 128
Digitalis toxicity, 59-83
  accelerated idiojunctional rhythm and, 74-75
  accelerated idioventricular rhythm and, 80
  arrhythmia and, 174
  atrial fibrillation and, 78-79
  atrial tachycardia with block and, 62-66
  atrioventricular Wenckebach period and, 78
  basis for dysrhythmia and, 60
  bidirectional ventricular tachycardia and,
    70-71
  cellular basis for dysrhythmia and, 60

Digitalis toxicity—cont'd
  delayed afterdepolarization and, 53
  double tachycardia and, 76
  drug interactions and, 61
  fascicular ventricular tachycardia and,
    66-69
  inotropy and, 59
  mortality and, 59
  potassium and, 61
  QRS tachycardia and, 245
  sinus bradycardia and, 77, 80
  temporary pacemaker and, 54
  ventricular bigeminy and, 72
  ventricular tachycardia and, 75
Digoxin, 61
Diltiazem, 61
Discharge rate in parasystole, 289
Disopyramide, 187
Dissociation
  atrioventricular, 224
  block/acceleration, 264
Diuretic, 53
Double tachycardia, 76
Dropped beat, 248
Drug
  arrhythmia caused by, 174-191; *see also*
    Antiarrhythmic drug, proarrhythmic
    action of
  atrioventricular node reentry and, 128

E
Early afterdepolarization, 54-55
Early beat, 369-372; *see also* Premature beat
Ectopic beat
  atrial, 206
  slow response action potential and, 87
  ventricular
    bigeminy and, 275
    fusion and, 270
    laddergram and, 353
    paired, 305
    reciprocal beat and, 133
Ectopic mechanism
  junctional, 347-353
  supraventricular, 340-344
Electrophysiology, cellular, 19-44; *see also*
  Cellular electrophysiology
Encainide
  drug-induced arrhythmia and, 189
  ventricular tachycardia and, 184
Enhanced normal automaticity, 46, 48, 52, 56
  early afterdepolarization and, 55
  overdrive suppression and, 49, 52
Entrance block, 289-293, 302

Escape rhythm
  junctional
    digitalis toxicity and, 68
    laddergram and, 350
    sinoatrial Wenckebach conduction and,
      346-347
  ventricular, 282
Excitability
  digitalis dysrhythmia and, 62
  supernormal, 328
Exit block
  parasystole and, 294-295, 300
  Wenckebach, 351-352
Extrasystole
  atrial, 107
    nonconducted, 373
    sinus node and, 107
  bigeminy and, 378
  concealed bigeminy and, 101
  concealed conduction and
    retrograde, 315-318
  concealed junctional, 318-320, 375
    supernormal conduction and, 332
  reentry and, 98-99
  sinus rhythm and, 382
  ventricular fusion and, 272, 273

F
Fascicular ventricular tachycardia, 66-69, 75
Fast response, depressed, 87
Fast response action potential, 87
Fast sodium channel blockade, 176-177
Fiber
  abnormal automaticity and, 47
  Mahaim
    Lown-Ganong-Levine syndrome and,
      170
    preexcitement with conduction over,
      68
  Purkinje, 47
    automaticity and, 46, 47, 56
    reentry and, 94-95
    reflection and, 91
Fibrillation
  atrial
    aberrancy in, 210-211
    accessory pathway and, 241
    atrioventricular node reentry and, 128
    concealed conduction in, 313-314
    digitalis toxicity and, 78
    sick sinus syndrome and, 114
    Wolff-Parkinson-White syndrome and,
      164-167
  ventricular, drug-induced, 189

Fixed coupling
  classical ventricular parasystole and,
    295
  parasystole and, 293, 304-305
Fixed-rate pacemaker, 296
Flecainide, 184
Flecamide, 189
Flutter, atrial
  aberrancy in, 213
  bigeminy and, 379
  laddergram and, 343, 344
  Wenckebach period and, 382
Fusion, 268-287
  accelerated idioventricular rhythm and, 276,
    278-279
  atrial, 268, 286-287
    laddergram and, 355
  classical ventricular parasystole and,
    295
  paced beats and, 284
  parasystole and, 276
  QRS tachycardia and, 224
  ventricular, 270-276
    laddergram and, 354-355
    preexcitation and, 285
  ventricular escape beats and, 282-283
  ventricular tachycardia and, 280-281

G

Gap phenomenon, 334-336
Gate, m or h, 175
Group beating, 381

H

h gate, 175
Haystack principle, 386
Heart failure, 53
Hemodynamic status, 220
High-grade atrioventricular block, 256, 257
  misconceptions about, 262-263
His bundle
  branching portion of, 8-10
  electrogram of, 12-18
  reentry within, 102
His-Purkinje cell, 48
HV interval, 15
Hypercalcemia, 53
Hyperthermia, 107
Hypokalemia
  delayed afterdepolarization and, 53
  digitalis toxicity and, 61
Hypomagnesemia, 53
Hypothermia, 107

I

IC drugs, 188
Idiojunctional pacemaker, 323
Idiojunctional rhythm, accelerated
  digitalis toxicity and, 74-75, 78
  Wenckebach exit block and, 351-352
Idioventricular rhythm
  accelerated
    digitalis toxicity and, 80
    drug-induced, 184, 185
    fusion and, 276, 278-279
    parasystolic, 303
    reciprocal beat and, 134
    ventricular fusion and, 273
  enhanced normal automaticity and, 49, 52
Impulse formation
  abnormal, 45; *see also* Automaticity, altered
  concealed conduction and, 321-325
  parasystole and, 288-289
Infarction, myocardial
  conduction in, 99
  depressed fast response and, 88
  digitalis toxicity and, 68, 69
  reentry and, 97
  sick sinus syndrome and, 113
Inhibition, definition of, 90
Interectopic interval, 295
Intermittent parasystole, 302
  entrance block and, 291
Internodal conduction, 4
Interpolated ventricular extrasystole,
    315-318
Intoxication
  digitalis; *see also* Digitalis toxicity
Intoxication, digitalis, 59-83
Intraventricular reentry, 94-104
  concealed, 100
  concealed bigeminy and, 101
  extrasystolic, 98-99
  ischemic myocardial tissue and, 95-97
  macroreentry and, 102-103
  Purkinje fiber and, 94-95
Invasive studies, 219
Ionized form of drug, 176
Ischemia
  cardiac action potential and, 179
  delayed after depolarization and, 53
  reentry and, 95-99

J

Jellyfish studies, 86
Junctional beat, concealed, 353
Junctional ectopic mechanism, 347-353

Junctional escape rhythm
  digitalis toxicity and, 68
  laddergram and, 350
    sinoatrial Wenckebach conduction and,
      346-347
Junctional extrasystole, concealed, 318-320, 375
  supernormal conduction and, 332
Junctional tachycardia
  bigeminy and, 379
  digitalis toxicity and, 74-75

L

Laddergram, 338-361
  junctional ectopic mechanism and, 348-353
  sinoatrial block and, 345-347
  supraventricular ectopic mechanism and,
    340-344
  ventricular ectopic beat and, 353-356
LBBB; *see* Left bundle branch block
Leads, 362-368
  QRS tachycardia and, 220
Left bundle branch
  development of, 8-9
  reentry within, 102
Left bundle branch block
  aberration and, 205
  alternating aberrancy and, 214-215
  digitalis toxicity and, 70, 71
  fusion and, 279
  phase 3 aberration and, 197
  rate-dependent, 201
LGL syndrome; *see* Lown-Ganong-Levine
    syndrome
Lidocaine
  abnormal conduction and, 180
  drug-induced arrhythmia and, 177
Lidocaine reflex, 218
Local anesthetic, 189
  fast sodium channel blockade and, 176-177
Lown-Ganong-Levine syndrome, 169-170

M

m gate, 175
Mahaim fiber
  digitalis toxicity and, 68
  Lown-Ganong-Levine syndrome and, 170
Masking by Wolff-Parkinson-White syndrome, 157
Membrane channel, 175-176
Membrane potential
  altered automaticity and, 46-48
  early afterdepolarization and, 54-55
  resting
    slow conduction and, 87
    unidirectional block and, 88

Microelectrode techniques, 288-289
Microreentry, 85
  laddergram and, 356
Mimicking
  of supernormal conduction, 332-336
  by Wolff-Parkinson-White syndrome,
    157
Modulated ventricular parasystole, 301
Monitoring, principles of, 362-368
Moricizine, 184
Myocardial fiber, 47
Myocardial infarction
  conduction in, 99
  depressed fast response and, 88
  digitalis toxicity and, 68, 69
  reentry and, 97
  sick sinus syndrome and, 113
Myocardial tissue
  ischemic, 95-99
  reflection and, 91

N

Nervous system, autonomic, 107
Node
  AV; *see* Atrioventricular node
  SA; *see* Sinoatrial node
Nonconducted atrial bigeminy, 377
  sinus rhythm and, 372
Nonconducted atrial extrasystole, 373
Nonconducted beat
  atrial premature, 341
  atrioventricular block and, 247-248
Noninvasive His bundle electrogram, 16
Nonionized form of drug, 176

O

Occlusion, coronary, 88; *see* Myocardial
    infarction
One-way conduction block, 89
Orthodromic circus movement tachycardia, 154,
    157, 159, 161-162
Overdrive pacing, 48
Overdrive suppression, 48, 49, 52

P

P wave, 387
  atrial tachycardia and, 63, 64
  atrioventricular dissociation and, 224
  laddergram and, 339
  paroxysmal sinus tachycardia and, 109
  sinoatrial block and, 112
  sinoatrial reentry and, 117
  sinus, 106
  skipped, 256

P′ wave
  atrioventricular node reentry and, 125
  Wolff-Parkinson-White syndrome and, 159,
    160-161, 162
PA interval, 15
Paced beat, 284
Pacemaker
  fixed-rate, 296
  idiojunctional, 323
  pauses and, 375
  sinoatrial node and, 105-109
  temporary, 54
Pacemaker cell, 47
Pacing, overdrive, 48
Paired ectopic ventricular beats, 305
Paradoxical critical rate, 198
  supernormal conduction and, 333
Parasystole, 288-311, 371
  accelerated idioventricular rhythm and,
    303
  atrial, 305-307
    laddergram and, 355
  bigeminy and, 378
  classical
    with exit block, 300
    without exit block, 295-299
  clinical significance of, 308
  concealed, 301
  entrance block and, 289-293
  exit block and, 294-295, 300
  fixed coupling in, 304-305
  fusion and, 276, 277
  intermittent, 302
  mechanism of, 288-289
  paired ectopic ventricular beats and, 305
  rate of discharge and, 289
  ventricular
    artificial, 292
    classical, 294-300
    modulated, 301
Paroxysmal sinus tachycardia, 108-109
Paroxysmal supraventricular tachycardia, 117
  atrioventricular node reentry and, 122
  sinoatrial node reentry and, 108-109
  Wolff-Parkinson-White syndrome and,
    159-162
Persistent circus movement tachycardia, 162
Potassium
  delayed afterdepolarization and, 53
  digitalis toxicity and, 61
Potential
  action; *see* Action potential
  membrane; *see* Membrane potential
  sinus node and, 106

Potential—cont'd
  transmembrane
    delayed afterdepolarization and, 52
    early afterdepolarization and, 54-55
PP interval
  atrial tachycardia and, 62
  sinoatrial block and, 110
  sinoatrial reentry and, 117
PR interval
  atrioventricular block and, 247
    misdiagnosis and, 263
  atrioventricular node reentry and, 122
  Lown-Ganong-Levine syndrome, 169-170
  ventricular fusion and, 270, 271
P′R interval
  atrioventricular node reentry and, 125
  Wolff-Parkinson-White syndrome and,
    161
Preexcitation
  conduction over Mahaim fibers and, 68
  ventricular fusion and, 285
Premature beat
  atrial, 366, 370
    aberration and, 193
    atrioventricular node reentry and,
     122
    concealed conduction and, 324-325
    laddergram and, 340, 341
    nonconducted, 341
    sinoatrial node reentry and, 108
  ventricular, 369
    atrioventricular node reentry and,
     124
    concealed retrograde conduction and,
     317-318
    reciprocal beat and, 132
    ventricular fusion and, 271
Procainamide
  atrioventricular node reentry and, 128
  torsades de pointes and, 187
  ventricular tachycardia and, 184
Propafenone, 184
Propranolol
  atrial flutter and, 213
  atrioventricular node reentry and, 128
PSVT; *see* Paroxysmal supraventricular
    tachycardia
Pump
  sodium, 60
  sodium-potassium ATPase, 53
Purkinje fiber
  automaticity and, 46, 47, 56
  reentry and, 94-95
  reflection and, 91

Q

QRS alternans, 161
QRS complex; *see also* QRS tachycardia
  atrioventricular node reentry and, 123,
    125-126
  digitalis toxicity and, 67
  laddergram and, 339
  left bundle branch block and, 205
  Lown-Ganong-Levine syndrome and, 169
  torsades de pointes and, 187
  Wolff-Parkinson-White syndrome and, 159,
    169
QRS tachycardia, 218-246
  clinical application and, 226-240
  differential diagnosis of, 220-226
  exceptions in, 241-245
  hemodynamic status and, 220
  lidocaine reflex and, 218
  new findings in, 219
  overdiagnosis of aberration and, 218
QT interval
  digitalis toxicity and, 75
  torsades de pointes and, 187
Quadrigeminal grouping, 98
Quinidine
  atrioventricular node reentry and, 128
  digoxin and, 61
  torsades de pointes and, 187
  ventricular tachycardia and, 184

R

r' wave, 125
Rate-dependent bundle branch block, 200, 201
RBBB; *see* Right bundle branch block
Reciprocal beat, 372
  atrioventricular node reentry and, 129-138
  bigeminy and, 380
  junctional rhythm and, 348, 349
Reciprocity, RP/PR, 252-253
Reentry, 84-93
  atrioventricular node and
    dual pathways and, 120
    laddergram and, 342-343
    mechanism of, 122-124
    reciprocal beats and tachycardia and,
      129-138
    supraventricular tachycardia and, 129
    tachycardia and, 125-126
    uncommon forms of, 126-128
  concealed, 100
    supernormal conduction and, 334, 335
  historical background on, 86
  inhibition and, 90

Reentry—cont'd
  intraventricular
    concealed, 100
    concealed bigeminy and, 101
    extrasystolic, 98-99
    ischemia myocardial tissue and, 95-97
    macroreentry and, 102-103
    Purkinje fiber and, 94-95
  reflection and, 91
  sinoatrial node and, 105-109
  slow conduction and, 87-88
  summation and, 89
  supernormal conduction and, 335
  unidirectional block and, 88
Reflection, 91
Refractory period
  atrioventricular node reentry and, 120
  drug-induced arrhythmia and, 182-183
  exit block versus, 294
  supernormality and, 328
Reperfusion, 53
Repetitive paroxysmal sinus tachycardia, 109
Resting membrane potential
  slow conduction and, 87
  unidirectional block and, 88
Retrograde conduction
  atrioventricular node reentry and, 123
  concealed, 315-318
  reciprocal beat and, 133
Right bundle branch
  aberration and, 193
    supraventricular tachycardia and, 365
  development of, 10
  reentry within, 102
Right bundle branch block, 368
  aberration and, 202
  alternating aberrancy and, 214-215
  deflection and, 207
  digitalis toxicity and, 70
  phase 3 aberration and, 196
  QRS complex and, 205
  sinus beat and, 364
  sinus rhythm and, 242
  supernormal conduction and, 330
  ventricular fusion and, 275
Ring, cardiac tube, 1
RP/PR reciprocity, 252-253

S

SA node; *see* Sinoatrial node
Schutzblockierung, 289
Second-in-a-row anomaly, 208-209
Sick sinus syndrome, 113-117, 374, 376
Silent zone of surface electrocardiogram, 12-13

Sinoatrial block, 110-113
  laddergram and, 345-347
Sinoatrial node
  conduction time of, 14
  reentry and, 105-109
  Wenckebach period and, 77
Sinoatrial ring, 1
Sinoatrial Wenckebach period, 77
Sinus bradycardia, 376
  digitalis toxicity and, 77, 81
Sinus node
  abnormal automaticity and, 48
  conduction velocity and, 107
  electrogram of, 12-18
  origin of, 2, 3
Sinus P wave, 106
Sinus rhythm
  extrasystole and, 382
  nonconducted atrial bigeminy and, 372
  right bundle branch block and, 242, 364
  Wolff-Parkinson-White syndrome and, 166, 167
Sinus tachycardia
  digitalis toxicity and, 68
  paroxysmal, 108-109
Skipped P wave, 256
Slow conduction, 87-88
Slow response action potential, 87, 88
Sodium, 87
Sodium-potassium ATPase pump, 53
Sodium pump, 60
ST segment
  digitalis toxicity and, 65
  Wolff-Parkinson-White syndrome and, 159
Subumbrella tissue, 86
Summation, 89
Superior vena cava, 3
Supernormal conduction, 328-337
  atrioventricular block and, 371
Suppression
  digitalis dysrhythmia and, 62
  overdrive, automaticity and, 48, 49, 52
Supraventricular arrhythmia, drug-induced, 183
Supraventricular ectopic mechanism, 340-344
Supraventricular tachycardia
  atrioventricular node reentry and, 122, 129
  bundle branch block and, 242, 243
  paroxysmal, 117, 122
    sinoatrial node reentry and, 108-109
    Wolff-Parkinson-White syndrome and, 159-162
  QRS tachycardia and, 221, 223
  right bundle branch aberration and, 365
  second-in-a-row anomaly, 208
  Wenckebach period and, 381

Surface electrocardiogram, 12-13
SVT; *see* Supraventricular tachycardia
Sympathetic stimulation, 107
Syncope, 113

T

Tachyarrhythmia
  drug-induced, 183-189
  Wolff-Parkinson-White syndrome and, 107
Tachycardia
  accelerated idiojunctional rhythm and, 74-75
  atrial
    aberrancy in, 212-213
    digitalis toxicity and, 62
  atrioventricular node reentry and, 125
  circus movement
    antidromic, 163-164, 241
    atrioventricular, 367
    atrioventricular node reentry and, 129
    orthodromic, 154, 157, 159, 161-162
    persistent, 162
  double, 76
  junctional, 379
    bigeminy and, 379
    digitalis toxicity and, 74-75
  paroxysmal sinus, 108-109
  QRS, 218-246; *see also* QRS tachycardia
  sick sinus syndrome and, 114
  sinus, 68
    digitalis toxicity and, 68
    paroxysmal, 108-109
  supraventricular; *see* Supraventricular tachycardia
  ventricular; *see* Ventricular tachycardia
  Wolff-Parkinson-White syndrome and
    circus movement and, 161-164
    digitalis toxicity and, 62, 66, 70-71, 74-75, 76, 162
    paroxysmal supraventricular, 159-162
Temperature, 107
Temporary pacemaker, 54
Tension, wall, 53
Torsades de pointes
  digitalis toxicity and, 75
  drug-induced, 186-188
Toxicity
  antiarrhythmic drug and, 174-189; *see also* Antiarrhythmic drug, proarrhythmic action of
  digitalis, 59-83; *see also* Digitalis toxicity
Transmembrane ionic channels, 177
Transmembrane potential
  delayed afterdepolarization and, 52
  early afterdepolarization and, 54-55

Tricyclic antidepressant, 184
Trigeminal grouping, 98
Triggered activity, 52-55, 56
  digitalis toxicity and, 60
Tube, cardiac, 1
Two to one atrioventricular block, 254-255
  misconceptions about, 262

U

Unidirectional block, 88
  parasystole and, 289

V

V-A-V sequence, 131
Vagal stimulation
  atrioventricular node reentry and, 128
  sinus node and, 107
Velocity, conduction
  aberrant ventricular conduction and, 193
  drug-induced arrhythmia and, 178
  Purkinje fibers and, 94
  sinus node and, 107
Ventricular asystole, 258, 259
Ventricular bigeminy
  digitalis toxicity and, 72
  ventricular fusion and, 272, 275
Ventricular cell, 47
Ventricular conduction, aberrant, 192-217
  alternating, 214, 215
  atrioventricular block and, 200
  bundle branch block and, 200
  clues to, 205-209
  mechanism of, 193
  morphology of, 202-204
  phase 3, 195-197
  phase 4, 198-199
  Wolff-Parkinson-White syndrome and, 161
Ventricular ectopic rhythm
  bigeminal; *see* Ventricular bigeminy
  laddergram and, 353
  paired, 305
  reciprocal beat and, 133
Ventricular escape beat, 282
Ventricular extrasystole, 315-318
Ventricular fibrillation, drug-induced, 189
Ventricular fusion, 268, 269, 270-276, 277; *see
    also* Fusion
  laddergram and, 354-355
  preexcitation and, 285
Ventricular microreentry, 356
Ventricular parasystole
  artificial, 292
  classical, 294-300
  modulated, 301

Ventricular premature beat, 369
  atrioventricular node reentry and, 124
  concealed retrograde conduction and,
      315
  reciprocal beat and, 132
  ventricular fusion and, 271
Ventricular tachyarrhythmia, drug-induced,
    183-189
Ventricular tachycardia
  abnormal automaticity and, 47
  atrioventricular dissociation and, 224
  bedside diagnosis of, 226
  bidirectional, 70-71
  bundle branch block and, 242, 243
  digitalis toxicity and, 75, 245
    fascicular, 66
  fusion in diagnosis of, 280-281
  QRS tachycardia and, 220-221
Verapamil
  atrioventricular node reentry and, 128
  digoxin and, 61
VPB; *see* Ventricular premature beat

W

Wall tension, 53
Wandering atrial pacemaker, 106-107
Wave
  delta, 154-157
  P; *see* P wave
  P′
    atrioventricular node reentry and, 125
    Wolff-Parkinson-White syndrome and,
      159
Wenckebach conduction
  atrial flutter and, 343
  conduction delay and, 98
Wenckebach exit block, 351-352
  atrial fibrillation and, 78
Wenckebach period
  atrioventricular block and, 248-249,
      252-253
  bigeminy and, 379, 380
  digitalis toxicity and, 78
  reciprocal beat and, 133
  sinoatrial
    digitalis toxicity and, 77
    laddergram and, 345, 346-347
  sinoatrial block and, 110, 111
  supraventricular tachycardia, 381
Wolff-Parkinson-White syndrome
  atrioventricular node reentry and, 123
  tachyarrhythmia and, 107
WPW syndrome; *see* Wolff-Parkinson-White
      syndrome